Angiogenesis in Health and Disease

Angiogenesis in Health and Disease

Editor: June Wade

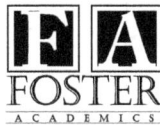

FOSTER
ACADEMICS

www.fosteracademics.com

www.fosteracademics.com

FA FOSTER ACADEMICS

Cataloging-in-Publication Data

Angiogenesis in health and disease / edited by June Wade.
     p. cm.
Includes bibliographical references and index.
ISBN 978-1-63242-930-8
1. Neovascularization. 2. Blood-vessels--Growth. 3. Cardiology. I. Wade, June.
QP106.6 .A54 2020
612.13--dc23

Foster Academics,
118-35 Queens Blvd., Suite 400,
Forest Hills, NY 11375, USA

ISBN 978-1-63242-930-8 (Hardback)

Contents

Permissions

List of Contributors

Index

Preface

Over the recent decade, advancements and applications have progressed exponentially. This has led to the increased interest in this field and projects are being conducted to enhance knowledge. The main objective of this book is to present some of the critical challenges and provide insights into possible solutions. This book will answer the varied questions that arise in the field and also provide an increased scope for furthering studies.

Angiogenesis is the physiological process of the generation of new blood vessels from pre-existing vessels that were formed during vasculogenesis. By sprouting and splitting, angiogenesis perpetuates the growth of the vasculature. It is a vital process in growth and development, as well as in the formation of granulation tissue and wound healing. However, it has a major role in the transition of benign tumors into malignant ones. Some diseases are characterized by abnormal vasculature. Therefore, such diseases are combated by inhibiting or inducing the creation of new blood vessels. The principle of angiogenesis can be applied clinically in two main areas- anti-angiogenic therapies and pro-angiogenic therapies. Anti-angiogenic therapies are employed to fight cancer and other malignancies, while pro-angiogenic therapies are potent against cardiovascular diseases. This book includes some of the vital pieces of work being conducted across the world, on various topics related to the role of angiogenesis in health and disease. It presents the complex subject of angiogenesis in the most comprehensible and easy to understand language. It is meant for students who are looking for an elaborate reference text on angiogenesis.

I hope that this book, with its visionary approach, will be a valuable addition and will promote interest among readers. Each of the authors has provided their extraordinary competence in their specific fields by providing different perspectives as they come from diverse nations and regions. I thank them for their contributions.

Editor

Unique Phenotypes of Endothelial Cells in Developing Arteries

Norika Mengchia Liu and Susumu Minamisawa

Abstract

Endothelial cells (ECs) play a critical role in regulating vascular pathophysiology. Various growth factors and relaxation factors such as vascular endothelial growth factor (VEGF) and nitric oxide (NO), which are derived from ECs, are known to maintain homeostasis and regulate vessel remodeling. Although the inner lumens of all types of vessels are covered by an EC monolayer, the characteristics of ECs differ in each tissue and developing stage of a vessel. Previously, we identified the heterogeneity of ECs of the ductus arteriosus (DA) by analyzing its gene profiles. The DA is a fetal artery that closes immediately after birth due to the changes in concentrations of oxygen and vasoactive factors such as NO and prostaglandin E. Studying the unique gene profile of ECs in the DA can therefore uncover the novel key genes involved in developing vascular function and morphology such as O_2 sensitivity and physiological vascular remodeling. A comprehensive gene analysis identified a number of genes related to morphogenesis and development in the DA. In this chapter, we discuss the heterogeneity of vascular ECs in the developing vessel in the DA.

Keywords: vascular endothelial cells, ductus arteriosus, vascular remodeling, comprehensive gene analysis, oxygen, vitamin A

1. Introduction

The endothelial cells (ECs) in vessels control the vascular tone, permeability, attraction of blood cells, which exhibit both innate and adaptive immunity, and migration/proliferation of underlying cells such as pericytes and smooth muscle cells (SMCs). To accomplish these roles, vascular ECs exhibit phenotypic heterogeneity during development in a time- and tissue-specific manner. The most significant diversity of ECs involves the differences between arteries and veins as well as between large and small vessels. ECs undergo constant changes in phenotype depending on different situations, both physiological and pathological. Physiological angiogenesis occurs during development and repair processes. Many events in vascular development during gestation are reciprocated in the adult neovascularization that takes place in wound healing and ischemic disease treatment. In these cases, ECs must express pro-angiogenic factors. Pathological angiogenesis is often implicated as the abnormal proliferation of ECs such as that seen in tumorigenesis. Accordingly, many cancer studies have focused on vascular endothelial growth factor (VEGF), a pro-angiogenic factor produced from ECs. Endothelial damage and dysfunction causes cardiovascular diseases. For example, endothelial dysfunction reduces nitric oxide (NO) production, which decreases vasodilatory effects on SMCs. In addition, a decrease in NO production is also involved in the attraction of leucocytes and the production of various growth factors that leads to unregulated intimal thickening (**Figure 1**). Therefore, ECs play a central role in modifying the phenotypes of vessels. ECs have different roles depending on where they are located. For instance, in a developing vessel, ECs become tip cells or other stalk cells to regulate different molecular signaling to guide vessel sprouting [1]. Endothelial tip cells coordinate to have less proliferative activity by repressing Notch activity, thus upregulating VEGFR-2 (Flk-1) and other downstream

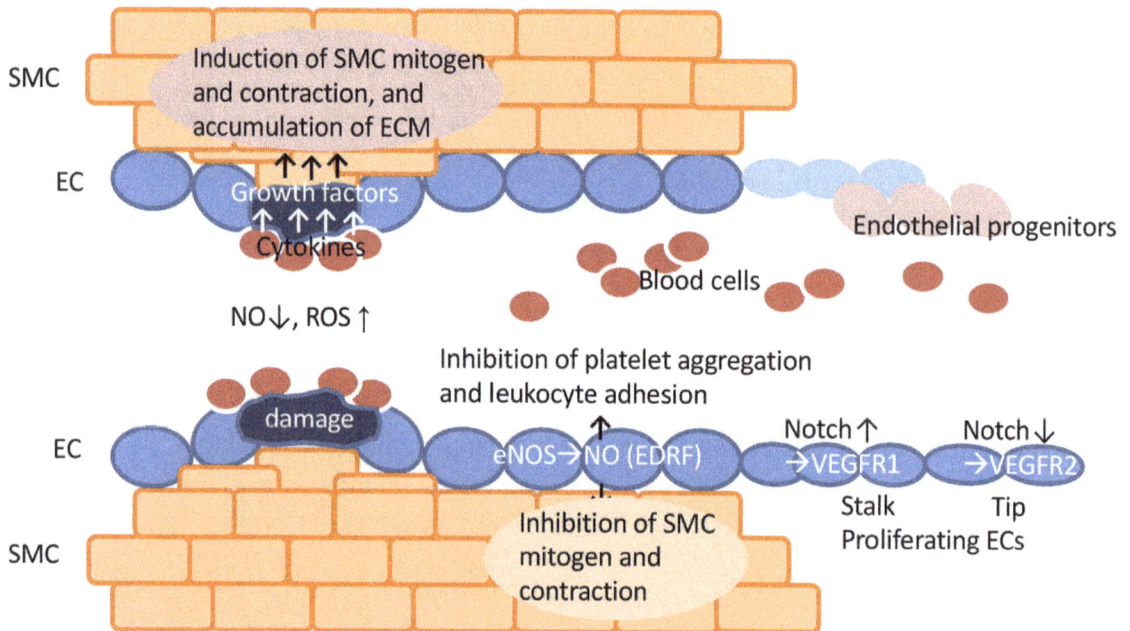

Figure 1. Summarized pathological and physiological vessel response. Damaged ECs are shown in dark blue. Due to the damage, there is a reduction of NO and an increase of ROS, which leads to platelet aggregation or leukocyte adhesion to the intima. Cytokines produced from platelets or leukocytes induce growth factor production and cause SMC hyperplasia and contraction. By contrast, healthy ECs constantly produce EDRF such as NO, so that SMC mitogen and contraction are absent. In developing vessels, ECs are proliferating or deriving from progenitor cells. Proliferating ECs can be distinguished into stalk cells and tip cells, which have different downstream VEGF pathways depending on Notch activity.

Notch transcription factors such as HASER1 [2]. By contrast, Notch signaling is more active and VEGFR-1 (Flt-1) expression is upregulated in stalk ECs. Although Notch and VEGF signals are greatly conserved in vessel sprouting among various tissues and species, how widespread it is in terms of tissue specificity remains to be elucidated (**Figure 1**). Increasing evidence shows that different signaling rules influence tissue-specific vessel sprouting—one study demonstrated that bone morphogenetic protein (BMP) signaling provides the cue for vein-specific angiogenesis during early development, and is independent from canonical VEGF-A signaling [3]. Casanello et al. reported that endothelial diversity is also present in the umbilico-placental vasculature, and emphasized that the heterogeneity of ECs is complicated and cannot be explained simply by comparing the differences between micro- and macro-vasculature, or artery versus vein [4]. Thus, EC shows great heterogeneity in health and disease, and studying the mechanisms of EC heterogeneity would contribute to the understanding of both vascular physiology and pathology.

We previously revealed the unique gene profile of ductus arteriosus (DA)-specific ECs. The DA, a fetal artery that connects the pulmonary artery (PA) and the aorta, is essential for fetuses to bypass the oxygenated blood delivered from the placenta directly to the descending aorta and not through the lung. The DA experiences a dramatic morphological change along with environmental factors after birth, though other connecting arteries remain unchanged. Therefore, even under similar physiological stresses underlying the DA and its connecting arteries, heterogeneity of ECs must exist. In this chapter, we focus on reviewing the unique identified gene profile of DA ECs, which should provide novel insights into heterogeneity in vascular ECs.

Moreover, investigating DA remodeling would potentially help the understanding of diseased vessels, just like other animal models in cardiovascular diseases. For instance, a wire injury model is used for studying pathology of endothelial injury/dysfunction [5]; low-density lipoprotein receptor-deficient mice [6] and apolipoprotein E-deficient mice [7] are commonly used as atherosclerosis models; calcium chloride [8], elastase [9], angiotensin II [10], or microRNA-21 [11] are infused to create an abdominal aortic aneurysms model. Developing a disease model occupies a great deal of scientific findings on pathophysiology, and so the existing models should always open to be refined. The DA can be an alternate model of an occluding vessel, an extracellular matrix (ECM)-enriched vessel, or an oxygen-sensitive vessel. Thus, studying DA ECs would be valuable for understanding an irregular angiogenic pathophysiology.

1.1. Embryonic vasculogenesis

Vasculogenesis and angiogenesis are nomenclaturally similar as they both refer to the genesis of blood vessels [12]. Vasculogenesis is the de novo formation of blood vessels differentiated from mesodermal cells. Angiogenesis is the sprouting of blood vessels that occurs as a result of the proliferation of existing vascular ECs. Despite the difference in these two processes, vasculogenesis and angiogenesis are often compared to further understand their underlying molecular mechanisms. Indeed, a significant amount of knowledge on tumor angiogenesis was achieved by studying embryonic vasculogenesis [13]. Therefore, it is important to study developmental vascular biology and to understand vessel-specific heterogeneity. Moreover, determining the heterogenic diversity of ECs would help open up more options in clinical therapy, ultimately enabling individually designed therapeutic treatments.

The vascular network is the first functional system established in the embryo. A primitive vascular network is formed shortly after gastrulation by deriving endothelial progenitor cells from the mesoderm. This first process is called the formation of angioblasts. Angioblasts then differentiate into ECs by expressing various transcription factors and pan endothelial markers for tubular formation, which is called the primitive vascular plexus [13]. Some of the homeobox (Hox) transcription factors are known to be involved in this process. For instance, Hox A9 regulates the expressions of endothelial NO synthase (eNOS), VEGF-receptor 2 (VEGFR2), and vascular endothelial-cadherin (VE-cadherin), and is responsible for the tubulogenesis of mature ECs [14]. Hox B3 also plays a role in tubulogenesis [15]. Hox D3 induces the differentiation of ECs from angioblasts [16]. The primitive vascular plexus then undergoes complex remodeling accompanied by specification among arteries, veins, and capillaries to become the functional vascular system [13]. Sry-related HMG box (Soxs)-F subgroups Sox7, Sox17, and Sox18, along with vascular endothelial zinc finger-1 (Vezf-1), were found to be essential to the remodeling process [17, 18]. Thus, vasculogenesis in general consists of three steps: formation of angioblasts, formation of the primitive vascular plexus, and vascular remodeling. During these steps, the heterogeneity of vascular ECs is established.

1.2. Physiology of the DA

After the vascular system appears during embryonic development, the heart starts to function, and fetal circulation is established. Fetal circulation is different from adult circulation since the blood is oxygenated in the placenta instead of the lung. Prenatal lungs do not yet need to function so the DA bypasses the pulmonary artery and the descending aorta to send most blood to the body instead of the lungs. Patency of the DA is maintained due to the low oxygen level and high concentration of prostaglandin E_2 (PGE_2) in the blood circulated from the placenta, as well as the production of NO from ECs of the DA. Once the infant has been delivered and lung ventilation has begun, the DA must close properly to enable the transformation to adult circulation. Normal closure happens in two steps: functional closure and anatomical occlusion [19]. The first closure is triggered by an increase in pO_2 and a drop in PGE_2, as well as a drop in blood pressure within the DA caused by the reduction in pulmonary vascular resistance. This functional closure causes the loss of blood flow which therefore induces hypoxia and extensive intimal thickening, followed by fibrosis. The hypoxia on the vessel wall further inhibits endogenous prostaglandin and NO production, which leads to an irreversible closure. Two to three weeks later, the sealed DA eventually becomes a fibrous band called the ligamentum arteriosum (**Figure 2**) [19]. Failed DA closure after birth is a condition called patent DA (PDA), and occurs frequently in premature infants. Medical or surgical treatment of PDA is required when the left-to-right blood shunt is significant.

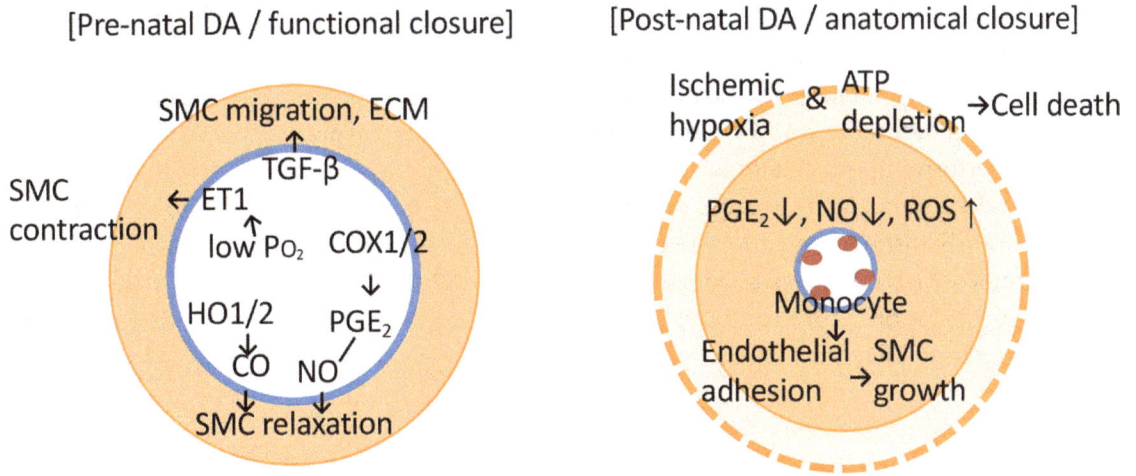

Figure 2. Representative pathways during DA remodeling. In early gestation, the DA remained open due to the high concentration of PGE$_2$ from placental circulation, and by producing EDHF (NO and CO in the figure). Low oxygen concentration induced ET-1 signaling and TGF-β expression in ECs, leading to functional closure. Postnatal DA is exposed to oxygenated blood that has reduced concentrations of PGE$_2$ and NO. Due to reduced NO production, ROS are produced and monocytes are attracted to the intima. Monocyte-endothelial interaction induces cytokine and growth factor upregulation, thus promoting SMC growth. Extensive neointimal formation at a later stage causes ischemic hypoxia and ATP depletion, and eventual cell death.

2. Endothelial heterogeneity in terms of the DA

2.1. Current methodologies to study the heterogeneity of DA-specific ECs

The DA is a small shunt vessel in fetuses or neonates. The size of the tissue has always been a study limitation in small mammals such as rodent models. Therefore, although many previous studies used larger mammals such as lamb or pig fetuses, they are inefficient for conducting primary-level research due to the difficulty in handling, low number of offspring, and long gestational period. Rodents overcome these disadvantages, and experimental tools of molecular biology are more available for rodents. Thanks to advancements in technology, there are now more options than ever to overcome the limitation of tissue size in rodents.

2.1.1. Isolation of ECs of the rat DA

DA researchers have used different species, including baboon, pig, sheep, rabbit, chicken, rat, and mouse [20]. These studies focused on a specific population of the cells in the DA and always faced limitations in using rodent animals due to the small size of the fetal tissue. To date, there are only three studies in which pure ECs were successfully isolated from rat DA, including ours. Weber et al. applied a magnetic-activated cell sorting (MACS) method to purify the ECs from collagenase-digested DA tissue [20]. They used von Willebrand factor (vWF) polyclonal antibody in MACS for the isolation. With their experimental method, they succeeded in passaging a pure population of ECs up to three times, which overcame the small number of primary-cultured ECs for further experiments. Following the isolation, they confirmed the purification by flow cytometry and immunohistochemistry analyses. In our previous study, we used a florescence-activated cell sorter (FACS) to purify ECs from collagenase-digested DA tissues [21]. In this experiment, we incubated pooled fresh cells with fluorescein isothiocyanate (FITC)-conjugated anti-CD31 and APC/Cy7-conjugated anti-CD45 antibodies to separate EC and hematopoietic derivation cells, respectively. We confirmed the purity by performing quantitative reverse transcription polymerase chain reaction (RT-PCR) for Tie2 and gamma2-actin expressions, which are markers of ECs and SMCs, respectively. After the FACS sorting, we proceeded directly to RNA isolation from the collected ECs for application to a DNA microarray experiment, which minimized differentiation of the isolated ECs after purification. More recently, a study focused on the heterogeneity of tissue-specific cells that separated ECs and SMCs from the DA using laser-capture microdissection [22].

2.1.2. Comprehensive gene expression analysis of DA tissues

During the past decade, several groups, including ours, have studied comprehensive gene expression in the DA using DNA microarray analysis. One study used human DA specimens, with a broad range of ages [23]. Because of the difficulty involved with human samples of the DA, they could not group the samples with biologic replicates. They found a tendency of expressing more genes that relate to ECM synthesis, which implied the presence of active neointimal proliferation in PDA. Other microarray studies used only rat vessels. Costa et al. compared rat DA samples from embryonic day 19 (E19) and 3 h after birth, examining the effects of oxygen [24]. Our group examined the expression profiles of rat DA and aorta at E19 and E21, and reported that the growth hormone (GH)-receptor signal is predominant in the SMCs of the DA [25]. We also investigated the effect of vitamin A maternal administration on the gene expression pattern of the DA at E19, E21 (full term), and 3–6 h after birth [26]. Moreover, our group utilized the unique phenotype of the Brown-Norway (BN) rat—this strain has been characterized as a novel animal model for PDA possibly due to systemic elastin-related impairments—to compare with vessels of its control strain Fisher 344 [27]. Although all of these studies reported somewhat overlapping results, none could determine the EC-specific gene profiles. As discussed above, the EC layer is maintained to form a single layer; the majority of genes that appear on microarray analysis using whole tissue are therefore from SMC origin.

Because the analysis of the expression profiles of the vascular ECs of the DA is challenging, only two studies have been published to date, including ours [21, 22]. It is difficult to compare these two studies because we used pooled DA ECs purified by FACS, whereas Bokenkamp et al. used laser-capture microdissection to isolate DA ECs from a frozen sample. Accordingly, some of the study results are inconsistent. For example, Bokenkamp et al. demonstrated that the expression of Rgs5 mRNA was higher in the DA compared to the aorta [22], whereas we did not find a difference in Rgs5 expression between DA ECs and aortic ECs. In our study, we divided samples into four groups: the DA and aorta of E21 fetals (F group) and neonates 30 min after birth (N group) rats. We further categorized the microarray data with GeneGo MetaCore software to clarify the meaning of enriched gene expressions. Interestingly, the majority of the identified DA-dominant genes had not previously been reported in previous DA-related studies. We review the unique gene profiles of DA-specific ECs in the following sections.

2.2. Characteristics of DA-specific ECs in DA remodeling

As mentioned in the earlier section, the DA has special remodeling processes that differ from other vessels. Most research on DA remodeling has been conducted using the whole tissue or its SMCs. The importance of signals generated from blood or ECs has, however, begun to be realized.

2.2.1. Extracellular matrix remodeling of the DA

In the late 1980s, Rabinovitch's group discovered that the intimal cushion formation of the DA is attributed to a special character in its cells [28, 29]. Using *in vitro* cells from lamb tissues, they demonstrated that there are 10-fold and five-fold increased incorporations of hyaluronan and heparansulfate in the ECM of DA ECs, respectively, compared to cells of the adjacent aorta or pulmonary artery (PA). They further found that this remodeling, which involves the increased hyaluronan accumulation in DA ECs, contributes to the migration of DA SMCs [30], and is transforming growth factor-beta (TGF-β)-dependent [31]. About a decade later, the same group reported that TGF-β1 expression in DA ECs was upregulated in the early gestation of fetal lambs compared to aortic ECs, but was downregulated to the same level as aortic ECs by late gestation [32]. This dynamic modification in the DA EC was explained to relate to stability in the translation and transcription of its mRNA. This second study provided some of the first evidence showing that there are tissue-specific and developmental patterns of expression in DA ECs.

The comprehensive gene analysis study identified significantly high expressions of N-deacetylase/N-sulfotransferase (Ndst3), Glipican 3(Gpc3), and heparan-sulfate 6-O-sulfo-transferase 2 (Hs6st2), all of which are involved in heparasulfate synthesis, in DA ECs in both full-term fetal and neonatal periods [21]. Ndst3 is the most important heparin-sulfate synthase among the three members of the NDST family [33]. Other genes that are known to relate to ECM, especially collagen synthesis, were also found to show higher expression levels in DA ECs than aortic ECs: the glycosyltransferase25 domain containing 2 (Glt25d2), which is known to strengthen collagen activity [34]; growth differentiation factor (Gdf6), and micro-fibrillar-associated protein 5 (Mfap5), which promotes collagen production [35, 36]; Mfap4, which stabilizes collagen activity [37]; anthrax toxin receptor 1 (Antxr1), which provides a link between collagen I and actin cytoskeleton [38]; and prolyl 4-hydroxylase-alpha polypep-tide (P4ha1), which is related to the procollagen process [39]. ADAM metallopeptidase with thrombospondin type 1 motif-17 preproprotein (Adamts17), plasminogen activator tissue (Plat), and fibrillin 1 (Fbn1), which are also categorized as related to ECM formation, were upregulated in DA ECs [21]. Interestingly, connective tissue growth factor (CTGF) was found to show higher expression in DA ECs than in aortic ECs in the postnatal period, whereas there was no difference in the fetal period [21]. CTGF is a well-known downstream mediator of TGF-β1 in various cells and it exhibits diverse functions, such as cell proliferation, apoptosis, cell adhesion, ECM or collagen production, and angiogenesis [40, 41]. Moreover, a recent study demonstrated that, via stimulation of TGF-β1, CTGF binds to VEGF, and that the complex inhibited VEGF-mediated angiogenesis in cardiac cells [42]. Although further studies are needed, these results imply that there are intricate regulations among TGF-β1, CTGF, and VEGF in the DA remodeling after birth.

2.2.2. PGE$_2$, endothelial-derived relaxation, and hyperpolarizing factors in the DA

PGE$_2$ is a potent vasodilator for the DA. It is generated by the enzyme cyclooxygenase (COX). There are two isoforms, COX-1 and COX-2. Although COX-2 is an inducible isoform that requires cytokine, both COX-1 and COX-2 are known to be involved in fetal development [43]. The expression levels of these two vary among species as well as the term of gestation. For instance, COX-2 is barely detected in the DA of fetal pig, but more dominantly regulates DA tone in fetal lamb by expressing it in ECs [43]. Another study found that there is a cooperative interaction between PGE$_2$ and NO, an endothelial-derived relaxation factor (EDRF) [44]. Several studies showed that NO is more potent than PGE$_2$ in the preterm DA, whereas the opposite relationship is seen at term [45–47]. Another EDRF that is found to be related to controlling DA tone is carbon monoxide (CO). CO is naturally formed in the body from the enzymatic activity of heme oxygenase (HO-1/2). Coceani et al. demonstrated that CO formed by HO (ECs of DA only express HO-1 in rat and pig fetuses) interfered with the reaction with the cytochrome P450-based monooxygenase and inhibited the synthesis of endothelin-1 (ET-1), which is a potent vasoconstrictor that is also critical in DA tone [48–50]. CO generated from HO-1, but not HO-2, is known to have a protective effect on ECs of various vessels [51], and induces angiogenesis [52]. Importantly, compensatory mechanisms among PGE$_2$, NO, and CO were elucidated by using eNOS, COX, or HO-2-mutant mice [53]. The study showed that there is no narrowing of the DA in each mutant, and that endothelial-derived hyperpolarizing factor (EDHF) additionally exhibits a large reciprocal effect [53]. In addition to bradykinin, which has been shown to have the same relaxation effect as EDHF, there could be more agents potentially qualified as EDHF. A more recent study reported that hydrogen sulfide (H$_2$S) also acts as EDHF by expressing its synthetic enzymes cystathionine-γ-lyase (CSE) and cystathionine-β-synthase (CBS) in the intima, likely ECs of the DA [54].

2.2.3. Inflammatory response in DA ECs during anatomic remodeling

Anatomic remodeling of the full-term DA shares similar features of inflammatory vascular disorders such as atherosclerosis. As a consequence of the functional closure of the DA, ischemic hypoxia of the muscle media is induced due to the loss of luminal and vasa vasorum blood flow. Therefore, ATP depletion causes cell death [55, 56] and VEGF induction increases the penetration of vasa vasorum into the DA muscle media [57]. Clyman's group examined the inflammatory processes involved in the postnatal constriction of the DA [58]. They found that VLA4 integrin expressing mononuclear cells (CD14$^+$/CD163$^+$ cells [59]), in which the ligand is vascular cell adhesion molecule-1 (VCAM-1) in ECs, increased to adhere to the lumen of the DA after birth. Along with the increased monocytes recruitment, VCAM-1 and E-selectin expressions were also elevated in DA ECs after birth [58]. Unlike the pathophysiology of atherosclerosis, the upregulation of P-selectin and intracellular adhesion molecule-1 (ICAM-1) induced by monocytes adhesion was not seen in the DA. Interestingly, VLA4$^+$ mononuclear cell adhesion was found to predominantly regulate the extent of neointimal remodeling of the DA after birth, with T-lymphocyte adhesion to a lesser extent, but no neutrophil or platelet adhesion [58]. VCAM-1 and E-selectin were also induced by VEGF and several cytokines, such as TNF-α, IFN-γ, and CD154, likely due to the profound hypoxia in the DA wall after birth. These responses are also seen in atherosclerotic remodeling, but the pattern of gene expression modification seemed less in DA closure since IL-1 and MCP-1 were not expressed in the closing DA [58]. Some researchers argue, however, that the inflammatory response during DA closure may cause a failure in constriction after birth [58], because TNF-α and IL-6 are known to have potent vasodilatory effects [60–63].

The monocyte-endothelial cell interaction has been implicated to play a critical role in vascular pathogenesis by inducing platelet-derived growth factor (PDGF) secretion that promotes the migration of SMCs into neointima [64]. Indeed, PDGF-B chain expression upregulation was confirmed in DA tissues after birth, and was inhibited by blocking monocyte adhesion using anti-VLA-4 monoclonal antibody treatment [59]. Moreover, the regulator of G-protein signaling 5 (Rgs5) that was found to be enriched in both ECs and SMCs of DA at full-term gestation compared to adjacent aortic cells [22] was suggested to be negatively regulated by PDGF [65]. PDGF-dependent repression of Rgs5 leads to SMC migration and G protein-coupled receptor-mediated-signaling pathways, such as mitogen-activated protein kinase activation, thus contributing to vessel contraction and remodeling [65]. The Rgs5 expression level in DA tissue after birth has not been studied, but it is reasonable to hypothesize that it would be decreased, likely due to increased PDGF secretion after birth. Further studies are required to elucidate the intricate effects of DA remodeling.

2.2.4. Epithelial/endothelial-to-mesenchymal transition-related gene expressions in the DA

Recent studies have suggested that epithelial/endothelial-to-mesenchymal transition (EMT/EndMT)-related genes play an important role in DA closure [21, 66]. Our microarray study on FACS isolated ECs from rat DA revealed that Tgfb2, actin alpha 2 smooth muscle aorta (ACTA2), N-cadherin (cadherin 2 or Cdh2), and met proto-oncogene (hepatocyte growth factor receptor or Met), which are known to be related to the EMT process, are significantly expressed compared to the aortic ECs [21]. In accordance with this finding, ACTA2 mutation is well characterized in PDA [67]. Another study that showed the importance of BMP9 and BMP10 as circulating growth factors in DA postnatal closure also found that they induced expressions of EMT/EndMT-initiating transcription factors SNAI1, SNAI2, ZEB2, TWIST1, and FOXC2 in ECs [66]. The study found that treatment with a neutralizing anti-BMP10 antibody on BMP9 knockout mice led to reopening of the DA. BMP9 and BMP10 are members of the TGF-β family, and are known to be elevated in mice around birth [68]. They have high affinity to bind to activin receptor-like kinase 1(ALK1), which is an EC-specific receptor [69], and additionally upregulate the expressions of BMPR2, ActR2A, and the co-receptor endoglin as well in the DA [66]. Moreover, BMP9 is reported to upregulate COX-2 and hyaluronic acid synthase 2 (HAS2) expressions, but not COX-1 [66, 70, 71]. Therefore, EMT or EndMT induced by BMP9 and BMP10 is thought to be a necessary process for anatomical closure of the DA.

Although it remains to be proved whether ECs at the lumen of closing DA would differentiate into mesenchymal cells, Levet et al. observed that there is a loss of EC-specific marker (PECAM or CD31)-positive cells at the lumen [66]. Since those cells at the lumen had an autophagic appearance, the authors speculated that the loss of ECs is at least partially due to cell death. However, it is also reasonable to assume that the EC loss is attributed to EndMT which resulted in loss of the EC characteristics.

2.3. Genetic responses to external stimuli on the DA and other vessels

The DA encounters great environmental changes during the perinatal period. Interestingly, the DA dramatically changes its morphology despite other neighboring arteries remaining unchanged. Therefore, it is reasonable to assume that the DA is sensitive to external or internal stimuli, which are primarily received by cells at the lumen, more than other neighboring arteries.

2.3.1. Response to oxygen

In fetal life when the lungs are not yet ventilated, the resistance of pulmonary vessels is high. Therefore, most of the blood that is oxygenated from the placenta passes to the descending aorta through the DA. At birth, in accordance with lung expansion, the blood passing via the DA is reduced, since the resistance of the pulmonary arteries is lower than that of the systemic arteries. In addition, an increase in oxygen concentration of the blood and a decrease in PGE_2 levels trigger the contraction of the DA. Our previous study demonstrated that $\alpha 1G$, a T-type voltage-dependent Ca^{2+} channel, mediates oxygenation-induced closure of the DA after birth [72].

Furthermore, as the neonatal period progresses, the DA constricts more and the vascular cells undergo hypoxic changes. As a result of hypoxia, reactive oxygen species (ROS) are generated by converting O_2 to $O_2^{\bullet-}$ by NADPH oxidase in ECs. Further activated redox-signaling pathways increase the tyrosine and serine/threonine phosphorylation of proteins, and result in various physiological and pathophysiological responses that are reviewed elsewhere [73]. VEGF is one of the best known genes that are elevated in response to hypoxia in the DA, which contributes to the ingrowth of vasa vasorum and neointimal proliferation [57].

Our microarray analysis identified a significant number of genes that more closely relate to oxygen in DA ECs than in aortic ECs. Aldehyde dehydrogenase 1 family-member A1 (Aldh1a1), aldolase C-fructose-bisphosphate (Aldoc), and CD38 are oxygen-related enzymes, and Vegfa, Tgfb2, and Ctgf are oxygen-related receptor ligands [21]. CD38 has been recently implicated to regulate Ca^{2+} signaling in response to ROS generation in pulmonary arterial SMCs [74]. Therefore, it would be interesting to examine the importance of CD38 in the DA.

2.3.2. Response to retinoic acid

Retinoic acid (RA), a metabolite of vitamin A, plays a critical role in organogenesis, such as the formation of the face, heart, eyes, limbs, and nervous systems [75]. Vitamin A maternal administration has been proven to increase the activities of vessel-contractile proteins and to accelerate the development of the O_2-sensing mechanism in the DA [76]. Yokoyama et al. compared gene expression profiles by microarray in the DA in the presence or absence of maternal vitamin A administration at different developmental stages, and found that 91 genes in total responded to the treatment [26]. In addition to the genes that were previously demonstrated to be induced by RA, such as fibronectin-1 and HAS2, the study also found that vitamin A treatment promoted the maturation of functions and structure of the DA. They also identified that VEGFA was increased by vitamin A administration.

Our microarray study on ECs from the DA versus the aorta also revealed the response to vitamin A to be one of the most dominant biological processes that worked in DA ECs [21]. TGF-beta 2, CD38, Ald1a1, Sp100, paired-like homeodomain 2-transcript variant 2 (Pitx2), fatty acid desaturase 1 (Fads1), and dickkopf homolog 1 (Dkk1) were listed in the category. Although the MetaCore system did not mention it, lecithin-retinol acyltransferase (Lrat) was also increased in DA ECs. Indeed, Lrat was identified as one of the most significant expressions in DA ECs, as it had a more than five-fold increase compared to aortic ECs. Given the fact that Lrat is the predominant enzyme in retinoid absorption [77], it is reasonable to think that this gene could play a great role in the DA having higher sensitivity to RA.

2.4. Other genes uniquely expressed in DA ECs

Our previous study identified more than 80 genes that were expressed more than two-fold or greater in ECs of the DA compared to those of the aorta, in both terms (F and N) [21]. In this section, DA EC-unique genes that were not mentioned in the earlier section will be summarized.

2.4.1. Neural crest cell-related genes during development

The DA derives from neural crest cells that are located in the sixth pharyngeal arch artery [78, 79], which is one of the progenitors of the second heart field [78, 79]. We identified that Tbx1, a major transcriptional factor in the second heart field, was expressed approximately four-fold more in DA ECs compared to aortic ECs. Pitx2 and Fgf10, which are known to co-express with Tbx1 [80, 81], also showed more than two-fold expressions in DA ECs than in aortic ECs. Indeed, Momma suggested that the deletion of human chromosome 22q11.2, where Tbx1 is, increased DA anomalies [82]. Moreover, cadherin 2 (Cdh2), which is known to work downstream of Pitx2 [83], and Ephrin B1 (Efnb1), Hs6st2, and Isl1, which are known to be in the Fgf10 signaling pathway [84–86], were also expressed dominantly in DA ECs [21].

2.4.2. Solute carrier family 38, member 1 (Slc38a1)

Slc38a1 is a highly homologous protein subtype of placental system A, a Na$^+$-dependent amino acid transporter that contributes to nutrient fetal growth, by expressing in the placenta [87]. Placental system A activity increases along with the progression of pregnancy and therefore coincides with demands of fetal nutrient [88]. Slc38a1 was found to be one of the most dominant genes in DA ECs compared to aortic ECs [21]. Slc38a1 itself has not been fully characterized yet and has not been implicated in studies in the DA. Recently, using siRNA technology on cytotrophoblast cells, Slc38a1 was revealed to be a key contributor to total system A activity in term placenta [87]. Hence, the fact that Slc38a1 expressed approximately seven-fold more in DA ECs than in aortic ECs at full-term gestation implies its involvement in the vascular remodeling of the DA. Further study is needed to identify the role of Slc38a1 in the DA during development.

2.4.3. Calpain-6

The calpain family is a calcium-dependent cysteine protease that is ubiquitously expressed in human tissues. Calpain-6 was identified about two decades ago; it has special features that make it stand out from other family members [89]. Calpain-6 is the only family member that lacks a calmodulin-like domain; it therefore has no protease active site [89]. Calpain-6 was exclusively but highly expressed during embryogenesis [90] and in placenta in 50 adult tissues [89] (no DA examination). Our microarray study identified that calpain-6 was also one of the most strongly expressed genes in DA ECs compared to aortic ECs, especially in fetal tissue [21]. Calpain-6 was recently implicated in tumor angiogenesis. Specifically, calpain-6 is suggested to play an important role in bone tumorigenesis and metastasis [91]. In the study, calpain-6 was found to be upregulated by ET-1, and to provide a protective effect against cell apoptosis and promote cell proliferation [91]. As mentioned earlier, ET-1 is increased in the DA to regulate its vasoconstriction [48–50]. Therefore, calpain-6 might be a newly identified gene in ET-1 signaling generated in DA ECs.

3. Conclusion

Studying EC heterogeneity aids our understanding of the physiology and pathophysiology of angiogenesis. It also has great potential to identify novel ways to regulate angiogenesis for treatment purposes. Comprehensive gene analysis using a microarray made it possible to reveal many genes that were previously functionally unidentified in tissue or disease. Molecular analyses using whole tissues hinder the data on specific cell types. ECs are the key cells responsible for primarily generating signaling pathways to modulate the functions or structure of a vessel. Vessels mainly consist of a medial layer (the majority of which is composed of SMCs), and a single layer of ECs. The separation of ECs would therefore be the first hurdle to overcome in order to acquire data on ECs.

This chapter focused on reviewing the current knowledge of DA ECs, since we believe that the DA could be utilized as a vessel model for studying the mechanisms of both neointimal formation and apoptosis in addition to embryonic vasculogenesis. DA-specific ECs are highly unique compared to aortic ECs in terms of their heterogeneity. DA ECs have a great number of specific genes related to ECM formation, inflammatory response, EMT or EndMT, and oxygen and retinoic acid response. DA ECs also have more genes that are conserved from embryogenesis compared to adjacent aortic ECs. In our previous study, Slac38a1, Capn6, and Lrat were found to be the most significantly expressed genes in DA ECs. Although much more research is required to validate the importance of these newly identified dominant genes in DA ECs, we expect that these findings will promote further studies on PDA, therapeutic angiogenesis, and cancer treatment.

Acknowledgements

We would like to thank Dr. Hua Cai for supporting N.M. Liu's continuing research at the University of California, Los Angeles, as well as the fellowship support from the American Heart Association, Western States Affiliate Winter 2014 Predoctoral Fellowship (Award#14PRE20380184), and the American Association of Japanese University Women 2016. This work was also supported by grants from the Ministry of Education, Culture, Sports, Science and Technology of Japan (S.M.), the Vehicle Racing Commemorative Foundation (S.M.), The Jikei University Graduate Research Fund (SM) and the Miyata Cardiology Research Promotion Foundation (S.M.).

Author details

Norika Mengchia Liu[1] and Susumu Minamisawa[2]*

*Address all correspondence to: sminamis@jikei.ac.jp

1 University of California, Los Angeles, CA, USA

2 The Jikei Medical University, Tokyo, Japan

References

[1] Chappell JC, Wiley DM, Bautch VL. (2011) Regulation of blood vessel sprouting. *Seminars in Cell & Developmental Biology* **22:** 1005–1011.

[2] Holderfield MT, Henderson Anderson AM, Kokubo H, Chin MT, Johnson RL, Hughes CC. (2006) HESR1/CHF2 suppresses VEGFR2 transcription independent of binding to E-boxes. *Biochemical and Biophysical Research Communications* **346:** 637–648.

[3] Wiley DM, Kim JD, Hao J, Hong CC, Bautch VL, Jin SW. (2011) Distinct signalling pathways regulate sprouting angiogenesis from the dorsal aorta and the axial vein. *Nature Cell Biology* **13:** 686–692.

[4] Casanello P, Schneider D, Herrera EA, Uauy R, Krause BJ. (2014) Endothelial heterogeneity in the umbilico-placental unit: DNA methylation as an innuendo of epigenetic diversity. *Frontiers in Pharmacology* **5:** 49.

[5] Sata M, Maejima Y, Adachi F, et al. (2000) A mouse model of vascular injury that induces rapid onset of medial cell apoptosis followed by reproducible neointimal hyperplasia. *Journal of Molecular and Cellular Cardiology* **32:** 2097–2104.

[6] Bentzon JF, Falk E. (2010) Atherosclerotic lesions in mouse and man: is it the same disease? *Current Opinion in Lipidology* **21:** 434–440.

[7] Zhang SH, Reddick RL, Piedrahita JA, Maeda N. (1992) Spontaneous hypercholesterolemia and arterial lesions in mice lacking apolipoprotein E. *Science* **258:** 468–471.

[8] Freest-one T, Turner RJ, Higman DJ, Lever MJ, Powell JT. (1997) Influence of hypercholesterolemia and adventitial inflammation on the development of aortic aneurysm in rabbits. *Arteriosclerosis, Thrombosis, and Vascular Biology* **17:** 10–17.

[9] Pyo R, Lee JK, Shipley JM, et al. (2000) Targeted gene disruption of matrix metalloproteinase-9 (gelatinase B) suppresses development of experimental abdominal aortic aneurysms. *The Journal of Clinical Investigation* **105:** 1641–1649.

[10] Daugherty A, Cassis LA. (2004) Mouse models of abdominal aortic aneurysms. *Arteriosclerosis, Thrombosis, and Vascular Biology* **24:** 429–434.

[11] Maegdefessel L, Azuma J, Toh R, et al. (2012) MicroRNA-21 blocks abdominal aortic aneurysm development and nicotine-augmented expansion. *Science Translational Medicine* **4:** 122ra122.

[12] Drake CJ. (2003) Embryonic and adult vasculogenesis. *Birth Defects Research. Part C, Embryo Today: Reviews* **69:** 73–82.

[13] Dejana E, Taddei A, Randi AM. (2007) Foxs and Ets in the transcriptional regulation of endothelial cell differentiation and angiogenesis. *Biochimica et Biophysica Acta* **1775:** 298–312.

[14] Rossig L, Urbich C, Bruhl T, et al. (2005) Histone deacetylase activity is essential for the expression of HoxA9 and for endothelial commitment of progenitor cells. *Journal of Experimental Medicine* **201:** 1825–1835.

[15] Myers C, Charboneau A, Boudreau N. (2000) Homeobox B3 promotes capillary morphogenesis and angiogenesis. *The Journal of Cell Biology* **148:** 343–351.

[16] Gorski DH, Walsh K. (2000) The role of homeobox genes in vascular remodeling and angiogenesis. *Circulation Research* **87:** 865–872.

[17] Downes M, Koopman P. (2001) SOX18 and the transcriptional regulation of blood vessel development. *Trends in Cardiovascular Medicine* **11:** 318–324.

[18] Kuhnert F, Campagnolo L, Xiong JW, et al. (2005) Dosage-dependent requirement for mouse Vezf1 in vascular system development. *Developmental Biology* **283:** 140–156.

[19] Gournay V. (2011) The ductus arteriosus: physiology, regulation, and functional and congenital anomalies. *Archives of Cardiovascular Diseases* **104:** 578–585.

[20] Weber SC, Gratopp A, Akanbi S, et al. (2011) Isolation and culture of fibroblasts, vascular smooth muscle, and endothelial cells from the fetal rat ductus arteriosus. *Pediatric Research* **70:** 236–241.

[21] Liu NM, Yokota T, Maekawa S, et al. (2013) Transcription profiles of endothelial cells in the rat ductus arteriosus during a perinatal period. *PloS One* **8:** e73685.

[22] Bokenkamp R, van Brempt R, van Munsteren JC, et al. (2014) Dlx1 and Rgs5 in the ductus arteriosus: vessel-specific genes identified by transcriptional profiling of laser-capture microdissected endothelial and smooth muscle cells. *PLoS One* **9:** e86892.

[23] Mueller PP, Drynda A, Goltz D, Hoehn R, Hauser H, Peuster M. (2009) Common signatures for gene expression in postnatal patients with patent arterial ducts and stented arteries. *Cardiology in the Young* **19:** 352–359.

[24] Costa M, Barogi S, Socci ND, et al. (2006) Gene expression in ductus arteriosus and aorta: comparison of birth and oxygen effects. *Physiological Genomics* **25:** 250–262.

[25] Jin MH, Yokoyama U, Sato Y, et al. (2011) DNA microarray profiling identified a new role of growth hormone in vascular remodeling of rat ductus arteriosus. *The Journal of Physiological Sciences: JPS* **61:** 167–179.

[26] Yokoyama U, Sato Y, Akaike T, et al. (2007) Maternal vitamin A alters gene profiles and structural maturation of the rat ductus arteriosus. *Physiological Genomics* **31:** 139–157.

[27] Hsieh YT, Liu NM, Ohmori E, et al. (2014) Transcription profiles of the ductus arteriosus in Brown-Norway rats with irregular elastic fiber formation. *Circulation Journal: Official Journal of the Japanese Circulation Society* **78:** 1224–1233.

[28] Rabinovitch M, Beharry S, Bothwell T, Jackowski G. (1988) Qualitative and quantitative differences in protein synthesis comparing fetal lamb ductus arteriosus endothelium and smooth muscle with cells from adjacent vascular sites. *Developmental Biology* **130:** 250–258.

[29] Rabinovitch M, Boudreau N, Vella G, Coceani F, Olley PM. (1989) Oxygen-related prostaglandin synthesis in ductus arteriosus and other vascular cells. *Pediatric Research* **26:** 330–335.

[30] Boudreau N, Turley E, Rabinovitch M. (1991) Fibronectin, hyaluronan, and a hyaluronan binding protein contribute to increased ductus arteriosus smooth muscle cell migration. *Developmental Biology* **143:** 235–247.

[31] Boudreau N, Clausell N, Boyle J, Rabinovitch M. (1992) Transforming growth factor-beta regulates increased ductus arteriosus endothelial glycosaminoglycan synthesis and a post-transcriptional mechanism controls increased smooth muscle fibronectin, features associated with intimal proliferation. *Laboratory Investigation; A Journal of Technical Methods and Pathology* **67:** 350–359.

[32] Zhou B, Coulber C, Rabinovitch M. (1998) Tissue-specific and developmental regulation of transforming growth factor-beta1 expression in fetal lamb ductus arteriosus endothelial cells. *Pediatric Research* **44:** 865–872.

[33] Pallerla SR, Lawrence R, Lewejohann L, et al. (2008) Altered heparan sulfate structure in mice with deleted NDST3 gene function. *The Journal of Biological Chemistry* **283:** 16885–16894.

[34] Schegg B, Hulsmeier AJ, Rutschmann C, Maag C, Hennet T. (2009) Core glycosylation of collagen is initiated by two beta(1-O)galactosyltransferases. *Molecular and Cellular Biology* **29:** 943–952.

[35] Albig AR, Becenti DJ, Roy TG, Schiemann WP. (2008) Microfibril-associate glycoprotein-2 (MAGP-2) promotes angiogenic cell sprouting by blocking notch signaling in endothelial cells. *Microvascular Research* **76:** 7–14.

[36] Mikic B, Rossmeier K, Bierwert L. (2009) Identification of a tendon phenotype in GDF6 deficient mice. *Anatomical Record* **292:** 396–400.

[37] Lausen M, Lynch N, Schlosser A, et al. (1999) Microfibril-associated protein 4 is present in lung washings and binds to the collagen region of lung surfactant protein D. *The Journal of Biological Chemistry* **274:** 32234–32240.

[38] Garlick KM, Batty S, Mogridge J. (2012) Binding of filamentous actin to anthrax toxin receptor 1 decreases its association with protective antigen. *Biochemistry* **51:** 1249–1256.

[39] Li L, Zhang K, Cai XJ, Feng M, Zhang Y, Zhang M. (2011) Adiponectin upregulates pro-lyl-4-hydroxylase alpha1 expression in interleukin 6-stimulated human aortic smooth muscle cells by regulating ERK 1/2 and Sp1. *PLoS One* **6:** e22819.

[40] Chen MM, Lam A, Abraham JA, Schreiner GF, Joly AH. (2000) CTGF expression is induced by TGF- beta in cardiac fibroblasts and cardiac myocytes: a potential role in heart fibrosis. *Journal of Molecular and Cellular Cardiology* **32:** 1805–1819.

[41] Szeto CC, Lai KB, Chow KM, Szeto CY, Wong TY, Li PK. (2005) Differential effects of transforming growth factor-beta on the synthesis of connective tissue growth factor and vascular endothelial growth factor by peritoneal mesothelial cell. *Nephron. Experimental Nephrology* **99:** e95–e104.

[42] Lai KB, Sanderson JE, Yu CM. (2013) The regulatory effect of norepinephrine on connective tissue growth factor (CTGF) and vascular endothelial growth factor (VEGF) expression in cultured cardiac fibroblasts. *International Journal of Cardiology* **163:** 183–189.

[43] Clyman RI, Hardy P, Waleh N, et al. (1999) Cyclooxygenase-2 plays a significant role in regulating the tone of the fetal lamb ductus arteriosus. *The American Journal of Physiology* **276:** R913–921.

[44] Baragatti B, Brizzi F, Ackerley C, Barogi S, Ballou LR, Coceani F. (2003) Cyclooxygenase-1 and cyclooxygenase-2 in the mouse ductus arteriosus: individual activity and functional coupling with nitric oxide synthase. *British Journal of Pharmacology* **139:** 1505–1515.

[45] Momma K, Toyono M. (1999) The role of nitric oxide in dilating the fetal ductus arteriosus in rats. *Pediatric Research* **46:** 311–315.

[46] Richard C, Gao J, LaFleur B, et al. (2004) Patency of the preterm fetal ductus arteriosus is regulated by endothelial nitric oxide synthase and is independent of vasa vasorum in the mouse. *American Journal of Physiology. Regulatory, Integrative and Comparative Physiology* **287:** R652–660.

[47] Takizawa T, Kihara T, Kamata A. (2001) Increased constriction of the ductus arteriosus with combined administration of indomethacin and L-NAME in fetal rats. *Biology of the Neonate* **80:** 64–67.

[48] Coceani F, Kelsey L, Seidlitz E. (1996) Carbon monoxide-induced relaxation of the ductus arteriosus in the lamb: evidence against the prime role of guanylyl cyclase. *British Journal of Pharmacology* **118:** 1689–1696.

[49] Coceani F, Kelsey L, Seidlitz E, Korzekwa K. (1996) Inhibition of the contraction of the ductus arteriosus to oxygen by 1-aminobenzotriazole, a mechanism-based inactivator of cytochrome P450. *British Journal of Pharmacology* **117:** 1586–1592.

[50] Coceani F, Kelsey L, Seidlitz E, et al. (1997) Carbon monoxide formation in the ductus arteriosus in the lamb: implications for the regulation of muscle tone. *British Journal of Pharmacology* **120:** 599–608.

[51] Brouard S, Otterbein LE, Anrather J, et al. (2000) Carbon monoxide generated by heme oxygenase 1 suppresses endothelial cell apoptosis. The *Journal of Experimental Medicine* **192:** 1015–1025.

[52] Li Volti G, Sacerdoti D, Sangras B, et al. (2005) Carbon monoxide signaling in promoting angiogenesis in human microvessel endothelial cells. *Antioxidants & Redox Signaling* **7:** 704–710.

[53] Baragatti B, Brizzi F, Barogi S, et al. (2007) Interactions between NO, CO and an endothelium-derived hyperpolarizing factor (EDHF) in maintaining patency of the ductus arteriosus in the mouse. *British Journal of Pharmacology* **151:** 54–62.

[54] Baragatti B, Ciofini E, Sodini D, Luin S, Scebba F, Coceani F. (2013) Hydrogen sulfide in the mouse ductus arteriosus: a naturally occurring relaxant with potential EDHF function. *American Journal of Physiology. Heart and Circulatory Physiology* **304:** H927–934.

[55] Goldbarg S, Quinn T, Waleh N, et al. (2003) Effects of hypoxia, hypoglycemia, and muscle shortening on cell death in the sheep ductus arteriosus. *Pediatric Research* **54:** 204–211.

[56] Levin M, Goldbarg S, Lindqvist A, et al. (2005) ATP depletion and cell death in the neonatal lamb ductus arteriosus. *Pediatric Research* **57:** 801–805.

[57] Clyman RI, Seidner SR, Kajino H, et al. (2002) VEGF regulates remodeling during permanent anatomic closure of the ductus arteriosus. *American Journal of Physiology. Regulatory, Integrative and Comparative Physiology* **282:** R199–206.

[58] Waleh N, Seidner S, McCurnin D, et al. (2005) The role of monocyte-derived cells and inflammation in baboon ductus arteriosus remodeling. *Pediatric Research* **57:** 254–262.

[59] Waleh N, Seidner S, McCurnin D, et al. (2011) Anatomic closure of the premature patent ductus arteriosus: the role of CD14+/CD163+ mononuclear cells and VEGF in neointimal mound formation. *Pediatric Research* **70:** 332–338.

[60] Hollenberg SM, Cunnion RE, Parrillo JE. (1991) The effect of tumor necrosis factor on vascular smooth muscle. In vitro studies using rat aortic rings. *Chest* **100:** 1133–1137.

[61] Johns DG, Webb RC. (1998) TNF-alpha-induced endothelium-independent vasodilation: a role for phospholipase A2-dependent ceramide signaling. *The American Journal of Physiology* **275:** H1592–1598.

[62] Minghini A, Britt LD, Hill MA. (1998) Interleukin-1 and interleukin-6 mediated skeletal muscle arteriolar vasodilation: in vitro versus in vivo studies. *Shock* **9:** 210–215.

[63] Patel JN, Jager A, Schalkwijk C, et al. (2002) Effects of tumour necrosis factor-alpha in the human forearm: blood flow and endothelin-1 release. *Clinical Science* **103:** 409–415.

[64] Funayama H, Ikeda U, Takahashi M, et al. (1998) Human monocyte-endothelial cell interaction induces platelet-derived growth factor expression. *Cardiovascular Research* **37:** 216–224.

[65] Gunaje JJ, Bahrami AJ, Schwartz SM, Daum G, Mahoney WM, Jr. (2011) PDGF-dependent regulation of regulator of G protein signaling-5 expression and vascular smooth muscle cell functionality. *American Journal of Physiology. Cell Physiology* **301:** C478–489.

[66] Levet S, Ouarne M, Ciais D, et al. (2015) BMP9 and BMP10 are necessary for proper closure of the ductus arteriosus. *Proceedings of the National Academy of Sciences of the United States of America* **112:** E3207–3215.

[67] Hajj H, Dagle JM. (2012) Genetics of patent ductus arteriosus susceptibility and treatment. *Seminars in Perinatology* **36:** 98–104.

[68] Ricard N, Ciais D, Levet S, et al. (2012) BMP9 and BMP10 are critical for postnatal retinal vascular remodeling. *Blood* **119:** 6162–6171.

[69] David L, Mallet C, Mazerbourg S, Feige JJ, Bailly S. (2007) Identification of BMP9 and BMP10 as functional activators of the orphan activin receptor-like kinase 1 (ALK1) in endothelial cells. *Blood* **109:** 1953–1961.

[70] Loftin CD, Trivedi DB, Tiano HF, et al. (2001) Failure of ductus arteriosus closure and remodeling in neonatal mice deficient in cyclooxygenase-1 and cyclooxygenase-2. *Proceedings of the National Academy of Sciences of the United States of America* **98:** 1059–1064.

[71] Yokoyama U, Minamisawa S, Quan H, et al. (2006) Chronic activation of the prostaglandin receptor EP4 promotes hyaluronan-mediated neointimal formation in the ductus arteriosus. *The Journal of Clinical Investigation* **116:** 3026–3034.

[72] Akaike T, Jin MH, Yokoyama U, et al. (2009) T-type Ca2+ channels promote oxygenation-induced closure of the rat ductus arteriosus not only by vasoconstriction but also by neointima formation. *The Journal of Biological Chemistry* **284:** 24025–24034.

[73] Frey RS, Ushio-Fukai M, Malik AB. (2009) NADPH oxidase-dependent signaling in endothelial cells: role in physiology and pathophysiology. *Antioxidants & Redox Signaling* **11:** 791–810.

[74] Lee S, Paudel O, Jiang Y, Yang XR, Sham JS. (2015) CD38 mediates angiotensin II-induced intracellular Ca^{2+} release in rat pulmonary arterial smooth muscle cells. *American Journal of Respiratory Cell and Molecular Biology* **52:** 332–341.

[75] Smith SM, Dickman ED, Power SC, Lancman J. (1998) Retinoids and their receptors in vertebrate embryogenesis. *The Journal of Nutrition* **128:** 467S–470S.

[76] Wu GR, Jing S, Momma K, Nakanishi T. (2001) The effect of vitamin A on contraction of the ductus arteriosus in fetal rat. *Pediatric Research* **49:** 747–754.

[77] O'Byrne SM, Wongsiriroj N, Libien J, et al. (2005) Retinoid absorption and storage is impaired in mice lacking lecithin:retinol acyltransferase (LRAT). *The Journal of Biological Chemistry* **280:** 35647–35657.

[78] Bergwerff M, DeRuiter MC, Gittenberger-de Groot AC. (1999) Comparative anatomy and ontogeny of the ductus arteriosus, a vascular outsider. *Anatomy and Embryology* **200:** 559–571.

[79] Ivey KN, Sutcliffe D, Richardson J, Clyman RI, Garcia JA, Srivastava D. (2008) Transcriptional regulation during development of the ductus arteriosus. *Circulation Research* **103:** 388–395.

[80] Hu T, Yamagishi H, Maeda J, McAnally J, Yamagishi C, Srivastava D. (2004) Tbx1 regulates fibroblast growth factors in the anterior heart field through a reinforcing autoregulatory loop involving forkhead transcription factors. *Development* **131:** 5491–5502.

[81] Nowotschin S, Liao J, Gage PJ, Epstein JA, Campione M, Morrow BE. (2006) Tbx1 affects asymmetric cardiac morphogenesis by regulating Pitx2 in the secondary heart field. *Development* **133:** 1565–1573.

[82] Momma K. (2010) Cardiovascular anomalies associated with chromosome 22q11.2 deletion syndrome. *The American Journal of Cardiology* **105:** 1617–1624.

[83] Plageman TF, Jr., Zacharias AL, Gage PJ, Lang RA. (2011) Shroom3 and a Pitx2-N-cadherin pathway function cooperatively to generate asymmetric cell shape changes during gut morphogenesis. *Developmental Biology* **357:** 227–234.

[84] Golzio C, Havis E, Daubas P, et al. (2012) ISL1 directly regulates FGF10 transcription during human cardiac outflow formation. *PLoS One* **7:** e30677.

[85] Morriss-Kay GM, Wilkie AO. (2005) Growth of the normal skull vault and its alteration in craniosynostosis: insights from human genetics and experimental studies. *Journal of Anatomy* **207:** 637–653.

[86] Qu X, Carbe C, Tao C, et al. (2011) Lacrimal gland development and Fgf10-Fgfr2b signaling are controlled by 2-O- and 6-O-sulfated heparan sulfate. *The Journal of Biological Chemistry* **286:** 14435–14444.

[87] Desforges M, Greenwood SL, Glazier JD, Westwood M, Sibley CP. (2010) The contribution of SNAT1 to system A amino acid transporter activity in human placental trophoblast. *Biochemical and Biophysical Research Communications* **398:** 130–134.

[88] Mahendran D, Byrne S, Donnai P, et al. (1994) Na+ transport, H+ concentration gradient dissipation, and system A amino acid transporter activity in purified microvillous plasma membrane isolated from first-trimester human placenta: comparison with the term microvillous membrane. *American Journal of Obstetrics and Gynecology* **171:** 1534–1540.

[89] Dear N, Matena K, Vingron M, Boehm T. (1997) A new subfamily of vertebrate calpains lacking a calmodulin-like domain: implications for calpain regulation and evolution. *Genomics* **45:** 175–184.

[90] Dear TN, Boehm T. (1999) Diverse mRNA expression patterns of the mouse calpain genes Capn5, Capn6 and Capn11 during development. *Mechanisms of Development* **89:** 201–209.

[91] Marion A, Dieudonne FX, Patino-Garcia A, Lecanda F, Marie PJ, Modrowski D. (2012) Calpain-6 is an endothelin-1 signaling dependent protective factor in chemoresistant osteosarcoma. *International Journal of Cancer* **130:** 2514–2525.

2

Pathogenic Angiogenic Mechanisms in Alzheimer's Disease

Chaahat Singh, Cheryl G. Pfeifer and
Wilfred A. Jefferies

Abstract

Vascular dysfunction is a crucial pathological hallmark of Alzheimer's disease (AD). Studies have reported that beta amyloid (Aβ) causes increased blood vessel growth in the brains of AD mouse models, a phenomenon that is also seen in AD patients. This has given way to an alternative angiogenesis hypothesis according to which, increased leakiness in the blood vessels disrupts the blood-brain barrier (BBB) and allows unwanted blood products to enter the brain causing progression of disease pathology, promoting amyloid clumping and aggregation along with impaired cerebral blood flow. Furthermore, the expression of melanotransferrin in AD model and patients may contribute to angiogenesis. The objective of this chapter is to attempt to establish a link between the vascular damage and AD pathology. Curbing the vascular changes and resulting damage seen in the brains of AD model mice and improving their cognition by treating with FDA-approved anti-angiogenic drugs may expedite the translational potential of this research into clinical trials in human patients. This direction into targeting angiogenesis will facilitate new preventive and therapeutic interventions for AD and related vascular diseases.

Keywords: Alzheimer's disease, amyloid beta, blood-brain barrier, angiogenesis

1. Introduction: history of vascular dysfunction in Alzheimer's disease

Alzheimer's disease (AD) presents itself as a progressive neurological disorder, which is the major cause of dementia leading to death in the elderly. It affects thinking, orientation and memory, causing impairment in cognition, social behaviour and motivation [1]. Approximately 47.5 million people worldwide have dementia, of which the most common contributor is AD with 60–70% [1]. In 2010, the total global societal costs were estimated to be US \$604 billion corresponding to 1.0% of the worldwide gross domestic product [1].

In 1906, Dr. Alois Alzheimer [2] noted two microscopic neuropathological findings, which were further characterized and eventually established as the hallmarks of AD: senile neuritic plaques, which are aggregates that are primarily composed of beta-amyloid (Aβ) peptides; [3, 4] and neurofibrillary tangles, which are primarily composed of intra-neuronal hyperphosphorylated tau aggregates [5]. Aβ, a 4 kDa peptide, is a proteolytic cleavage product of the amyloid precursor protein (APP) by the action of α and γ secretase enzymes [6, 7]. Mutations either in the *APP* gene or in the secretase enzyme complex lead to a β secretase cleavage, forming a pathogenic Aβ species (Aβ1-42). These Aβ molecules aggregate to form oligomers, which multimerize into protofibrils, followed by the formation of dense core amyloid plaques [8–10].

1.1. Initial clinical observations linking AD and vascular disease

Post-mortem analysis has established that 50–84% of the brains of persons, who die aged 80–90+ years, show appreciable cerebrovascular lesions and although there is a debate around their impact on AD pathology, it is suggested that the independent dementia caused by vascular and AD-type pathologies may have additive or synergistic effect on cognitive impairment [11]. Vascular pathologies that have been seen in the aged human brain include: cerebral amyloid angiopathy (CAA), cerebral atherosclerosis, small vessel disease in most cases caused by hypertensive vasculopathy or microvascular degeneration, blood-brain barrier (BBB) dysfunction causing white matter lesions, microinfarctions, lacunar infarcts and microbleeds [11]. Studies in post-mortem of human brains also found evidence of increased angiogenesis in the hippocampus, midfrontal cortex, substantia nigra pars compacta, and locus coeruleus of AD brains compared to control brains suggesting that vascular dysfunction is an inherent part of AD pathology [12, 13].

1.2. Genetic risk factors linking AD and vascular disease

Epidemiological studies have identified risk factors for AD that are similar to those for cardiovascular disease (CVD) [14] such as hypertension during midlife, diabetes mellitus, smoking, apolipoprotein E (APOE) 4 isoforms, hypercholesterolemia, homocysteinemia and, in particular, age [1]. Familial AD is caused most commonly by presenilin 1 (*PSEN1*) or presenilin 2 (*PSEN2*) mutations. It is also seen that the presenilins are expressed in the heart and are critical to cardiac development. The work by Li *et al.* indicated that *PSEN1* and *PSEN2* mutations are associated with dilated cardiomyopathy (DCM) and heart failure and implicate novel mechanisms of myocardial disease [15]. Amyloid is a known vasculotrope and an increased amyloid aggregation in AD brains is seen to be in interaction with the angiogenic and CAA positive vessels [14]. Apolipoprotein 3 (APOE3) is responsible for normal lipid metabolism; however, the APOE4 isoforms is strongly associated with the late onset of AD [13]. Carriers of this isoform show a decreased cerebral blood flow and have also been linked to disorders associated with elevated cholesterol levels or lipid derangements (*i.e.* hyperlipoproteinemia type III, coronary heart disease, strokes, peripheral artery disease and diabetes mellitus) [15]. These overlapping genetic risk factors might give us a direction for understanding the mechanisms of the disease-related pathways.

1.3. Factors linked to AD and increased angiogenesis: melanotransferrin (p97), VEGF, transglutaminases (factor XIIIa and tTG)

Melanotransferrin (also known as p97 or melanoma tumour antigen) is a member of the transferrin family and is responsible for the cellular uptake of iron. P97 was shown to be present in the capillary endothelium in a normal brain, in contrast to the brain from patients with AD, where it is found to be localized in microglia cells, associated with senile plaques [16, 17]. Serum normally contains very low levels of p97; however, it is reported to increase by five- and six-fold in patients with AD [18, 19]. From this observation, it was proposed that serum p97 could be a potential biochemical marker for this disease. It was further demonstrated that melanotransferrin exerts an angiogenic response quantitatively similar to that elicited by fibroblast growth factor 2 [20], and hypervascularity has been shown to be a feature in the brains of AD patients [12]. Overexpression of vascular endothelial growth factor (VEGF) receptor 2 was observed in newly formed vessels, suggesting that the angiogenic activity of melanotransferrin may depend on activation of endogenous VEGF [20]. VEGF is the major player in pathological/dysfunctional blood vessel formation. It is shown that VEGF is highly up-regulated in AD brains via the inflammatory pathway and also that VEGF co-aggregates with Aβ in AD brains [13]. The role of transglutaminases in AD is highly debated; however, it is shown that the activity of these enzymes might contribute to both angiogenesis and in the formation of protein aggregates in the AD brain [21, 22].

2. Alzheimer's disease and the blood-brain barrier pathogenesis: angiogenesis and inflammation

A physical seal is present between the vasculature in the brain and the central nervous system that restricts fluid and entrained molecules from being transported into the brain from the systemic circulation [13, 23]. Dysfunction of the BBB was originally seen in animal models of AD [24] and was later established as a prominent, but unexplained clinical feature of AD in patients [23]. Though it is unknown where the BBB dysfunction stems from, it is, however, argued that Aβ may be directly involved in this process [25, 26]. Leakiness of the BBB has been demonstrated in a number of AD transgenic animal models that have overexpression of *APP*, including the Tg2576, which manifests a form of early-onset AD [24, 25]. Studies show that BBB integrity is compromised in this mouse model as early as 4 months of age, much before the onset of other disease pathology, such as the consolidated amyloid plaques [24, 27]. Hence, the mechanism leading to the BBB disruption is a potential target for AD therapy.

2.1. Tight junction disruption in mouse models

The brain has a unique structure termed as the blood-brain barrier (BBB), which is a specialized physical seal that precludes the transport of various, large and/or hydrophilic, peripheral blood molecules from entering the brain parenchyma [13, 25]. This restricted exchange protects the brain from indiscriminate exposure to peptides, macromolecules and potentially toxic molecules [13, 25]. The integrity of the BBB is maintained by inter-endothelial complexes called tight junctions (TJ), in the brain capillaries, that are composed of a variety of plasma membrane spanning proteins (occludin), scaffold proteins (zonula occludens protein-1; ZO-1) and the actin cytoskeleton [12, 13, 25]. The peripheral membrane protein, ZO-1, localizes along blood vessels in the brain parenchyma and along with claudins and occludin ensures the intactness and permeability of the BBB [26, 28]. A second barrier is presented by the basal lamina, composed of type IV collagen, fibronectin and heparan sulphate along with other molecules, which operates as a molecular weight filter [26]. Lastly, there are cells that interact to protect the BBB, known as the neurovascular unit (NVU). This is composed of neurons, cerebral endothelial cells, basal lamina, astrocytic foot processes (containing proteases and neurotransmitters) and perivascular macrophages called pericytes [26].

Since the BBB plays crucial role in maintaining central nervous system (CNS) homeostasis, its dysfunction proves deleterious for the smooth working of the brain. The BBB dysfunction includes: (1) BBB disruption, resulting in the discharge of potentially neurotoxic circulating substances into the CNS; (2) transporter dysfunction, which consequently creates deficiency of nutrient supply and amplify toxic substances in the CNS; and (3) altered protein expression and NVU cell secretions, potentially resulting in inflammatory activation, oxidative stress and neuronal damage [28]. The three effects stated above have been reported in AD patients, although the scope of this chapter pertains only to BBB disruption.

The compromised integrity of the BBB has been indicated by increased CSF/serum albumin ratios seen in AD patients [28]. Albumin is a macromolecule that is unable to cross an intact BBB [27, 28]. Histological studies have also revealed the presence of albumin staining around microvessels that shows co-localization of amyloid plaques and angiopathy [12, 13, 26]. It is suggested that this staining is a result of an affinity of extravasated albumin for amyloid [28].

Prothrombin is seen at elevated levels particularly around the microvessels in the brains of AD patients [29]. Highest levels of the protein were observed in people scoring higher in the Braak staging [30, 31].

The increased vesicularization of brain endothelial cells damages the BBB by altering the tight junction function. This is consistent with increased transcytotic disruption of the BBB initiated by the release of inflammatory cytokines that are angiogenic triggers, promoting paracellular leakage [28].

2.2. CBF impairment: a road to hypervascularity in mouse models and humans

Vascular dysfunction is a crucial pathological hallmark of AD [12, 32]. The two key precursors to neurodegenerative changes and Aβ deposition in AD are the BBB breakdown [12, 32] and cerebral blood flow (CBF) impairment [33]. Various studies with the help of a non-invasive imaging technique (arterial spin labelling MRI) have shown that AD is associated with a global, as well as a regional CBF impairment, also known as cerebral hypoperfusion [34]. While AD patients exhibit a global decrease in blood flow (averaged 40%), compared to healthy controls, the CBF reduction is seen only in specific regions that are usually implicated in the disease state [14, 34]. It is, however, argued whether a diminished blood flow in AD is a cause or consequence of the disease.

Hypoperfusion is associated with both structural and functional changes in the brain and hence plays a pivotal role in influencing the permeability of the BBB [34]. Severe reductions in CBF have been seen in the elderly at a high risk for cognitive decline and AD [34]. Individuals that are carriers of the major AD risk allele, (APOE4), have a more impacted regional deteriorated CBF than non-carriers of the allele [35, 36]. AD-related vascular pathology impairs cerebral autoregulation and causes cerebrovascular insufficiency [37]. This impaired CBF and compromised BBB result in the accumulation of potentially neurotoxic molecules (e.g. increased Aβ concentration) in the brain along with the entry of unwanted blood products via peripheral circulation [38, 39]. Data obtained from structural MRI scans show atrophy in different regions of the brain, and an overall change in cortical thickness is observed due to hypoperfusion in AD patients [34]. The thickness of the cortex is an important predictive measure of evolution to AD for subjects with mild cognitive impairment [34]. Carriers of the APOE4 allele, a demographic reported to have glucose hypo-metabolism, demonstrate hastened cortical thinning in areas most vulnerable to aging (medial prefrontal and peri-central cortices) as well as in areas associated with AD and amyloid-aggregation (e.g. occipito-temporal, basal temporal cortices and hippocampus) [34]. Ageing is the leading risk factor for the development of late-onset AD. Aberrations in vascular ultrastructure, vascular reactivity, resting cerebral blood flow and oxygen metabolism are all associated with age and act as a catalyst for cerebrovascular diseases and subsequent cognitive deficits [40]. To cope with the decrease in blood flow, the brain has evolved a compensatory mechanism whereby it increases the formation of blood vessels resulting in hypervascularity, a phenomenon which is seen not only in mouse models [40–43] but also in post-mortem samples of AD patients [43].

2.3. Involvement of angiogenesis and not apoptosis

The 'vascular hypothesis' as stated currently, defends that the vascular damage is a consequence of diminished blood perfusion of the brain, leading to hypoperfusion/hypoxia causing the BBB dysfunction [44]. A subsequent amalgamation of accumulated Aβ, neuro-inflammation, and the eventual disintegration of the neurovascular unit is seen, culminating in vascular death [13, 25, 45]. In a state of hypoperfusion, the hypoxia-inducible factors initiate angiogenesis (the formation of blood vessels) through the up-regulation of pro-angiogenic factors [25]. The main player in this blood vessel formation is VEGF, which induces differentiation and proliferation of endothelial cells from its progenitors, the hemangioblast and the angioblast

[46]. This forms an inefficiently differentiated primitive vascular plexus (vasculogenesis) [47]. The vascular plexus undergoes remodelling, that is triggered by the angiopoietin-1 (Ang-1), into a hierarchically structured mature vascular system established through endothelial cell sprouting, trimming differentiation and pericyte recruitment (normal angiogenesis) [48]. In contrast to these events in AD, it is observed that, a downstream cell signalling molecule to VEGF, angiopoietin-2 (Ang-2), destabilizes the vessel wall of mature vessels [32, 49–51]. The quiescent endothelial cells become sensitive to VEGF (and other angiogenic factors), proliferate indiscriminately, migrate to form new vessels that are not able to mature and eventually lead to the establishment of a leaky network of blood vessels [32]. This phenomenon is termed as pathological angiogenesis, which is a common occurrence seen during the evolution of tumours. In accordance with the current version of the 'vascular hypothesis', the BBB disruption is due to vascular cell death caused by apoptosis and angiogenesis would only be required to ensure tissue regeneration and likely be limited to replacing the damaged tissues and ensuring oxygenation of brain tissues [12, 13]. However, this role of apoptosis in BBB dysfunction is highly debated. Recent studies have shown that endothelial cell proliferation, during pathological angiogenesis, results in hypervascularity [12]. As a compensatory mechanism to the decreased blood flow caused by the leaky blood vessel network, vascular remodelling and structural changes take place in the physical arrangement of the tight junction proteins, resulting in compromised BBB integrity [12, 52]. The work of Biron *et al.* characterized the relationship between amyloidogenesis and BBB integrity, through changes in the TJ morphology in the Tg2576 AD mouse. They reported that the Tg2576 AD mice exhibit no apparent vascular apoptosis but have significant TJ disruption, which was seen directly linked to pathological angiogenesis, resulting in a significant increase in vascular density in AD brain [12]. Hence, it can be said that these data support the model that TJ disruption results from increased vascular permeability that takes place during extreme neovascularization in AD.

2.4. Angiogenesis: inflammation and vascular activation

Increasing evidence suggest that the vascular perturbation appears as a common feature in AD pathology as its hallmarks: amyloid plaques and neurofibrillary tangles. Over the years, emphasis has still been given to the accumulation of Aβ in AD, which, as a result of its impaired clearance from the brain, is thought to be responsible for the onset of cognitive decline [39, 53–55]. Paradoxical to this hypothesis, aggregated Aβ can be extensively present in the human brain in the absence of AD symptoms [56–58]. Although Aβ plays a crucial role in AD, it is neither necessary nor by itself sufficient to cause full AD pathology [27]. The alternate idea is that the mere production of Aβ (amyloidogenesis), promotes extensive pathological angiogenesis, leading to the redistribution of TJs, which then causes disruption to the BBB integrity, thereby increasing vascular permeability, subsequent hypervascularization and eventual AD pathology. This alternate 'vascular hypothesis' stems from a body of data that now establishes hypervascularization as a mechanistic explanation for amyloid-associated TJ pathology [12]. It provides new modalities for therapeutic intervention that target the restoration of the BBB by modulating angiogenesis, thereby possibly preventing AD onset and potentially repairing damage in the AD brain. A second study by Biron *et al.* demonstrated that immunization with Aβ peptides neutralized the amyloid trigger that causes pathological angiogenesis and thereby reverses hypervascularity in Tg2576 AD mice [59]. The Aβ plaques were seen to be dissolved, solubilized Aβ removed from the brain parenchyma along perivascular drainage routes, which resulted in a decrease in the hypervascularity [59]. This supports a vascular angiogenesis model for AD pathophysiology and provides the first evidence that modulating angiogenesis repairs damage in the AD brain.

Pathological angiogenesis and hypervascularization in an AD brain occurs in response to impaired cerebral perfusion (oligaemia) and inflammatory response to vascular injury [60]. We have already discussed the impaired perfusion in Section 2.2. In this section, we will look at the inflammatory activation of angiogenesis. Morphological and biochemical evidences present themselves in the form of regionally increased capillary density, unresolved vascular sprouting, glomeruloid vascular structure formation, and up-regulated expression of angiogenic factors: VEGF, transforming growth factor β (TGF β) and tumour necrosis factor α (TNF α) [60]. In AD, inflammatory pathways, when stimulated, cause the release of angiogenic cytokines such as thrombin and VEGF, contributing to pathological angiogenesis [60]. It is hypothesized that a thrombogenic region develops in the endothelial cells of the vessel wall, leading to intra-vascular accumulation of thrombin. This thrombin activates the vascular endothelial cells to secrete amyloid precursor protein via a receptor-mediated protein kinase C-dependent pathway [60]. Progressive deposition of amyloid precursor protein leads to accumulation of the Aβ plaques, which generates more reactive oxygen species and induces further endothelial damage in a cycle of neurotoxic insult. This establishes a cycle of neurotoxicity and death, instituted by the discharge of thrombin following Aβ-induced neuroinflammatory responses [60]. Other studies further support the interaction of Aβ with thrombin and fibrin throughout the clotting cascade, to increase neurovascular damage and neuroinflammation [61–63]. Astrocytes, cultured in vitro and stimulated with Aβ, showed a release of neuroinflammatory cytokines that resulted in the increased expression of VEGF [49, 50]. Other pro-inflammatory cytokines, such as interleukin-1β are increased during AD and known to induce VEGF and growth of new blood vessels [52, 64].

Consequential evidence is present implicating Aβ as a vasculotrope, modulating blood vessel density and vascular remodelling through angiogenic mechanisms. Brain microvessels have been shown to be closely associated with Aβ plaques with the aid of ultrastructural studies. It was observed that that AD brain capillaries contained pre-amyloid deposits [60]. Aβ stimulates angiogenesis in a highly conserved manner, which is speculated to be mediated through γ-secretase activity and Notch signalling [60, 65]. The in vitro studies of human umbilical vein endothelial cells (hUVEC), exposed directly to Aβ1-40 and Aβ1-42, show an angiogenic effect on the hUVEC, which exhibited an increase in the number of tip cells and branching [60].

The indication for Aβ-related angiogenesis has been extended in vivo as well, which can be observed with the chick embryo chorioallantoic membrane assay [65]. Aβ1-40 and Aβ1-42 stimulated embryos illustrated escalated vascular growth [65]. In vivo studies, using various APP mutant AD mouse models that have an overproduction of Aβ, show modifications in brain vasculature compared to the wild-type animals [12, 25]. APP23 AD model mice exhibit significant blood flow alterations correlated with structural modifications of blood vessels [51].

A study using three-dimensional architectural analysis [51], revealed significant changes to be accelerated only in the amyloid positive vessels [64]. Interestingly, brain homogenates taken from Aβ-overexpressing AD model mice, demonstrated an increase in the formation of new vessels in an *in vivo* angiogenesis assay [52]. This increase in vessels was blocked on exposure to a VEGF antagonist [52]. The vascular changes observed in these mice may be thought to be due to unrelated, 'off-target' effects of the APP mutation. However, the fact that the vascular changes observed in transgenic mice correlate well with vascular disturbances reported in human AD brains, it is safe to say that angiogenesis plays a crucial role in the establishment of AD pathology.

Post-mortem studies of human brains also show evidence of increased angiogenesis in the hippocampus, mid-frontal cortex, substantia nigra pars compacta, and locus coeruleus of AD brains compared to healthy individuals [43]. Further analysis found no correlation between the number of microglia (activation of apoptosis) and angiogenesis or microglia with vessel density, suggesting that it may be the presence of Aβ that is initiating angiogenesis (and not activation of apoptosis) and subsequently causing BBB dysfunction [66, 67].

It is seen that there are additional proteins at the BBB, which act to regulate brain Aβ levels and the disruption of which takes the brain towards up-regulated angiogenesis. The receptor for advanced glycation products (RAGE), a multi-ligand receptor, regulates the entry of peripheral Aβ to the brain [67–69]. Its expression is up-regulated by binding with ligands including Aβ and pro-inflammatory cytokine-like mediators [67]. This facilitates the entry of Aβ into the cerebral neurons, microglia and vasculature [69]. *In vitro* studies have also implicated RAGE in the vascular pathogenesis of AD, by suppressing the CBF, leading to hypoperfusion [67, 70].

3. Haemostatic mechanisms in relation to angiogenesis in AD

Maintenance of the fluidity of blood and limiting its loss upon blood vessel endothelium injury is a crucial physiological process known as haemostasis [71]. Haemostasis is possible due to the existence of a delicate balance between pro-coagulation and anti-coagulation along with numerous pathways and feedback loops [71, 72]. Haemostasis has three distinct phases— where the primary haemostasis is involved in adhering platelets to site of injury, forming a 'haemostatic or platelet plug' [71]; secondary haemostasis—which involves the activation of coagulation cascade, culminating in a fibrin clot; the last stage—which is fibrinolysis, or the dissolution of the clot [71]. Accompanied with vascular dysfunction, an altered haemostatic scenario is increasingly implicated in AD. Majority of the research, barring a few, support an association of pro-coagulation mechanism in AD. The proteins like transglutaminases are core components of the coagulation system that could be used as therapeutics to resolve the altered haemostasis in AD.

3.1. The involvement of haemostatic factors in angiogenesis: transglutaminases (factor XIIIa and tTG)

Transglutaminases (TG) are a family of enzymes, which catalyse irreversible post-translational modifications of proteins [22, 73]. Yamada *et al.* put forward the suggestion that TG activity might contribute to the formation of protein aggregates in AD brain [21]. Though this idea is debated, tau proteins have been shown to be in support of this hypothesis by being an appropriate *in vitro* substrate of TGs [22]. Studies also show that transglutaminase-catalysed cross-links, co-localize with pathological lesions in AD brain. More recently, amyloid β-protein oligomerization and aggregation, at physiologic levels *in vitro*, have seen to be induced by the activity of TGs [22]. By these molecular mechanisms, TGs could contribute to AD symptoms and progression. Though the studies mentioned above support the involvement of TG in neurodegeneration, they fail to indicate whether aberrant TG activity, *per se*, directly determines the disease's progression [22].

Factor XIII (FXIII), a plasma TG, besides clot stabilization, plays an important role in wound healing and embryo implantation—a process that involves angiogenesis [74]. Haemostasis and angiogenesis are inter-related as can be seen by the haemostatic proteins assisting the spatial localization and stabilization of endothelial cells, which is succeeded by growth and repair of damaged vessels [74]. Post clot stabilization, the coagulation and fibrinolytic proteins regulate angiogenesis [74]. Thrombin-activated FXIII promotes endothelial cell migration, proliferation and inhibits apoptosis [74]. It is known to bind endothelial cell integrin αvβ3. This binding enhances the integrin's interaction with VEGFR2, which then activates downstream, the Erk and Akt, thus augmenting cell proliferation [74]. This body of data suggests that there is an altered state of haemostasis that could contribute to AD pathology through angiogenesis.

4. Therapeutic modalities in treating pathogenic angiogenesis in AD

Angiogenesis, as stated by the studies mentioned in this chapter, can be viewed as that stage in AD pathology where all the different pathways (hypoperfusion, BBB dysfunction, inflammation) merge, leading to the AD pathology. Observations showing increased cerebrovascular permeability prior to the appearance of the hallmarks of AD, sprout a novel paradigm for integrating vascular remodelling (angiogenesis) with the pathophysiology of the disease. Targeting this integral step in the pathophysiology of AD and developing a novel therapeutic intervention using anti-angiogenic drugs can help to alleviate the global societal burden of AD.

4.1. Anti-angiogenics: small molecule tyrosine kinase inhibitors

Anti-angiogenics, including small molecule tyrosine kinase inhibitors have been tested and approved as anti-cancer therapeutics and have shown to maintain normal vascular [75–77]. Sunitinib is a broad spectrum tyrosine kinase inhibitor. This is known to inhibit the phosphorylation of multiple receptor tyrosine kinases and is a potent inhibitor of VEGF as well as platelet-derived growth factor (PDGF-β). Currently, it is in use for gastrointestinal stromal tumours, renal cell cancer and pancreatic cancer. Sunitinib was shown to decrease the amyloid burden and reverse cognitive decline in AD model mice, suggesting that if we target angiogenesis, we can revert the increase in the accumulation of Aβ and abate the cognitive decline associated with AD [76].

4.2. Biologics and small molecule VEGFR inhibitors

We now know that VEGF is the prime and central component of pathological blood vessel formation. There are biologics and small molecules that specifically target the ligand or its receptor. This specific-targeted therapy could prove more efficient and less deleterious due to avoidance of unwanted 'off target' effects. A potential therapeutic is Bexarotene, a retinoid X receptor agonist, is shown to facilitate Aβ clearance via activation of apolipoprotein (APOE) expression and promoting microglial phagocytosis [78]. Bexarotene counteracts VEGF-mediated angiogenesis by decreasing blood vessel density and reversing cognitive deficits in AD mice [78].

These are examples of some of the therapeutic routes that could target angiogenesis; however, understanding the molecular mechanism behind angiogenesis causing eventual AD pathology is of utmost importance in order to look for safe and effective novel therapeutics for AD and other vascular diseases.

5. Concluding remarks

As the Western world ages, AD represents an ailment that will place a significant burden on all the aspects of society. This burden, primarily placed on family caregivers, has been estimated to cost billions in lost productivity and healthcare costs (both direct and indirect). Currently, there is a lack of understanding regarding the cause(s) of the disease that translates into a lack of viable treatments or cures. Over the years, limited progress has been made with regards to the clinical translation of the popular amyloid hypothesis for treating AD and hence new thinking towards AD pathogenesis is required. Vascular risk factors and neurovascular dysfunction associated with hypotension, hypertension, cholesterol levels, type II diabetes mellitus, smoking, oxidative stress and iron overload have been found to play integral roles in the pathogenesis of stroke and AD. Observations showing increased cerebrovascular permeability prior to the appearance of the hallmarks of AD, sprout a novel paradigm for integrating vascular remodelling (angiogenesis) with the pathophysiology of the disease. Taking this into account, research focused on understanding the molecular mechanism behind the pathophysiology of angiogenesis leading to AD pathology will mediate in developing novel therapeutic interventions targeting this pathological blood vessel formation help to alleviate the global societal burden of AD.

Author details

Chaahat Singh[1,3], Cheryl G. Pfeifer[1] and Wilfred A. Jefferies[1,2,3,4,5,6*]

*Address all correspondence to: wilf@msl.ubc.ca

1 The Michael Smith Laboratories, University of British Columbia, Vancouver, Canada

2 Department of Microbiology & Immunology, University of British Columbia, Vancouver, Canada

3 Department of Medical Genetics, University of British Columbia, Vancouver, Canada

4 Department of Zoology, University of British Columbia, Vancouver, Canada

5 Centre for Blood Research, University of British Columbia, Vancouver, Canada

6 Djavad Mowafaghian Centre for Brain Health, University of British Columbia, Vancouver, Canada

References

[1] WHO: Dementia—Fact sheet. April 2016. http://www.who.int/mediacentre/factsheets/fs362/en/

[2] Alzheimer A: About a peculiar disease of the cerebral cortex. By Alois Alzheimer, 1907 (Translated by L. Jarvik and H. Greenson). Alzheimer Dis Assoc Disord 1987, 1:3–8.

[3] Glenner GG, Wong CW: Alzheimer's disease: initial report of the purification and characterization of a novel cerebrovascular amyloid protein. Biochem Biophys Res Commun 1984, 120:885–90.

[4] Glenner GG, Wong CW: Alzheimer's disease: initial report of the purification and characterization of a novel cerebrovascular amyloid protein. Biochem Biophys Res Commun 2012, 425:534–9.

[5] Gorevic PD, Goni F, Pons-Estel B, Alvarez F, Peress NS, Frangione B: Isolation and partial characterization of neurofibrillary tangles and amyloid plaque core in Alzheimer's disease: immunohistological studies. J Neuropathol Exp Neurol 1986, 45:647–64.

[6] Hardy JA, Higgins GA: Alzheimer's disease: the amyloid cascade hypothesis. Science 1992, 256:184–5.

[7] Thinakaran G, Koo EH: Amyloid precursor protein trafficking, processing, and function. J Biol Chem 2008, 283:29615–9.

[8] Citron M, Oltersdorf T, Haass C, McConlogue L, Hung AY, Seubert P, Vigo-Pelfrey C, Lieberburg I, Selkoe DJ: Mutation of the beta-amyloid precursor protein in familial Alzheimer's disease increases beta-protein production. Nature 1992, 360:672–4.

[9] Haass C, Lemere CA, Capell A, Citron M, Seubert P, Schenk D, Lannfelt L, Selkoe DJ: The Swedish mutation causes early-onset Alzheimer's disease by beta-secretase cleavage within the secretory pathway. Nat Med 1995, 1:1291–6.

[10] Haass C, De Strooper B: The presenilins in Alzheimer's disease—proteolysis holds the key. Science 1999, 286:916–9.

[11] Attems J, Jellinger KA: The overlap between vascular disease and Alzheimer's disease —lessons from pathology. BMC Med 2014, 12:206.

[12] Biron KE, Dickstein DL, Gopaul R, Jefferies WA: Amyloid triggers extensive cerebral angiogenesis causing blood brain barrier permeability and hypervascularity in Alzheimer's disease. PLoS One 2011, 6:e23789.

[13] Jefferies WA, Price KA, Biron KE, Fenninger F, Pfeifer CG, Dickstein DL: Adjusting the compass: new insights into the role of angiogenesis in Alzheimer's disease. Alzheimers Res Ther 2013, 5:64.

[14] Claassen JA, Zhang R: Cerebral autoregulation in Alzheimer's disease. J Cereb Blood Flow Metab 2011, 31:1572–7.

[15] Li D, Parks SB, Kushner JD, Nauman D, Burgess D, Ludwigsen S, Partain J, Nixon RR, Allen CN, Irwin RP, Jakobs PM, Litt M, Hershberger RE: Mutations of presenilin genes in dilated cardiomyopathy and heart failure. Am J Hum Genet 2006, 79:1030–9.

[16] Jefferies WA, Food MR, Gabathuler R, Rothenberger S, Yamada T, Yasuhara O, McGeer PL: Reactive microglia specifically associated with amyloid plaques in Alzheimer's disease brain tissue express melanotransferrin. Brain Res 1996, 712:122–6.

[17] Yamada T, Tsujioka Y, Taguchi J, Takahashi M, Tsuboi Y, Moroo I, Yang J, Jefferies WA: Melanotransferrin is produced by senile plaque-associated reactive microglia in Alzheimer's disease. Brain Res 1999, 845:1–5.

[18] Feldman H, Gabathuler R, Kennard M, Nurminen J, Levy D, Foti S, Foti D, Beattie BL, Jefferies WA: Serum p97 levels as an aid to identifying Alzheimer's disease. J Alzheimers Dis 2001, 3:507–16.

[19] Kennard ML, Feldman H, Yamada T, Jefferies WA: Serum levels of the iron binding protein p97 are elevated in Alzheimer's disease. Nat Med 1996, 2:1230–5.

[20] Sala R, Jefferies WA, Walker B, Yang J, Tiong J, Law S, Carlevaro MF, Di Marco E, Vacca A, Cancedda R: The human melanoma associated protein melanotransferrin promotes endothelial cell migration and angiogenesis in vivo. Eur J Cell Biol 2002, 81:599–607.

[21] Yamada T, Yoshiyama Y, Kawaguchi N, Ichinose A, Iwaki T, Hirose S, Jefferies W: Possible roles of transglutaminases in Alzheimer's disease. Dementia Geriatr Cogn Disorder 1998, 9:103–10.

[22] Martin A, De Vivo G, Gentile V: Possible role of the transglutaminases in the pathogenesis of Alzheimer's disease and other neurodegenerative diseases. Int J Alzheimers Dis 2011, 2011:865432.

[23] Rosenberg GA: Blood-brain barrier permeability in aging and Alzheimer's disease. J Prev Alzheimers Dis 2014, 1:138–9.

[24] Ujiie M, Dickstein D, Carlow D, Jefferies WA: Blood-brain barrier permeability precedes senile plaque formation in an Alzheimer disease model. Microcirculation 2003, 10:463–70.

[25] Kook SY, Seok Hong H, Moon M, Mook-Jung I: Disruption of blood-brain barrier in Alzheimer disease pathogenesis. Tissue Barriers 2013, 1:e23993.

[26] Erickson MA, Banks WA: Blood-brain barrier dysfunction as a cause and consequence of Alzheimer's disease. J Cereb Blood Flow Metab 2013, 33:1500–13.

[27] Vagnucci AH, Jr., Li WW: Alzheimer's disease and angiogenesis. Lancet 2003, 361:605–8.

[28] Banks WA, Gray AM, Erickson MA, Salameh TS, Damodarasamy M, Sheibani N, Meabon JS, Wing EE, Morofuji Y, Cook DG, Reed MJ: Lipopolysaccharide-induced blood-brain barrier disruption: roles of cyclooxygenase, oxidative stress, neuroinflammation, and elements of the neurovascular unit. J Neuroinflamm 2015, 12:223.

[29] Arai T, Miklossy J, Klegeris A, Guo JP, McGeer PL: Thrombin and prothrombin are expressed by neurons and glial cells and accumulate in neurofibrillary tangles in Alzheimer disease brain. J Neuropathol Exp Neurol 2006, 65:19–25.

[30] Zipser BD, Johanson CE, Gonzalez L, Berzin TM, Tavares R, Hulette CM, Vitek MP, Hovanesian V, Stopa EG: Microvascular injury and blood-brain barrier leakage in Alzheimer's disease. Neurobiol Aging 2007, 28:977–86.

[31] Lewczuk P, Wiltfang J, Lange M, Jahn H, Reiber H, Ehrenreich H: Prothrombin concentration in the cerebrospinal fluid is not altered in Alzheimer's disease. Neurochem Res 1999, 24:1531–4.

[32] Desai BS, Schneider JA, Li JL, Carvey PM, Hendey B: Evidence of angiogenic vessels in Alzheimer's disease. J Neural Transm 2009, 116:587–97.

[33] Austin BP, Nair VA, Meier TB, Xu G, Rowley HA, Carlsson CM, Johnson SC, Prabhakaran V: Effects of hypoperfusion in Alzheimer's disease. J Alzheimers Dis 2011, 26 Suppl 3:123–33.

[34] Thomas T, Miners S, Love S: Post-mortem assessment of hypoperfusion of cerebral cortex in Alzheimer's disease and vascular dementia. Brain 2015, 138:1059–69.

[35] Olichney JM, Hansen LA, Galasko D, Saitoh T, Hofstetter CR, Katzman R, Thal LJ: The apolipoprotein E epsilon 4 allele is associated with increased neuritic plaques and

cerebral amyloid angiopathy in Alzheimer's disease and Lewy body variant. Neurology 1996, 47:190–6.

[36] Verghese PB, Castellano JM, Holtzman DM: Apolipoprotein E in Alzheimer's disease and other neurological disorders. Lancet Neurol 2011, 10:241–52.

[37] Zlokovic BV: The blood-brain barrier in health and chronic neurodegenerative disorders. Neuron 2008, 57:178–201.

[38] D'Esposito M, Jagust W, Gazzaley A: Methodological and conceptual issues in the study of the aging brain: Oxford University Press, Oxford, UK, 2009.

[39] Selkoe DJ: Toward a comprehensive theory for Alzheimer's disease. Hypothesis: Alzheimer's disease is caused by the cerebral accumulation and cytotoxicity of amyloid beta-protein. Ann N Y Acad Sci 2000, 924:17–25.

[40] Kara F, Dongen ES, Schliebs R, Buchem MA, Groot HJ, Alia A: Monitoring blood flow alterations in the Tg2576 mouse model of Alzheimer's disease by *in vivo* magnetic resonance angiography at 17.6 T. Neuroimage 2012, 60:958–66.

[41] Beckmann N, Schuler A, Mueggler T, Meyer EP, Wiederhold KH, Staufenbiel M, Krucker T: Age-dependent cerebrovascular abnormalities and blood flow disturbances in APP23 mice modeling Alzheimer's disease. J Neurosci 2003, 23:8453–9.

[42] Thal DR, Capetillo-Zarate E, Larionov S, Staufenbiel M, Zurbruegg S, Beckmann N: Capillary cerebral amyloid angiopathy is associated with vessel occlusion and cerebral blood flow disturbances. Neurobiol Aging 2009, 30:1936–48.

[43] Pfeifer LA, White LR, Ross GW, Petrovitch H, Launer LJ: Cerebral amyloid angiopathy and cognitive function: the HAAS autopsy study. Neurology 2002, 58:1629–34.

[44] de la Torre JC, Mussivand T: Can disturbed brain microcirculation cause Alzheimer's disease? Neurol Res 1993, 15:146–53.

[45] de la Torre JC: How do heart disease and stroke become risk factors for Alzheimer's disease? Neurol Res 2006, 28:637–44.

[46] Rose JA, Erzurum S, Asosingh K: Biology and flow cytometry of proangiogenic hematopoietic progenitors cells. Cytometry A 2015, 87:5–19.

[47] Patan S: Vasculogenesis and angiogenesis. Cancer Treat Res 2004, 117:3–32.

[48] Herbert SP, Stainier DY: Molecular control of endothelial cell behaviour during blood vessel morphogenesis. Nat Rev Mol Cell Biol 2011, 12:551–64.

[49] Chiarini A, Whitfield J, Bonafini C, Chakravarthy B, Armato U, Dal Pra I: Amyloid-beta (25–35), an amyloid-beta (1–42) surrogate, and proinflammatory cytokines stimulate VEGF-A secretion by cultured, early passage, normoxic adult human cerebral astrocytes. J Alzheimers Dis 2010, 21:915–26.

[50] Pogue AI, Lukiw WJ: Angiogenic signaling in Alzheimer's disease. Neuroreport 2004, 15:1507–10.

[51] Meyer EP, Ulmann-Schuler A, Staufenbiel M, Krucker T: Altered morphology and 3D architecture of brain vasculature in a mouse model for Alzheimer's disease. Proc Natl Acad Sci U S A 2008, 105:3587–92.

[52] Schultheiss C, Blechert B, Gaertner FC, Drecoll E, Mueller J, Weber GF, Drzezga A, Essler M: *In vivo* characterization of endothelial cell activation in a transgenic mouse model of Alzheimer's disease. Angiogenesis 2006, 9:59–65.

[53] Selkoe DJ: The cell biology of beta-amyloid precursor protein and presenilin in Alzheimer's disease. Trends Cell Biol 1998, 8:447–53.

[54] Selkoe DJ: Translating cell biology into therapeutic advances in Alzheimer's disease. Nature 1999, 399:A23–31.

[55] de la Torre JC: Alzheimer's disease: how does it start? J Alzheimers Dis 2002, 4:497–512.

[56] Mielke R, Schroder R, Fink GR, Kessler J, Herholz K, Heiss WD: Regional cerebral glucose metabolism and postmortem pathology in Alzheimer's disease. Acta Neuropathol 1996, 91:174–9.

[57] Davis DG, Schmitt FA, Wekstein DR, Markesbery WR: Alzheimer neuropathologic alterations in aged cognitively normal subjects. J Neuropathol Exp Neurol 1999, 58:376–88.

[58] Morris GP, Clark IA, Vissel B: Inconsistencies and controversies surrounding the amyloid hypothesis of Alzheimer's disease. Acta Neuropathol Commun 2014, 2:135.

[59] Biron KE, Dickstein DL, Gopaul R, Fenninger F, Jefferies WA: Cessation of neoangiogenesis in Alzheimer's disease follows amyloid-beta immunization. Sci Rep 2013, 3:1354.

[60] Cortes-Canteli M, Paul J, Norris EH, Bronstein R, Ahn HJ, Zamolodchikov D, Bhuvanendran S, Fenz KM, Strickland S: Fibrinogen and beta-amyloid association alters thrombosis and fibrinolysis: a possible contributing factor to Alzheimer's disease. Neuron 2010, 66:695–709.

[61] Zamolodchikov D, Strickland S: Abeta delays fibrin clot lysis by altering fibrin structure and attenuating plasminogen binding to fibrin. Blood 2012, 119:3342–51.

[62] Paul J, Strickland S, Melchor JP: Fibrin deposition accelerates neurovascular damage and neuroinflammation in mouse models of Alzheimer's disease. J Exp Med 2007, 204:1999–2008.

[63] Fioravanzo L, Venturini M, Di Liddo R, Marchi F, Grandi C, Parnigotto PP, Folin M: Involvement of rat hippocampal astrocytes in beta-amyloid-induced angiogenesis and neuroinflammation. Curr Alzheimer Res 2010, 7:591–601.

[64] Boulton ME, Cai J, Grant MB: gamma-Secretase: a multifaceted regulator of angiogenesis. J Cell Mol Med 2008, 12:781–95.

[65] Boscolo E, Folin M, Nico B, Grandi C, Mangieri D, Longo V, Scienza R, Zampieri P, Conconi MT, Parnigotto PP, Ribatti D: Beta amyloid angiogenic activity *in vitro* and *in vivo*. Int J Mol Med 2007, 19:581–7.

[66] Johnston H, Boutin H, Allan SM: Assessing the contribution of inflammation in models of Alzheimer's disease. Biochem Soc Trans 2011, 39:886–90.

[67] Yan SD, Chen X, Fu J, Chen M, Zhu H, Roher A, Slattery T, Zhao L, Nagashima M, Morser J, Migheli A, Nawroth P, Stern D, Schmidt AM: RAGE and amyloid-beta peptide neurotoxicity in Alzheimer's disease. Nature 1996, 382:685–91.

[68] Mackic JB, Stins M, McComb JG, Calero M, Ghiso J, Kim KS, Yan SD, Stern D, Schmidt AM, Frangione B, Zlokovic BV: Human blood-brain barrier receptors for Alzheimer's amyloid-beta 1–40. Asymmetrical binding, endocytosis, and transcytosis at the apical side of brain microvascular endothelial cell monolayer. J Clin Invest 1998, 102:734–43.

[69] Stern D, Yan SD, Yan SF, Schmidt AM: Receptor for advanced glycation endproducts: a multiligand receptor magnifying cell stress in diverse pathologic settings. Adv Drug Deliv Rev 2002, 54:1615–25.

[70] Deane R, Du Yan S, Submamaryan RK, LaRue B, Jovanovic S, Hogg E, Welch D, Manness L, Lin C, Yu J, Zhu H, Ghiso J, Frangione B, Stern A, Schmidt AM, Armstrong DL, Arnold B, Liliensiek B, Nawroth P, Hofman F, Kindy M, Stern D, Zlokovic B: RAGE mediates amyloid-beta peptide transport across the blood-brain barrier and accumulation in brain. Nat Med 2003, 9:907–13.

[71] McMichael M: New models of hemostasis. Top Companion Anim Med 2012, 27:40–5.

[72] Versteeg HH, Heemskerk JW, Levi M, Reitsma PH: New fundamentals in hemostasis. Physiol Rev 2013, 93:327–58.

[73] Martin A, Giuliano A, Collaro D, De Vivo G, Sedia C, Serretiello E, Gentile V: Possible involvement of transglutaminase-catalyzed reactions in the physiopathology of neurodegenerative diseases. Amino Acids 2013, 44:111–8.

[74] Inbal A, Dardik R: Role of coagulation factor XIII (FXIII) in angiogenesis and tissue repair. Pathophysiol Haemost Thromb 2006, 35:162–5.

[75] Powles T, Chowdhury S, Jones R, Mantle M, Nathan P, Bex A, Lim L, Hutson T: Sunitinib and other targeted therapies for renal cell carcinoma. Br J Cancer 2011, 104:741–5.

[76] Grammas P, Martinez J, Sanchez A, Yin X, Riley J, Gay D, Desobry K, Tripathy D, Luo J, Evola M, Young A: A new paradigm for the treatment of Alzheimer's disease: targeting vascular activation. J Alzheimers Dis 2014, 40:619–30.

[77] Barrascout E, Medioni J, Scotte F, Ayllon J, Mejean A, Cuenod CA, Tartour E, Elaidi R, Oudard S: Angiogenesis inhibition: review of the activity of sorafenib, sunitinib and bevacizumab. Bull Cancer 2010, 97:29–43.

[78] Tousi B: The emerging role of bexarotene in the treatment of Alzheimer's disease: current evidence. Neuropsychiatr Dis Treat 2015, 11:311–5.

3

Vascular Repair and Remodeling

Nicolás F. Renna, Rodrigo Garcia, Jesica Ramirez and
Roberto M. Miatello

Abstract

Vascular remodeling is alterations in the structure of resistance vessels contributing to elevated systemic vascular resistance in hypertension. In this review, physiopathology of vascular remodeling is discussed, and the impact of antihypertensive drug treatment on remodeling is described, emphasizing on human data, fundamentally as an independent predictor of cardiovascular risk in hypertensive patients. Then we discussed a vascular repair by endothelial progenitor cells (EPCs) that play important roles in the regeneration of the vascular endothelial cells (ECs). The normal arterial vessel wall is mostly composed of ECs, vascular smooth muscle cells (VSMCs), and macrophages. Endothelial impairment is a major contributor to atherosclerosis and restenosis after percutaneous coronary intervention (PCI). Reendothelialization can effectively inhibit VSMC migration and proliferation and decrease neointimal thickening.

Keywords: endothelial progenitor cells, fructose-fed hypertensive rats, metabolic syndrome, hypertension, oxidative stress, vascular remodeling

1. Role of endothelial progenitor cells in vascular repair

Vascular diseases, including atherosclerosis, media calcification, and microangiopathy, are prevalent in patients with diabetes mellitus and are considered to be primary causes of death and disability in these individuals [1]. Atherosclerosis occurs earlier in patients with diabetes, frequently with greater severity and a more diffuse distribution. Patients with diabetes have increased prevalence of vascular disease and, as a result, increased morbimortality from acute myocardial infarction. Diabetes and metabolic syndrome (MS) are associated with vascular function abnormalities and ensuing morphological changes associated with vascular remodeling and atherosclerosis [2, 3].

The arterial vessel wall is mostly composed of endothelial cells (ECs), vascular smooth muscle cells (VSMCs), adventitial connective tissue and macrophages. Endothelial impairment is believed to be a major contributor to atherosclerosis or restenosis after percutaneous coronary intervention (PCI). Reendothelialization with ECs can effectively inhibit VSMC migration and proliferation and decrease neointimal thickening. It is for this reason that we studied a mechanism to achieve a rapid reendothelialization, through, for example, autologous translators of endothelial progenitor cells (EPC), mature or immature, as a fundamental hypothesis in the prevention of these two pathologies: atherosclerosis and restenosis, which derive in the same clinical entity: acute coronary syndrome.

EPCs are divided into different evolutionary stages from mother cells to mature ECs. Both early and late EPCs can repair blood vessels, but late EPCs that have a strong proliferation capacity are more involved in the formation of new vessels or angiogenesis. By measuring EPC in patients by flow cytometry in patients by flow cytometry, we found that in patients with atherosclerosis are decreased compared to control subjects without atherosclerosis [4–6]. Several studies show that EPCs can be recruited to sites of endothelial injury then mature in site, changing cluster of differentiation (CD), and playing a major role in reendothelialization [7–9].

Atherosclerosis is an inflammatory disease with leukocyte infiltration, accumulation of smooth muscle cells, and formation of neointima. Damage of the endothelial monolayer triggers the development of thrombosis with consequent occlusion versus arterial subocclusion. Recent studies demonstrated the recruitment and incorporation of EPC into atherosclerotic lesions and therefore provided evidence supporting the role of vascular cells in the pathophysiology of atherosclerosis. Moreover, there is evidence that EPC are capable of regenerating cells, vascular grafts, and native vessels [10, 11].

The EPCs can mediate vascular repair and attenuate atherosclerosis progression even in the continued presence of vascular injury. Although the mechanisms involved are still not clear, EPCs seem to contribute to the restoration of the endothelial monolayer [12]. In addition to bone marrow, spleen-derived EPCs also have the capacity to repair damaged endothelium [13]. EPCs derived from spleen homogenates also enhanced reendothelialization and reduce neointima formation after induction of endothelial cell damage using the carotid artery model [14].

Other models have also been used, such as the balloon injury model, mobilization of circulating EPCs, and accelerated repair of the nude endothelium [15]. In addition, autologous EPCs that overexpress endothelial nitric oxide synthase (eNOS) ameliorates endothelial integrity when transplanted into mice after carotid artery balloon injury. Increased NO bioavailability significantly strengthens the vasoprotective properties of the reconstituted endothelium, leading to inhibition of neointimal hyperplasia [16].

Transfer of progenitor cells is not always beneficial. ApoE KO mice receiving mononuclear bone marrow cells, following induced hind limb ischemia, showed increased neovascularization, accelerated atherosclerotic plaque formation, and lesion size compared to control groups [17]. In an alternate study, because of proinflammatory properties of these cells, as reduction in IL-10 levels in the atherosclerotic aortas was observed accelerated atherosclerosis along with reduced plaque stability [18]. Similarly, even though implantation of an arteriovenous anti-CD34-ePTFE graft in pigs, it also stimulated intimal hyperplasia [19, 20]. Besides obvious differences in various experimental models, it is difficult to reconcile these findings and it seems that excessive mobilization of progenitor cells may lead to restenosis, but its absence may impair reendothelialization [21]. It is important to mention term EPC is loosely used to describe a vastly heterogenic cell population that is consisted of different progenitors. Recent studies have highlighted the impact of cell isolation protocols on the functional capacity, that is, different phenotypes.

2. Flow cytometric characteristics of EPC

EPCs are identified by expression of CD34, CD133, or VEGFR2. Their accurate characterization is very difficult, because as these cells may originate from multiple precursors: the hemangioblast, nonhematopoietic mesenchymal precursors, such as the bone marrow, monocytic cells, and also tissue resident stem cells. Two methods for isolation of EPCs from the peripheral blood have been described [22]:

1. From isolated monocytic cells onto fibronectin-coated plates and cultured in the presence of growth factors, form colonies after 5–7 days, denominated endothelial cell colony-forming units (CFU-EC) [23].

2. From monocytic cells from peripheral blood plated onto collagen-I-coated plates in endothelial growth media (EGM-2) can give rise to CFU-EC after 14–21 days [24]. The expression of VEGFR2 on peripheral blood monocytes is essential for their endothelial-like function [25].

How was it exposed beforehand, there are two distinct phenotypes: early EPCs and late outgrowth EPCs [26, 27] which differ fundamentally from each other their proliferation potential. The first, that are derived from monocytic cells, have low proliferative capacity but express of eNOS and they fail to form perfused vessels in vivo. The late outgrowth EPCs have a high proliferation rate and can be maintained in culture extensively. These cells play a key role in angiogenesis [22]. Some studies further identified these cells as CD34$^+$CD45$^-$ precursors [28] and clarified their origin from the peripheral blood monocytes. CD14$^+$ cells seem to give rise to early EPCs, whereas late EPCs develop exclusively from the CD14$^-$ subpopulation [29].

In experimental studies, where EPCs are infused into ischemic lower limbs, only a small number of these can be seen in capillaries of the patient, although the perfusion improves considerably [30–33]. This suggests the potential release paracrine of angiogenic factors. This supportive function of EPCs may be crucial in ensuring the survival of tissue-residing cells and enhancing blood vessel formation and tissue repair. Early outgrowth EPCs produce higher levels of growth factors [34, 35]. To summary, it can say that EPC phenotype vary depending on their origin and their clutters of differentiation, with different functions:

1. immature EPCs that have proliferative ability

2. mature EPCs that can physically engraft into neoendothelial layer

3. supportive EPCs that produce growth factors to promote endothelial repair.

3. Angiogenesis in the vessel wall

An interesting question could be: How do the vessel wall progenitor cells migrate to the endothelial and intima layer of the vessel? The answer is the vasa vasorum. These play a significant role in transporting cells to the intimal region and have positively correlated with the development of atherosclerosis [35, 36]. In atherosclerotic lesions abundant microvessels can be observed. The vasa vasorum are considered to significantly contribute to:

1. atherosclerosis progression

2. plaque instability

3. also authors, support that contribute to plaque regression.

The real thing is that decreased blood supply through the adventitial vasa vasorum can trigger atherogenic intima thickening [37, 38]. Using the Lac-Z mice, Xu et al. [10] provided unique insights into the formation of these microvessels. It was clearly demonstrated that endothelial cells of microvessels within allografted vessels were derived from bone marrow progenitor cells (**Figure 1**). These results suggest a potentially dual role of EPCs in transplant atherosclerosis, protective through the repair of the denuded endothelium and promoting plaque

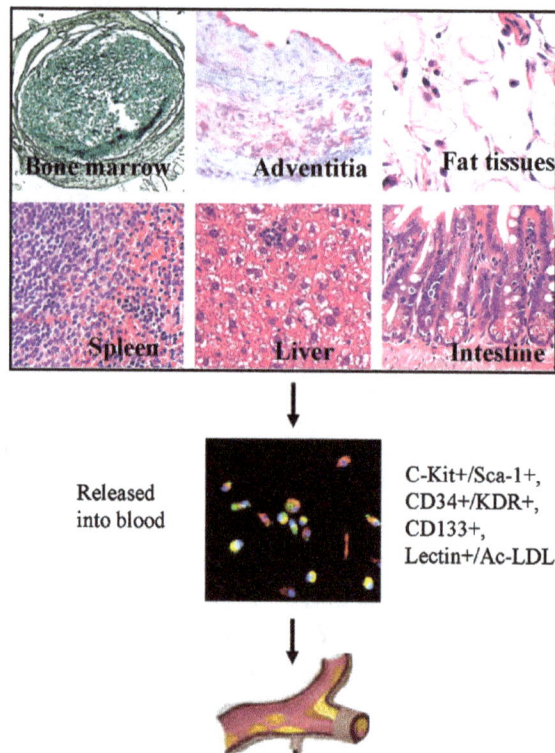

Figure 1. EPC origins. EPCs could be released from bone marrow, fat tissues, vessel wall, especially adventitia and spleen, liver, and intestine, where they form a circulating EPC pool. They can then contribute to the repair of damaged vessels in pathological conditions.

angiogenesis. Some studies have shown the potential detrimental EPC transplantation as lung cancer or multiple myeloma [38]. Additional experiments are required to fully delineate the functional significance of stem cell incorporation into the microvasculature and define the role of progenitors in tipping the balance between atheroprotection and atherogenesis.

4. Definition of vascular remodeling

The vascular wall is formed by endothelium cells, smooth muscle cells, and fibroblasts interacting to form an autocrine-paracrine complex. During vascularization, the vascular wall cells detects changes in the environment, releasing communication signals as growth factors, inflammation mediators, and paracrine mediators that influences on vascular structure and function. The results are vascular remodeling. This is an active process of structural change that involves changes in at least four cellular processes: cell growth, cell apoptosis, cell migration, and the synthesis or degradation of extracellular matrix.

Vascular remodeling is dependent on dynamic interactions between: (1) local growth factors, (2) vasoactive substances, and (3) hemodynamic stimuli, and is an active process that occurs in response to long-standing changes in afterload conditions; that it may subsequently contribute to the pathophysiology of vascular diseases and circulatory disorders [39].

Increased peripheral vascular resistance in hypertension was uniformly ascribed to a higher volume of wall material per unit length of vessel or "hypertrophy." It was always thought that the process of vascular hypertrophy was only due to increased muscle cells, as in the left ventricle, the term remodeling was first applied to the resistance vessels by Baumbach and Heistad to indicate a structural rearrangement of existing wall material around a smaller lumen [39–41].

Mulvany proposed that vascular remodeling should encompass any change in diameter noted in a fully relaxed vessel, not explained by a change in transmural pressure or compliance, and therefore due to structural factors [42–44]. With the objective of to be operational, the classification necessitates appropriate methods for the measurement of resistance vessels dimensions, supplying factors either removed or controlled for: (i) vascular tone, (ii) transmural pressure, and (iii) vessel compliance [38, 45].

5. Classification of vascular remodeling

Consideration of morphological changes has changed over time. Gibbons proposed a classification based on the response to increased blood pressure. These changes are displayed predominantly in media-to-lumen ratio (M/L), changing the vessel wall width for increased muscle mass (**Figure 2A**) or in the reorganization of cellular and noncellular elements (**Figure 2B**). These changes increase vascular reactivity, thus enhancing peripheral resistance. Another mechanism are mainly involves changes in the dimensions of the lumen (**Figure 2C** and **D**). In this case, the restructuring of the active components and cell signals does not

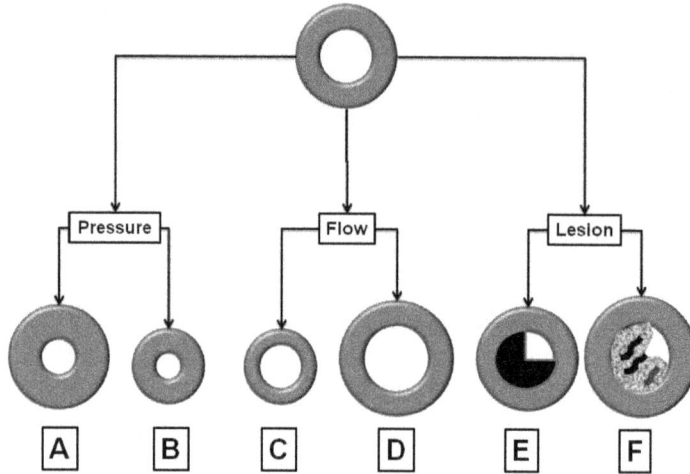

Figure 2. Changes are predominantly in media-to-lumen ratio (M/L), changing the vessel wall width for increased muscle mass (A) or in the reorganization of cellular and noncellular elements (B). Another mechanism of remodeling are mainly involves changes in the dimensions of the lumen (C) and (D). In this case, the restructuring of the active components and cell signals does not result in significant changes in the dimensions of the vascular lumen. Another form of vascular remodeling is microcirculation rarefaction (E) and (F).

result in significant changes in the dimensions of the vascular lumen; the changes in vessel wall thickness are relatively small. Clinical examples of this type of restructuring include the dilation of vascular remodeling associated with a constantly high blood flow (**Figure 2D**) (e.g. arteriovenous fistula) or the loss of cellularity and extracellular matrix proteolysis, resulting in the formation of an aneurysm. Equally, a reduction in the diameter of the vascular mass results from a long-term reduction in blood flow (**Figure 2C**). In fact, microcirculation rarefaction is another form of vascular remodeling that promotes hypertension and ischemic tissue. The vascular wall is also markedly changed in response to vascular injury (**Figure 2E and F**). In neointima, forms of reparative response to injury, as thrombosis, migration and vascular smooth muscle cells (VSMCs) proliferation, increased matrix production, and infiltration of inflammatory cells also exist.

Hypertension is associated with structural changes in the resistance vessels such as reduction in lumen diameter and increase in M/L ratio. This mode of structural change has been called "remodeling" [46].

Structural changes in resistance vessels are described as a rearrangement process to understand the pathogenesis of the disease and its therapeutic approach. However, it has been discussed that the term "remodeling" is not ideal because it is frequently used to describe any change in the structure of the vessel or myocardium. To avoid this difficulty, some authors make four proposals [47].

First, the term "remodeling" is limited to situations where there is a change in the lumen of a relaxed vessel, as measured under standard intravascular pressure. The changes in the characteristics of the wall material do not take into account the change in the vascular lumen.

Second, the process of changing the vessel wall without changes in the amount or characteristics of the materials are termed eutrophic remodeling. This process can be characteristic from situations involving an increase in the amount of material (hypertrophic remodeling) and those involving a reduction in the amount of material (hypotrophic remodeling).

Third, changes associated with decreased or an increased in lumen diameter should be classified as internal remodeling and external remodeling, respectively.

Finally, the remodeling process should be quantified. The term "remodeling index" refers to the variations of lumen referred to as eutrophic remodeling, depending on the changes in the wall section area.

The four proposals above allow for accurate terminology. Thus, the increase in the M/L ratio and decrease in the lumen diameter in resistance vessels of patients with essential hypertension without any change in the amount of wall material is called inner eutrophic remodeling. The decrease in the lumen diameter of the renal afferent arteriole with a decrease in the amount of wall material is called inner hypotrophic remodeling.

Chronic changes in hemodynamic forces structurally alter the vascular wall. In addition, hemodynamic changes are not the only production mechanisms of vascular remodeling. The inflammatory response and changes in the components of the matrix have been suggested as important mediators in the vascular adaptation process [48].

Figure 3 highlights schematically the adaptation of these changes in different pathologies, including structural changes to the intima layer that contribute to remodeling of the vascular wall. Thus, outward remodeling compensates for atherosclerotic plaque growth and delays the progression of blood flow limitation during stenosis, whereas during restenosis, intimal hyperplasia causes a narrowing of the lumen.

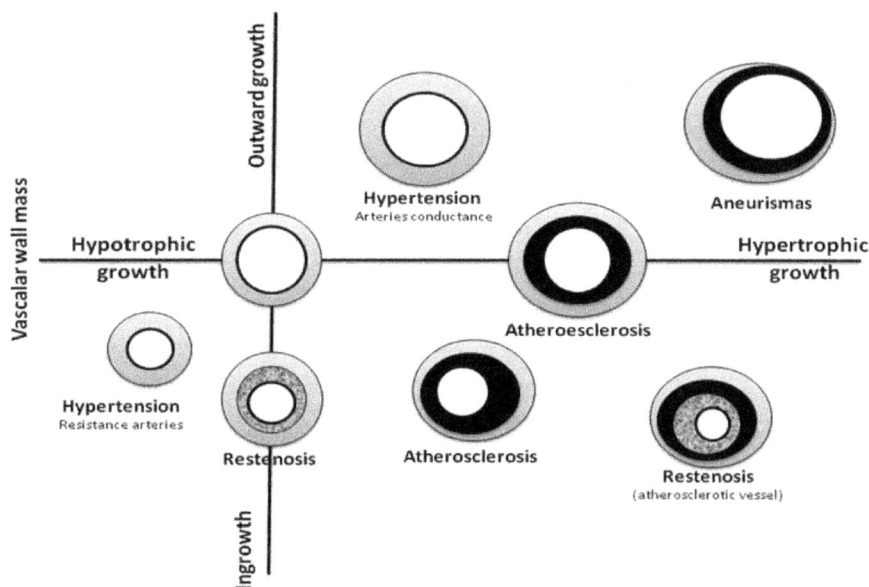

Figure 3. Schematic adaptation of changes in different pathologies, including structural changes to the intima layer that contribute to remodeling of the vascular wall. Thus, outward remodeling compensates for atherosclerotic plaque growth and delays the progression of blood flow limitation during stenosis, whereas during restenosis, intimal hyperplasia causes a narrowing of the lumen.

In summary, vascular wall remodeling is the result of changes in cellular and noncellular components, depending on the disease process causing the changes. Changes in the growth and migration of VSMC, endothelial dysfunction, inflammatory processes, and the synthesis or degradation of extracellular matrix components may be present during the disease process.

6. Pathophysiology of vascular remodeling in hypertension

6.1. Hypothesis of inflammatory and endothelial dysfunction

The traditional view of atherosclerosis as a lipid storage disease is crumbling with growing evidence that inflammation is involved during all stages, from the initial injury to the final stage of thrombotic complications. The narrowing of the arterial lumen is not necessarily a sign of myocardial infarction, and treating narrowed blood vessels does not prolong life. Although invasive procedures are needed in some cases, we understand that medical treatment and lifestyle modification (diet and physical activity) produce benefits that may result from reductions in inflammatory processes [49].

Usually, endothelial cells (EC) prevent leukocyte adhesion. However, the triggers of atherosclerosis can initiate the expression of adhesion molecules on EC, mediating leukocyte adhesion to the arterial wall. A key part of this interaction is VCAM-1. It is likely that oxidized lipids can induce gene expression via the pathway initiated by the nuclear transcription factor-kB (NF-kB), such as IL-1β and TNF-α [50].

This concept of vascular inflammatory disease allows a new approach for risk stratification and treatment. Increased levels of CAM are predictive of cardiac events and are an independent risk factor in men with coronary disease [51]. In our previous study, we demonstrated the presence of the endothelium as well as the products of NF-kB signaling and VCAM-1 in an experimental model of metabolic syndrome in hypertensive rats receiving a fructose-rich diet fructose-fed hypertensive rats (FFHR) [52].

Chemokines are low molecular weight cytokines responsible for mediating the maturation, differentiation, and migration of cells involved in the inflammatory response. In addition to this role, chemokines could promote reactive oxygen species (ROS) production and other cytokines during leukocyte infiltration of the vessel wall. Monocyte chemotactic protein-1 (MCP-1) is a chemokine that regulates the migration and infiltration of monocytes and macrophages into the site of inflammation. It is overexpressed in the presence of cardiovascular risk factors, especially in atherosclerotic lesions. Differential activation induces nuclear transcription factors such as NF-kB and AP-1, which leads to the release of IL-6 and the proliferation of VSMC [53].

Cytokines are soluble proteins that form a complex signaling network critical in the regulation of innate and adaptive inflammatory response. Cytokines modulate the inflammatory response through their influence on the growth, development and activation of leukocytes, and other inflammatory cells. TNF-α is a key mediator in systemic inflammation with a significant role in the Th1 inflammatory pathway. The activity of TNF-α is varied and includes the production of interleukin CAM expression, cell migration and activation, and activation of metalloproteinases (MMP) and COX activity, promoting the procoagulant state. TNF-α is detected in endothelial cells and smooth muscle cells at all stages of the formation of atheromatous plaques [54].

There are over 30 members of the interleukin family. They are subdivided by the similar structure or homology of the receptor. The transformation from a vascular homeostasis inflammatory state is influenced by an imbalance between the pro-inflammatory and anti-inflammatory activities of interleukins. The role of IL-1 includes the stimulation of CAM, chemokines, growth factors, tissue factor, and other cytokines. The expression levels of the receptor antagonist IL-1Ra significantly increase in unstable angina compared with stable angina. Decreased levels of IL-1Ra after coronary stent placement may be linked to a low association with recurrent ischemia [55]. IL-6 is a multifunctional cytokine with a central role in inflammation. Elevated levels of IL-6 increase the risk of myocardial infarction and mortality in patients with coronary heart disease [56].

IL-10 has pleiotropic properties and influences different cell populations. Its most important role is in inflammatory vascular disease as part of the Th2 response. The expression of IL-10 decreases the expression of inflammatory cytokines, decreasing the Th1 phenotype. IL-10 also decreases NF-kB signaling reducing synthesis of pro-inflammatory cytokines, CAM, chemoattractants, and growth factors [57, 58].

Endothelial dysfunction in FFHR causes an increase in the expression of NF-kB and AP-1 and the posttranscriptional product VCAM-1. The expression of NF-kB (p65) and AP-1 (c-fos) predominates throughout the vessel wall. Increased VCAM-1, as discussed in the literature, is a marker of vascular inflammation, vascular permeability, and endothelial dysfunction.

This experimental model produced an increased expression of several cytokines. This finding demonstrates that the vascular bed FFHR model presents a pro-inflammatory and proatherogenic microenvironment that favors vascular remodeling. C-reactive protein (CRP) was used to evaluate whether this local inflammatory process is also systemic and revealed significantly increased IL-6 expression in the liver.

The potential importance of vascular wall inflammation as a therapeutic target remains an area not yet fully explored, where understanding the involvement of inflammatory mediators in vascular remodeling is relevant. The data suggest that oxidative stress and the subsequent activation of genes involved in the inflammatory process are actively involved in organ damage at the vascular level.

6.2. Vascular remodeling and extracellular matrix metalloproteinases

MMPs are tools for maintaining the homeostasis of extracellular structures. Their synthesis is induced by cytokines as well as cell-cell and cell-matrix interactions. Acute coronary syndromes are an example of an increase in clinical conditions, specifically in the vulnerable region of the plaque [59]. Exposure to oxidized low-density lipoproteins or TNF-α induces the expression of MT3-MMP, a protease that degrades atherosclerotic plaques and is expressed in macrophages [60, 61].

MMPs with accessory signaling molecules can modulate cell-cell interactions through the activation of signal transmission and release of cytokines and chemokines. By these effects, accessory signaling molecules can propagate the inflammatory response.

6.3. Vascular remodeling and acute phase reactants

The production of acute phase reàctants is a normal physiological response to cytokine release in acute and chronic inflammatory conditions. Ultrasensitive quantification of CRP, when it is below the detection limits of the common assay, has a very important role in the detection of vascular inflammation and cardiovascular risk prediction. There is evidence that CRP is involved in atherosclerosis, especially during the early stages. It stimulates the production of pro-inflammatory cytokines in monocytes and macrophages [62] and mediates the expression of CAM, allowing for increased leukocyte adhesion and migration. Their increased expression suppresses endothelial nitric oxide synthase [34] and promotes a procoagulant state.

Multiple studies have determined that increases in CRP are an independent risk factor for developing atherosclerosis. Data from clinical studies indicate that this association is less important when viewed in healthy subjects and controls inflammatory markers such as IL-6 and fibrinogen [63, 64], whereas another study identified CRP as a predictor of diabetes mellitus independent of established risk factors. CRP also indicated a correlation with the risk of cardiovascular events in women with metabolic syndrome [65].

6.4. Vascular remodeling and the renin-angiotensin-aldosterone system

Another important pillar in the vascular remodeling process is the renin-angiotensin-aldosterone system (RAAS) [66, 67]. To evaluate its participation, we studied the expression of AT1R and AT2R at the vascular level. In the experimental model of FFHR, we observed increased expression of AT1R and decreased expression of AT2R, promoting growth, vascular hypertrophy, and endothelial dysfunction. The release of ROS and initiation of vascular inflammation through different intracellular signaling cascades foster interconnections with other routes such as NAD(P)H oxidase and the growth factor receptor associated with insulin (IGFR).

Figure 4 allows us to appreciate the AT1R-associated intracellular cascades. In this experimental model, the route associated with the satellite receptor and the IGFR subunit associated with NAD(P)H oxidase are the most important pathophysiological mechanisms. The FAK pathways PI3K and JAK2 generate stimuli and trigger contraction, migration and cell adhesion via intranuclear promoters that synthesize ICAM-1 and VCAM-1. Endothelial Growth Factor Receptor (EGFR) and Insulin Growth Factor Receptor (IGFR) amplified pathways are associated with cellular growth and hypertrophy as a result of insulinogenic stimuli and permit activation of collagenase, which modifies the extracellular matrix. Finally, the oxidative stress pathway stimulated by angiotensin activates redox-sensitive inflammatory molecules such as AP-1 and NF-kB, which amplify the inflammatory response by cytokines, chemokines, and lymphokines to ultimately induce more vascular inflammation.

Angiotensin II is the main effector of the RAAS in the homeostatic regulation of the cardiovascular system and in the pathogenesis of cardiovascular disease. Aldosterone interacts with mineralocorticoid receptors (MR), causing endothelial dysfunction, facilitating thrombosis,

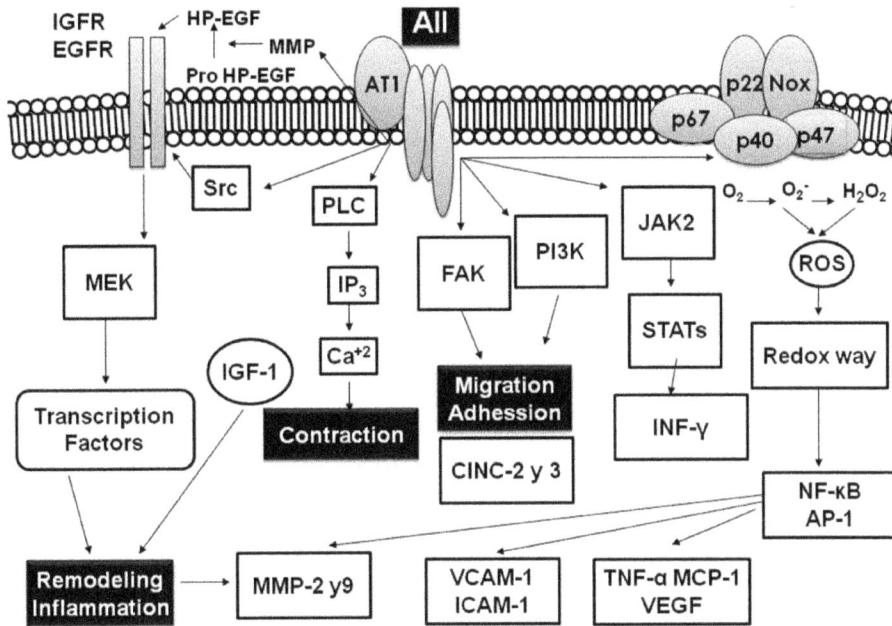

Figure 4. Associated intracellular cascades to physiopathology of vascular remodeling. In FFHR experimental model, the route associated with the satellite receptor and the IGFR subunit associated with NAD(P)H oxidase are the most important pathophysiological mechanisms. Also, the oxidative stress pathway stimulated by angiotensin activates redox-sensitive inflammatory molecules such as AP-1 and NF-kB, which amplify vascular inflammatory response.

reducing complacence, causing vascular hypertrophy and cardiac fibrosis, and generating pathological remodeling. Aldosterone also induces the growth and proliferation of VSMC. A classical genomic action of aldosterone on MR is the translocation of this Aldo-MR complex into the nucleus, where it interacts with promoters to post-transcriptionally regulate gene and protein expression. For this path, increased Ki-ras2A expression (small and monomeric GTP-binding protein), which is associated with cardiac remodeling, generates fibrosis, and cell proliferation by ERK1/2 possibly [68]. Recently, some authors have demonstrated that aldosterone stimulates EGFR intracellularly in CHO cells. The transactivation of this receptor has also been described as a crucial step in the cascade of MAPK signaling activated by angiotensin II. This pathway allows for "cross-talk" and mutual activation that allows the development of cardiovascular injury and subsequent remodeling. The latter route is via "fast" activation, which is different from genomic stimulation and stimulates MKP-1 and Ki-generated ras2A proliferation and vascular remodeling; this discovery explains the changes previously observed in other studies [69].

Noting the role of aldosterone in vascular remodeling in FFHR, we observed that chronic administration of spironolactone did not change the variables of metabolic syndrome that were partially reversed by oxidative stress. This can be explained by the relationship between aldosterone and the angiotensin II receptor AT1R, which sensitizes the effects and increased the post-receptor response [67].

In summary, abundant evidences indicate the involvement of the RAAS in the pathophysiology of vascular remodeling; our observations in experimental pathology highlight the structural and functional changes.

In this special issue, different authors have tried to demonstrate the involvement of different pathophysiological mechanisms to clarify the vascular changes associated with hypertension and metabolic syndrome.

7. Clinical data

The most feasible possibility for studies of resistance vessels in humans relies on the examination of small muscular arteries from biopsies of subcutaneous gluteal fat. Small arteries can also be obtained from omental fat [70–73]. The dissected vessels are mounted in a wire or pressure myograph, but due to the invasive character of these procedures, most relevant studies are of modest size [74–76]. In other cases, untreated hypertensives in place of patients newly diagnosed. In this studies, a data indicate that small subcutaneous arteries of nondiabetic hypertensives undergo inward eutrophic remodeling. Evidence suggests that diabetes, on top of essential hypertension, is associated with media hypertrophy (eutrophy remodeling). The same hypertrophy was also shown by one of these studies in normotensive diabetics, supporting a pressure-independent effect.

Finally, hypertension secondary as renovascular disease could promote media growth in arteries [77–80].

When evaluating the clinical data, there are two problems.

1. sampling problem.
2. subcutaneous vasculature is not necessarily representative of other vascular beds. In opposition to this idea, a positive correlation has been found in hypertensive patients between coronary flow reserve and the M/L ratio of subcutaneous arteries, indeed supporting that hypertensive changes of microvascular structure were not limited to the subcutis tissue.

Author details

Nicolás F. Renna[1,2]*, Rodrigo Garcia[2], Jesica Ramirez[3] and Roberto M. Miatello[1,2]

*Address all correspondence to: nicolasfede@gmail.com

1 Department of Pathology, School of Medicine, National University of Cuyo, Mendoza, Argentina

2 Institute of Experimental Medicine and Biology of Cuyo (IMBECU), CONICET, Mendoza, Argentina

3 Genetics Institute, School of Medicine, National University of Cuyo, Mendoza, Argentina

References

[1] Werner N, Nickenig G. Endothelial progenitor cells in health and atherosclerotic disease. Ann Med 2007;39:82–90.

[2] Tepper OM, Galiano RD, Capla JM, Kalka C, Gagne PJ, Jacobowitz GR, et al. Human endothelial progenitor cells from type II diabetics exhibit impaired proliferation, adhesion, and incorporation into vascular structures. Circulation 2002;106:2781–2786.

[3] Ghani U, Shuaib A, Salam A, Nasir A, Shuaib U, Jeerakathil T, et al. Endothelial progenitor cells during cerebrovascular disease. Stroke 2005;36:151–153.

[4] Cubbon RM, Rajwani A, Wheatcroft SB. The impact of insulin resistance on endothelial function, progenitor cells and repair. Diab Vasc Dis Res 2007;4:103–111.

[5] Xiao Q, Kiechl S, Patel S, Oberhollenzer F, Weger S, Mayr A, et al. Endothelial progenitor cells, cardiovascular risk factors, cytokine levels and atherosclerosis—results from a large population-based study. PLoS ONE 2007;2:e975.

[6] Fadini GP, Agostini C, Sartore S, Avogaro A. Endothelial progenitor cells in the natural history of atherosclerosis. Atherosclerosis 2007;194:46–54.

[7] Heiss C, Keymel S, Niesler U, Ziemann J, Kelm M, Kalka C. Impaired progenitor cell activity in age-related endothelial dysfunction. J Am Coll Cardiol 2005;45:1441–1448.

[8] Vasa M, Fichtlscherer S, Aicher A, Adler K, Urbich C, Martin H, et al. Number and migratory activity of circulating endothelial progenitor cells inversely correlate with risk factors for coronary artery disease. Circ Res 2001;89:E1–E7.

[9] Kissel CK, Lehmann R, Assmus B, Aicher A, Honold J, Fischer-Rasokat U, et al. Selective functional exhaustion of hematopoietic progenitor cells in the bone marrow of patients with postinfarction heart failure. J Am Coll Cardiol 2007;49:2341–2349.

[10] Xu Q Mouse models of arteriosclerosis: from arterial injuries to vascular grafts. Am J Pathol 2004;165:1–10.

[11] Hu Y, Davison F, Zhang ZG, Xu Q. Endothelial replacement and angiogenesis in arteriosclerotic lesions of allografts are contributed by circulating progenitor cells. Circulation 2003;108:3122–3127.

[12] Xu Q, Zhang Z, Davison F, Hu Y. Circulating progenitor cells regenerate endothelium of vein graft atherosclerosis, which is diminished in apoE-deficient mice. Circ Res 2003;93:e76–e86.

[13] Rauscher FM, Goldschmidt-Clermont PJ, Davis BH, Wang T, Gregg D, Ramaswami P, et al. Aging, progenitor cell exhaustion, and atherosclerosis. Circulation 2003;108:457–463.

[14] Wassmann S, Werner N, Czech T, Nickenig G. Improvement of endothelial function by systemic transfusion of vascular progenitor cells. Circ Res 2006;99:e74–e83.

[15] Werner N, Junk S, Laufs U, Link A, Walenta K, Bohm M, et al. Intravenous transfusion of endothelial progenitor cells reduces neointima formation after vascular injury. Circ Res 2003;93:e17–e24.

[16] Kong D, Melo LG, Gnecchi M, Zhang L, Mostoslavsky G, Liew CC, et al. Cytokine-induced mobilization of circulating endothelial progenitor cells enhances repair of injured arteries. Circulation 2004;110:2039–2046.

[17] Griese DP, Ehsan A, Melo LG, Kong D, Zhang L, Mann MJ, et al. Isolation and transplantation of autologous circulating endothelial cells into denuded vessels and prosthetic grafts: implications for cell-based vascular therapy. Circulation 2003;108:2710–2715.

[18] Silvestre JS, Gojova A, Brun V, Potteaux S, Esposito B, Duriez M, et al. Transplantation of bone marrow-derived mononuclear cells in ischemic apolipoprotein E-knockout mice accelerates atherosclerosis without altering plaque composition. Circulation 2003;108:2839–2842.

[19] George J, Afek A, Abashidze A, Shmilovich H, Deutsch V, Kopolovich J, et al. Transfer of endothelial progenitor and bone marrow cells influences atherosclerotic plaque size and composition in apolipoprotein E knockout mice. Arterioscler Thromb Vasc Biol 2005;25:2636–2641.

[20] Rotmans JI, Heyligers JM, Verhagen HJ, Velema E, Nagtegaal MM, de Kleijn DP, et al. In vivo cell seeding with anti-CD34 antibodies successfully accelerates endothelialization but stimulates intimal hyperplasia in porcine arteriovenous expanded polytetrafluoro-ethylene grafts. Circulation 2005;112:12–18.

[21] Yeh ET, Zhang S, Wu HD, Korbling M, Willerson JT, Estrov Z. Transdifferentiation of human peripheral blood CD34+-enriched cell population into cardiomyocytes, endothelial cells, and smooth muscle cells in vivo. Circulation 2003;108:2070–2073.

[22] Seeger FH, Tonn T, Krzossok N, Zeiher AM, Dimmeler S. Cell isolation procedures matter: a comparison of different isolation protocols of bone marrow mononuclear cells used for cell therapy in patients with acute myocardial infarction. Eur Heart J 2007;28:766–772.

[23] Yoder MC, Mead LE, Prater D, Krier TR, Mroueh KN, Li F, et al. Redefining endothelial progenitor cells via clonal analysis and hematopoietic stem/progenitor cell principals. Blood 2007;109:1801–1809.

[24] Hur J, Yang HM, Yoon CH, Lee CS, Park KW, Kim JH, et al. Identification of a novel role of T cells in postnatal vasculogenesis: characterization of endothelial progenitor cell colonies. Circulation 2007;116:1671–1682.

[25] Urbich C, Heeschen C, Aicher A, Dernbach E, Zeiher AM, Dimmeler S. Relevance of monocytic features for neovascularization capacity of circulating endothelial progenitor cells. Circulation 2003;108:2511–2516.

[26] Elsheikh E, Uzunel M, He Z, Holgersson J, Nowak G, Sumitran-Holgersson S. Only a specific subset of human peripheral-blood monocytes has endothelial-like functional capacity. Blood 2005;106:2347–2355.

[27] Gehling UM, Ergun S, Schumacher U, Wagener C, Pantel K, Otte M, et al. In vitro differentiation of endothelial cells from AC133-positive progenitor cells. Blood 2000;95:3106–3112.

[28] Lin Y, Weisdorf DJ, Solovey A, Hebbel RP. Origins of circulating endothelial cells and endothelial outgrowth from blood. J Clin Invest 2000;105:71–77.

[29] Timmermans F, Van Hauwermeiren F, De Smedt M, Raedt R, Plasschaert F, De Buyzere ML, et al. Endothelial outgrowth cells are not derived from CD133+ cells or CD45+ hematopoietic precursors. Arterioscler Thromb Vasc Biol 2007;27:1572–1579.

[30] Gulati R, Jevremovic D, Peterson TE, Chatterjee S, Shah V, Vile RG, et al. Diverse origin and function of cells with endothelial phenotype obtained from adult human blood. Circ Res 2003;93:1023–1025.

[31] Crosby JR, Kaminski WE, Schatteman G, Martin PJ, Raines EW, Seifert RA, et al. Endothelial cells of hematopoietic origin make a significant contribution to adult blood vessel formation. Circ Res 2000;87:728–730.

[32] Gothert JR, Gustin SE, van Eekelen JA, Schmidt U, Hall MA, Jane SM, et al. Genetically tagging endothelial cells in vivo: bone marrow-derived cells do not contribute to tumor endothelium. Blood 2004;104:1769–1777.

[33] Peters BA, Diaz LA, Polyak K, Meszler L, Romans K, Guinan EC, et al. Contribution of bone marrow-derived endothelial cells to human tumor vasculature. Nat Med 2005;11:261–262.

[34] Zentilin L, Tafuro S, Zacchigna S, Arsic N, Pattarini L, Sinigaglia M, et al. Bone marrow mononuclear cells are recruited to the sites of VEGF-induced neovascularization but are not incorporated into the newly formed vessels. Blood 2006;107:3546–3554.

[35] Calvi LM, Adams GB, Weibrecht KW, Weber JM, Olson DP, Knight MC, et al. Osteoblastic cells regulate the haematopoietic stem cell niche. Nature 2003;425:841–846.

[36] Asahara T, Takahashi T, Masuda H, Kalka C, Chen D, Iwaguro H, et al. VEGF contributes to postnatal neovascularization by mobilizing bone marrow-derived endothelial progenitor cells. Embo J 1999;18:3964–3972.

[37] Hanahan D, Folkman J. Patterns and emerging mechanisms of the angiogenic switch during tumorigenesis. Cell 1996;86:353–364.

[38] Baumbach GL, Heistad DD. Remodeling of cerebral arterioles in chronic hypertension. Hypertension 1989;13:968–972.

[39] Mulvany MJ. Vascular remodelling of resistance vessels: can we define this? Cardiovasc Res 1999;41:9–13.

[40] Bund SJ, Lee RM. Arterial structural changes in hypertension: a consideration of methodology, terminology and functional consequence. J Vasc Res 2003;40:547–557.

[41] Mulvany MJ. Structural abnormalities of the resistance vasculature in hypertension. J Vasc Res 2003;40:558–560.

[42] Dunn WR, Gardiner SM. Differential alteration in vascular structure of resistance arteries isolated from the cerebral and mesenteric vascular beds of transgenic [(mRen-2)27], hypertensive rats. Hypertension 1997;29:1140–1147.

[43] Hashimoto H, Prewitt RL, Efaw CW. Alterations in the microvasculature of one-kidney, one-clip hypertensive rats. Am J Physiol 1987;253: H933–H940.

[44] Korsgaard N, Mulvany MJ. Cellular hypertrophy in mesenteric resistance vessels from renal hypertensive rats. Hypertension 1988;12:162–167.

[45] Intengan HD, Deng LY, Li JS, Schiffrin EL. Mechanics and composition of human sub‐cutaneous resistance arteries in essential hypertension. Hypertension 1999;33:569–574.

[46] Heagerty AM, Aalkjaer C, Bund SJ, Korsgaard N, Mulvany MJ, Small artery structure in hypertension: dual processes of remodeling and growth. Hypertension 1993;21: 391–397.

[47] Pasterkamp, G, Galis ZS, de Kleijn DPV. Expansive arterial remodeling: location, location, location. Arterioscler Thromb Vasc Biol 2004;24(4):650–657.

[48] Libby, P. Inflammation and cardiovascular disease mechanisms. Am J Clin Nutr 2006;83(2):456S–460.

[49] Nakane, H, et al. Gene transfer of endothelial nitric oxide synthase reduces angiotensin II-induced endothelial dysfunction. Hypertension 2000;35(2):595–601.

[50] Lopez Garcia CM, Perez Gonzalez PA. Handbook on metabolic syndrome: classification, risk factors and health impact. 1 ed. Vascular Repair by Endothelial Progenitor Cells in an Experimental Model of Metabolic Syndrome, ed. Endocrinology Research and Clinical Developments, 2012. NY: Nova Science Publishers, Inc. 450.

[51] Viedt, C, et al. Monocyte chemoattractant protein-1 induces proliferation and interleukin-6 production in human smooth muscle cells by differential activation of nuclear factor-{kappa}b and activator protein-1. Arterioscler Thromb Vasc Biol 2002;22(6):914–920.

[52] Sack, M. Tumor necrosis factor-alpha in cardiovascular biology and the potential for anti-tumor necrosis factor-alpha therapy in heart disease. Pharmacol Ther 2002;94:123–135.

[53] Giuseppe, P, et al. Prognostic value of interleukin-1 receptor antagonist in patients undergoing percutaneous coronary intervention. Am J Cardiol 2002;89(4):372–376.

[54] Hernandez-Rodriguez, J, et al. Elevated production of interleukin-6 is associated with a lower incidence of disease-related ischemic events in patients with giant-cell arteritis: angiogenic activity of interleukin-6 as a potential protective mechanism. Circulation 2003;107(19):2428–2434.

[55] de Waal Malefyt, R, et al. Interleukin 10(IL-10) inhibits cytokine synthesis by human monocytes: an autoregulatory role of IL-10 produced by monocytes. J Exp Med 1991;174(5):1209–1220.

[56] Galis, ZS, et al. Increased expression of matrix metalloproteinases and matrix degrading activity in vulnerable regions of human atherosclerotic plaques. J Clin Investig 1994;94(6): 2493–2503.

[57] Uzui, H, et al. Increased expression of membrane type 3-matrix metalloproteinase in human atherosclerotic plaque: role of activated macrophages and inflammatory cytokines. Circulation 2002;106(24):3024–3030.

[58] Pasceri, V, Willerson JT, Yeh ETH. Direct proinflammatory effect of C-reactive protein on human endothelial cells. Circulation 2000;102(18):2165–2168.

[59] Venugopal, SK, et al. Demonstration that C-reactive protein decreases eNOS expression and bioactivity in human aortic endothelial cells. Circulation 2002;106(12):1439–1441.

[60] Luc, G, et al. C-reactive protein, interleukin-6, and fibrinogen as predictors of coronary heart disease: the PRIME study. Arterioscler Thromb Vasc Biol 2003;23(7):1255–1261.

[61] van der Meer, IM, et al. The value of C-reactive protein in cardiovascular risk prediction: the Rotterdam study. Arch Intern Med 2003;163(11):1323–1328.

[62] Freeman, DJ, et al. C-reactive protein is an independent predictor of risk for the development of diabetes in the West of Scotland Coronary Prevention Study. Diabetes 2002;51(5):1596–1600.

[63] Touyz, RM, et al. Differential activation of extracellular signal-regulated protein kinase 1/2 and p38 mitogen activated-protein kinase by AT1 receptors in vascular smooth muscle cells from Wistar-Kyoto rats and spontaneously hypertensive rats. J Hypertens 2001;19(3):553–559.

[64] Min, L-J, et al. Cross-talk between aldosterone and angiotensin II in vascular smooth muscle cell senescence. Cardio Res 2007;76(3):506–516.

[65] Min, L-J, et al. Aldosterone and angiotensin II synergistically induce mitogenic response in vascular smooth muscle cells. Circ Res 2005;97(5):434–442.

[66] Brown, NJ, Aldosterone and vascular inflammation. Hypertension 2008;51(2):161–167.

[67] Rizzoni D, Porteri E, Boari GE, De Ciuceis C, Sleiman I, Muiesan ML et al. Prognostic significance of small-artery structure in hypertension. Circulation 2003;108:2230–2235.

[68] Mathiassen ON, Buus NH, Sihm I, Thybo NK, Morn B, Schroeder AP et al. Small artery structure is an independent predictor of cardiovascular events in essential hypertension. J Hypertens 2007;25:1021–1026.

[69] Aalkjaer C, Heagerty AM, Bailey I, Mulvany MJ, Swales JD. Studies of isolated resistance vessels from offspring of essential hypertensive patients. Hypertension 1987;9:III155–III158.

[70] Korsgaard N, Aalkjaer C, Heagerty AM, Izzard AS, Mulvany MJ. Histology of subcutaneous small arteries from patients with essential hypertension. Hypertension 1993;22:523–526.

[71] Izzard AS, Cragoe EJ Jr, Heagerty AM. Intracellular pH in human resistance arteries in essential hypertension. Hypertension 1991;17:780–786.

[72] Thurmann PA, Stephens N, Heagerty AM, Kenedi P, Weidinger G,Rietbrock N. Influence of isradipine and spirapril on left ventricular hypertrophy and resistance arteries. Hypertension 1996;28:450–456.

[73] Schofield I, Malik R, Izzard A, Austin C, Heagerty A. Vascular structural and functional changes in type 2 diabetes mellitus: evidence for the roles of abnormal myogenic responsiveness and dyslipidemia. Circulation 2002;106:3037–3043.

[74] Kvist S, Mulvany MJ. Reduced medication and normalization of vascular structure, but continued hypertension in renovascular patients after revascularization. Cardiovasc Res 2001;52:136–142.

[75] Schiffrin EL, Deng LY. Structure and function of resistance arteries of hypertensive patients treated with a beta-blocker or a calcium channel antagonist. J Hypertens 1996;14:1247–1255.

[76] Schiffrin EL, Park JB, Intengan HD, Touyz RM. Correction of arterial structure and endothelial dysfunction in human essential hypertension by the angiotensin receptor antagonist losartan. Circulation 2000;101:1653–1659.

[77] Park JB, Schiffrin EL. Small artery remodeling is the most prevalent (earliest?) form of target organ damage in mild essential hypertension. J Hypertens 2001;19:921–930.

[78] Harazny JM, Ritt M, Baleanu D, Ott C, Heckmann J, Schlaich MP et al. Increased wall: lumen ratio of retinal arteriole s in male patients with a history of a cerebrovascular event. Hypertension 2007;50:623–629.

[79] Lee RM. Vascular changes at the prehypertensive phase in the mesenteric arteries from spontaneously hypertensive rats. Blood Vessels 1985;22:105–126.

[80] Takeshita A, Imaizumi T, Ashihara T, Yamamoto K, Hoka S, Nakamura M. Limited maximal vasodilator capacity of forearm resistance vessels in normotensive young men with a familial predisposition to hypertension. Circ Res 1982;50:671–677.

4

Hypoxia, Angiogenesis and Atherogenesis

Lamia Heikal and Gordon Ferns

Abstract

The balance between vascular oxygen supply and metabolic demand for oxygen within the vasculature is tightly regulated. An imbalance leads to hypoxia and a consequential cascade of cellular signals that attempt to offset the effects of hypoxia. Hypoxia is invariably associated with atherosclerosis, wound repair, inflammation and vascular disease. There is now substantial evidence that hypoxia plays an essential role in angiogenesis as well as plaque angiogenesis. It controls the metabolism, and responses of many of the cell types found within the developing plaque and whether the plaque will evolve into a stable or unstable phenotype. Hypoxia is characterized in molecular terms by the stabilization of hypoxia-inducible factor (HIF)-1α, a subunit of the heterodimeric nuclear transcriptional factor HIF-1 and a master regulator of oxygen homeostasis. The expression of HIF-1 is localized to perivascular tissues, inflammatory macrophages and smooth muscle cells where it regulates several genes that are important to vascular function including vascular endothelial growth factor, nitric oxide synthase, endothelin-1 and erythropoietin. This chapter summarizes the effects of hypoxia on the functions of cells involved in angiogenesis as well as atherogenesis (plaque angiogenesis) and the evidence for its potential importance from experimental models and clinical studies.

Keywords: hypoxia, HIF-1, proliferation, atherosclerosis, plaque formation, blood vessel

1. Introduction

The circulatory system develops early in mammalian embryogenesis. An oxygen supply is essential for normal tissue function, development and homeostasis. The vascular network within the cardiovascular system is essential for the delivery of oxygen, nutrients and other molecules to the tissues of the body [1]. Oxygen availability serves as an important regulator of the cardiovascular system. Oxygen balance may be perturbed if there is reduced oxygen diffusion, or increased oxygen consumption that may be a consequence of rapid cellular division during embryonic development, by tumour growth, or by vasculature dysfunction due to vessel occlusion or rupture [2].

Hypoxia is defined by a reduced oxygen tension relative to those normally extant within a particular tissue. It has multiple impacts on the vascular system and cell function [3]. The effects of moderate hypoxia (3–5% O_2) are usually reversible and are usually accompanied by adaptive physiological responses in the cells. A lower oxygen tension (0–1% O_2) contributes to the pathophysiology of tumour progression and cell apoptosis [4] and is a feature of conditions that include cancer, ischemic heart disease, peripheral artery disease, wound healing and neovascular retinopathy. Hypoxia promotes vessel growth by stimulating an upregulation of multiple proangiogenic pathways that mediate key aspects of endothelial, stromal and vascular support cell biology. The role of hypoxia in human disease is now becoming increasingly clear [5] including the association between hypoxia and endothelial dysfunction that affects several cellular processes and signal transduction.

Hypoxia can occur in several ways: (1) hypoxic hypoxia is caused by an insufficient oxygen concentration in the air in the lungs, which may occur during sleep apnea, when the diffusion of oxygen to the blood is reduced, or at high altitude; (2) hypoxemic hypoxia occurs when the blood has reduced transport capacity as seen in carbon monoxide poisoning when haemoglobin cannot carry oxygen at its normal concentrations; (3) stagnant hypoxia results when the cardiac output does not match the demands of the body and the flow is not sufficient to deliver enough oxygenated blood to the tissue and (4) histotoxic hypoxia occurs when cells cannot utilize the available oxygen, for example following cyanide poisoning when oxygen cannot be used to produce ATP as the mitochondrial electron transport is inhibited.

Chronic tissue hypoxia (an oxygen tension of 2–3% for a prolonged period of time) may cause uncontrolled proliferation of cells. When physiological oxygen concentrations are restored, the increased blood flow supplies excessive oxygen; this may then lead to increased free-radical generation, tissue damage and concomitant activation of stress-response genes; a condition known as 'reoxygenation injury'. In these circumstances, normal cells/tissues may not survive; but tumour cells are still able to proliferate despite the hypoxic milieu, as they have developed genetic and adaptive changes leading to resistance to hypoxia [6].

Hypoxia plays important roles in normal human physiology and development. For example, it is integral to normal embryonic development. Whatever the cause, or the severity of hypoxia, it leads to an induction of adaptive responses within the endothelial and vascular smooth muscle cells through the activation of genes that participate in angiogenesis, cell proliferation/survival and in glucose and iron metabolism [7].

In healthy vascular tissue, vascular smooth muscle cells (SMCs) and endothelial cells (ECs) proliferate at very low levels. However, SMCs and ECs can be stimulated to re-enter the cell cycle in response to several physiological and pathological stimuli. Hypoxia is considered an important stimulus of SMC and EC proliferation and is found in atherosclerotic lesions and rapidly growing tumours [4].

The proliferation of ECs is pivotal to the formation of new micro-vessels and is important during organ development in embryogenesis and tumour growth, and also contributes to diabetic retinopathy, psoriasis, rheumatoid arthritis and atherosclerosis. Abnormal SMC proliferation contributes to atherosclerosis, intimal hyperplasia after angioplasty and graft atherosclerosis after coronary transplantation [8, 9].

2. Consequences of hypoxia

Most cells are able to survive under hypoxic conditions through the transcriptional activation of a series of genes. The oxygen-sensitive transcriptional activator, hypoxia-inducible factor-1 (HIF-1) is the key transcriptional mediator of the hypoxic response and master regulator of O_2 homeostasis. It orchestrates the profound changes in cellular transcription that accompanies hypoxia by controlling the expression of numerous angiogenic, metabolic and cell cycle genes. Accordingly, the HIF pathway is currently viewed as a master regulator of angiogenesis [5].

HIF-1 is normally only found in hypoxic cells. It is a heterodimer that is composed of an O_2-regulated HIF-1α subunit and a constitutively expressed HIF-1β subunit [10]. In the α-subunit, there is an oxygen-dependent degradation (ODD) domain, where the 4-hydroxyproline formation is catalysed by proline-hydroxylase-2 (PHD-2). This leads to its ubiquitination by the von Hippel-Lindau E3 ubiquitin ligase (VHL) and subsequent proteasomal degradation under normoxic cellular conditions. This prevents the formation of a functional HIF dimer [11]. Since PHDs require oxygen for their catalytic activity, and function as cellular oxygen sensors, HIF degradation only occurs under normoxic conditions. Factor inhibiting HIF-1 (FIH) protein, which hydroxylates HIF-1, also contributes to HIF-1 inactivation in normoxic conditions, and thereby prevents the interaction of this subunit with the two transcriptional co-activators of HIF-1: p300 and CREB-binding protein (CBP) which are essential for HIF-1 transcription. Expression and stabilization of the HIF-1 complex is also regulated through feedback inhibition, as PHD-2 itself is activated by HIF-1 [12].

Under hypoxic conditions, HIF-1 protein is stable and active as the hydroxylase, VHL proteins, and FIH are all inhibited by a lack of oxygen. HIF-1 is then able to interact with its co-activators and can dimerize with its constitutively expressed β-subunit [12]. Once stabilized, the HIF-1 protein can bind to the regulatory regions of its target genes, inducing their expression; these target genes include VEGF (vascular endothelial growth factor) [13], erythropoietin [14] and nitric oxide synthase (NOS) [15, 16] and other proangiogenic factors such as PlGF (placental growth factor), or angiopoietins [12] (**Figure 1**).

It has been proposed that the induction of a pseudo-hypoxic response by inhibiting HIF prolyl 4-hydroxylases may provide a novel therapeutic target in the treatment of hypoxia-associated diseases [17].

Several small molecules, such as dimethyloxalyl glycine [18], Roxadustat (FG-4592) [19] and ZYAN1 [20], have been developed to inhibit prolyl hydroxylase domain-containing (PHD) enzymes, and cause HIF activation [21]. These agents have been applied to the treatment of renal anaemia in which there is a deficiency of erythropoietin [22, 23]. The administration of

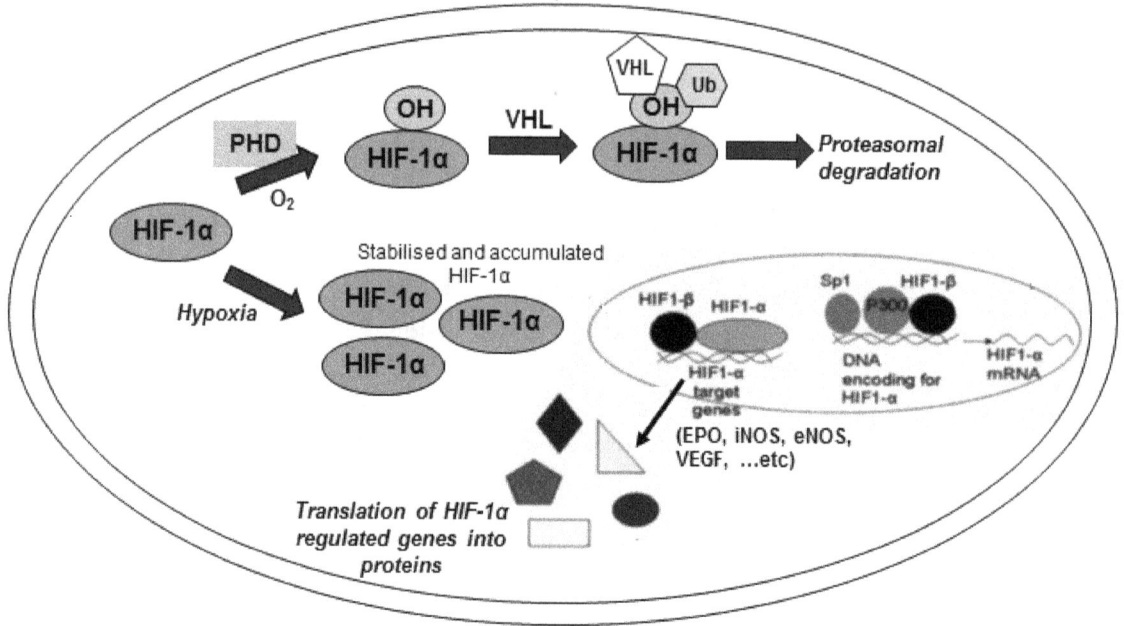

Figure 1. Regulation of the hypoxia-inducible transcription factor (HIF-1α) pathway. Under normal oxygen tensions (normoxia), prolyl hydroxylase (PHD) enzymes, von Hippel-Lindau protein (pVHL), the ubiquitin ligase complex (Ub) and factor inhibiting HIF-1 (FIH) are active leading to HIF-1α proteasomal degradation. Under hypoxic conditions, PHD, pVHL and Ub are not active leading to its cytoplasmic accumulation of HIF-1α. The HIF-1α gene is transcribed in the nucleus with the help of specificity protein (Sp) 1, P300, and HIF-1β leading to transcription of HIF target genes such as EPO, NOS and VEGF.

these compounds is associated with an improved iron profile and an increase of endogenous erythropoietin production to near the physiological range. The clinical trials currently underway aim to address whether PHD enzyme inhibitors will improve clinical end-points, including cardiovascular events [24]. PHD inhibitors have been reported to reduce blood pressure [22] and plasma cholesterol concentrations [19]. Hence, there is a good reason to believe that some PHD inhibitors will reduce cardiovascular endpoints in patients with renal disease. Whether they will benefit a broader category of patients with high risk of cardiovascular disease is difficult to predict.

Hydroxylase activity can be also rescued by mutating specific regions, or by adding cobalt ions to the cell, the latter of which presumably compete for iron-binding sites. Some hydroxylases in the prolyl family can be selectively inhibited by Adriamycin *in vitro*. Cobalt (II) and nickel (II) ions increase HIF-1 activity in cells, presumably because these ions displace iron from the active sites of 2-oxo-glutarate (2OG) hydroxylases [12].

It has been shown that HIF-1α can be regulated by non-hypoxic stimuli such as lipopolysaccharides (LPS), thrombin and angiotensin II (Ang II) [25]. Hormones such as angiotensin II and platelet-derived growth factor stimulate the HIF pathway by increasing HIF-1α protein levels through production of reactive oxygen species (ROS) within the cell. Although the exact mechanism for this is unclear, it appears to be entirely distinct from the hypoxia pathways.

Thrombin and other growth factors appear to increase angiogenesis through HIF-1α protein agonist mechanisms. Insulin similarly activates HIF-1α through the action of multiple protein kinases necessary for expression and function. p53 is responsible for promoting ubiquitination of HIF-1α, and may be an another possible target for enhancing HIF-1. Homozygous deletion of the p53 gene has been found to cause HIF-1 activation [26]. Gene therapy may eventually be used to increase HIF-1 levels and relieve complications of ischemia. For example, delivery of a stabilized, recombinant form of HIF-1α through adeno-associated virus (AAV) in order to overexpress HIF-1 has been shown to result in significantly increased capillary density in skeletal muscle [27]. While gene therapy approaches aimed at the process and effects of angiogenesis continue to be developed and studied, higher levels of success in pre-clinical trials currently are being sought before clinical applications are pursued. Amongst the remaining obstacles in using gene therapy for this purpose is the effective mode of delivery [12]. Inhibition of PHD2 using siRNA has been shown to decrease cardiac infarction size in murine models [28, 29].

In addition to HIF-1α, there are two other members of HIF superfamily that have been described: HIF-2 and HIF-3 [30]. Both are important regulators of the hypoxia response with similar actions as HIF-1 [31] and lead to the transcriptional activation of target genes in hypoxia [32]. However, Eubank et al demonstrated opposing roles for the HIFs in tumour angiogenesis, with HIF-1 exhibiting proangiogenic properties that act through its effects on VEGF secretion, whereas HIF-2 exhibits anti-angiogenic activity by inducing the production of the endogenous angiogenesis inhibitor, sVEGFR-1 [33]. HIF-3α has complementary functions, rather than redundant to HIF-1α induction in protection against hypoxic damage in alveolar epithelial cells in protection against hypoxic damage in alveolar epithelial cells [34].

Although the oxygen-sensing mechanism involving oxygen-dependent hydroxylation of the HIF-α subunits is probably a universal mechanism in cells, and has been highly conserved during evolution, additional regulatory steps appear to determine which of the alternative subunits is induced [34]. One of the best studied hypoxic responses that will be discussed in this chapter is the induction of angiogenic factors and growth factors, which lead to the formation and growth of new blood vessels.

3. Hypoxia and angiogenesis

Blood vessels formation occurs through two basic mechanisms: (1) vasculogenesis represents de novo formation of blood vessels, and is derived from endothelial progenitors and (2) angiogenesis and arteriogenesis (formation of blood vessels from pre-existing blood vessels).

Angiogenesis is a tightly regulated multi-step process that begins when cells within a tissue respond to hypoxia. When tissues grow beyond the physiological oxygen diffusion limit, the relative hypoxia triggers expansion of vascular beds by inducing angiogenic factors in the cells of the vascular beds, which are physiologically oxygenated by simple diffusion of oxygen. Angiogenesis may be a physiological process, as in the case in embryonic development, wound healing or vessel penetration into avascular regions. It may also be pathological, for example when it occurs during the formation of solid tumours, eye disease, chronic inflammatory disorders such as rheumatoid arthritis, psoriasis and periodontitis and atherosclerosis.

The regulation of angiogenesis (whether in physiological or pathological cases) by hypoxia is an important component of homeostatic mechanisms that link vascular oxygen supply to metabolic demand. An understanding of the processes involved in angiogenic, the role of the interacting proteins involved, and how all this is regulated by hypoxia through an ever-expanding number of pathways in multiple cell types may lead to the identification of novel therapies and modalities for ischemic vascular diseases as well as diseases characterized by excessive angiogenesis, such as rheumatoid arthritis, psoriasis, tumours, ischemic brain and heart attack [5, 6].

Angiogenesis in hypoxia is regulated by several pro- and anti-angiogenic factors [1]. HIF-1 has been established as the major inducer of angiogenesis [35]. It regulates the transcription of VEGF, a major regulator of angiogenesis which promotes endothelial cell migration towards the hypoxic area. During hypoxia, HIF-1 binds to the regulatory region of the VEGF gene, inducing its transcription and initiating its expression. VEGF is then secreted and binds to cognate receptor tyrosine kinases (VEGFR1 and VEGFR2) located on the surface of vascular endothelial cells triggering a cascade of intracellular signalling pathways that initiate angiogenesis [10]. These endothelial cells are recruited to form new blood vessels which ultimately supply the given area with oxygenated blood [12]. Interestingly, recent studies have shown that hypoxia influences additional aspects of angiogenesis, including vessel patterning, maturation and function [5].

Other factors such as angiopoietin-2/angiopoietin-1 [36, 37], angiopoietin receptor (Tie2) [38], platelet-derived growth factor (PDGF) [39], basic fibroblast growth factor (bFGF) [40] and monocyte chemoattractant protein 1 (MCP-1) [41] have also been reported to be responsible not only for increasing vascular permeability, endothelial sprouting, maintenance, differentiation and remodelling but also cell proliferation, migration, enhancement of endothelial assembly and lumen formation (**Figure 2**). In hypoxia, angiogenesis is also modulated by several factors that are secreted by leucocytes, which produce a high abundance of angiogenic factors, various interleukins such as TGF-β1 and MCP-1 and proteinases [42]. Thus, hypoxia provides an important environmental stimulus not only for angiogenesis but also for related phenomena in the hypoxic or surrounding area, suggesting that hypoxia is more than simply a regulator of angiogenesis [6].

Angiogenesis may be detrimental when it is excessive. Therefore, angiogenic factors must be highly active but also be tightly regulated. Angiogenesis that is associated with pathological consequences may exhibit differences in the responsible molecular pathways in comparison to physiological angiogenesis. Mutations in oncogenes and tumour suppressor genes and disruptions in growth factor activity play an important role in tumour angiogenesis. The activation of the most prominent proangiogenic factor VEGF might be due to physiological stimuli such as hypoxia or inflammation or due to oncogene activation and tumour suppression function loss. Physiological angiogenesis that occurs during embryonic development or wound healing seems to be dependent on VEGF signalling, whereas tumour angiogenesis adopts

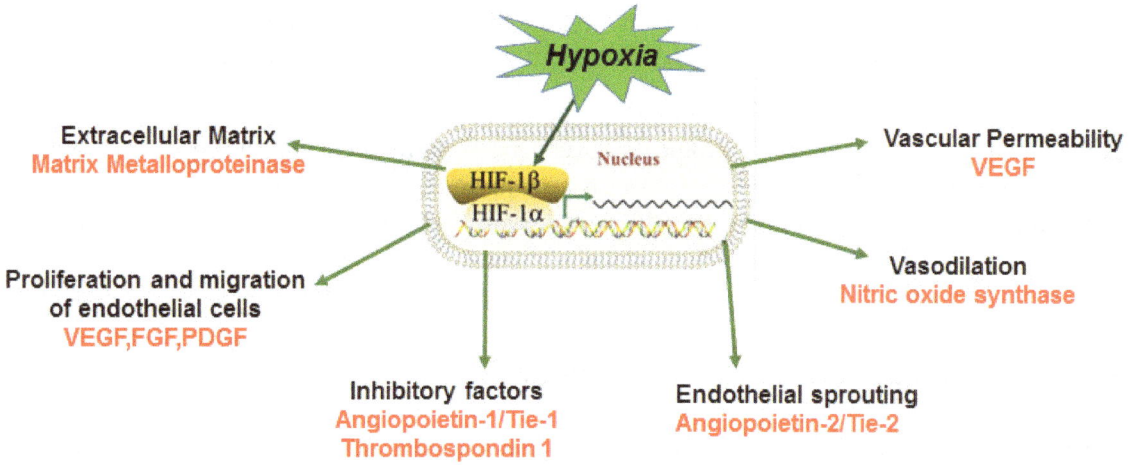

Figure 2. HIF-1α regulates factors involved in developmental and pathological angiogenesis. HIF-1α directly regulates genes involved in steps such as vasodilation, increased vascular permeability, extracellular matrix remodelling and proliferation.

the ability to shift its dependence from VEGF to other proangiogenic pathways, for example, through the recruitment of myeloid cells and the upregulation of alternative vascular growth factors (PlGF and FGF) [1].

The identification of alternative ways of inhibiting tumour growth by disrupting the growth-triggering mechanisms of increasing vascular supply through angiogenesis will depend on the understanding of how tumour cells develop their own vasculature. Other cofactors are essential to ensure maximum efficiency of the transcriptional machinery related to changes in oxygen availability within cells/tissues, and the roles of different HIFs in eliciting hypoxic responses seem to be more divergent as originally assumed. Chen et al. have shown new regulatory interactions of HIF-related mechanisms involving the interactions of basic HIFs, HIF-1α and HIF-2α with their regulatory binding proteins, histone deacetylase 7 (HDAC7) and translation initiation factor 6 (Int6), respectively [6]. Int6 induces HIF-2 degradation. In addition, silencing of *Int6* produces a potent, physiological induction of angiogenesis that may be useful in the treatment of diseases related to insufficient blood supply. The newly discovered binding proteins-HDAC7 for HIF-1 and Int6 for HIF-2 support the assumption that the 2 HIF isoforms play distinct roles in eliciting hypoxia-related responses. HIF-2 may be considered as one of the master switches for inducing angiogenic factors at least in some cell types [6].

The hypoxia/reoxygenation cycle leads to the formation of reactive oxygen species (ROS) that may subsequently regulate HIF-1 but in a rather complex manner. It has been suggested that ROS promote angiogenesis, either directly through stimulation of HIF-1 genes that are involved in stimulating angiogenesis, such as NOS and NADPH oxidase orthrough the generation of active oxidation products, including lipid peroxides. ROS are associated with the development of several chronic diseases that include atherosclerosis, type 2 diabetes mellitus, and cancer [43]. Although ROS have damaging effects on tissues, causing cell death at high concentrations, lesser degrees of oxidative stress may play a positive role during angiogenesis, or other pathophysiological processes. Angiogenesis induced by oxidative stress involves vascular endothelial growth factor (VEGF) signalling, although VEGF-independent pathways have also been identified [44].

The clinical importance of this biological process has become increasingly apparent over the last decade, and angiogenesis now represents a major focus for novel therapeutic approaches to the prevention and treatment of multiple diseases, most notably ischemic cardiovascular disease and cancer [10].

4. Atherosclerosis and plaque angiogenesis

Considering the important contributions of HIF-1 in angiogenesis, it may also be a promising target for treating ischaemic disease [1] and pressure-overload heart failure [45].

Atherosclerosis causes clinical disease through the occlusion of the arteries as a result of excessive build-up of plaque within the artery wall resulting from the accumulation of cholesterol, fatty material and extracellular matrix. This causes obstruction in the blood flow to the myocardium (coronary heart disease), brain (ischemic stroke) or lower extremities (peripheral vascular). The most common of these manifestations is coronary heart disease that includes stable angina pectoris and the acute coronary syndromes [46].

Coronary heart disease (CHD) is a major cause of mortality globally (1 in every 6 deaths annually). An estimated £2bn per annum is used to treat CHD and its co-morbidities [47]. Arterial injury plays a key role in the initiation and progression of CHD [48]. Treatments for CHD range from lifestyle changes and non-invasive medical therapies to pharmacological therapies and open surgical interventions. Despite the widespread use of drugs such as statins, there remains a significant proportion of individuals for whom response to therapy is sub-optimal, and who develop atherosclerosis [49, 50].

Atherosclerosis is a lipoprotein-driven disease affecting medium and large arteries that leads to plaque formation at specific sites of the arterial tree through intimal inflammation, necrosis, fibrosis and calcification. It is a chronic inflammatory process that involves increased oxidative stress, endothelial damage, and smooth muscle cell proliferation and migration. It is associated with several established risk factors, including hypertension, hyperglycaemia, ageing and dyslipidaemia [51]. It is important to control the factors involved in the progression of atherosclerosis because advanced atherosclerotic lesions are prone to rupture, leading to disability or death. Plaque at risk of rupture has been a major focus of research [52]. There is an emerging need for new therapies to stabilize atherosclerotic lesions. Further understanding of the effects of hypoxia in atherosclerotic lesions could indicate potential therapeutic targets [53, 54]. The presence of hypoxia in human carotid atherosclerotic lesions correlates with angiogenesis. Hypoxia plays a key role in the progression and development of advanced lesions by promoting lipid accumulation, increased inflammation, ATP depletion and angiogenesis. A recent study has convincingly demonstrated the presence of hypoxia in macrophage-rich regions of advanced human carotid atherosclerotic lesions [53].

4.1. Evidence for hypoxia within atherosclerotic plaque

Hypoxia in atherosclerotic plaques is now widely recognized, because of the use of specific probes in imaging studies [4]. Imaging plaque hypoxia could provide a means of assessing putative culprit lesions that are at risk of rupture, and are consequentially liable to adverse outcomes.

Hypoxia has been consistently found in atherosclerotic plaques *in vivo* in humans and animal models using different biomarkers [55]. The immunologically identifiable hypoxia marker, 7-(4″-(2-nitroimidazole-1-yl)-butyl)-theophylline (NITP), has been used to assess hypoxia in three murine models *in vivo*. NITP can bind to cells under low-oxygen conditions [56, 57].

Other non-invasive imaging techniques have also been applied, which directly target plaque hypoxia, and these techniques are now being further validated in human studies. The metabolic marker F-fluorodeoxyglucose (FDG) has been used to detect human atherosclerosis *in vivo* and may also serve as an indirect marker of plaque hypoxia as the enhanced glucose uptake in anaerobic metabolism results in an increased uptake of the labelled FDG [58]. F-18-fluoromisonidazole positron emission tomographic (PET) has been used for the *in vivo* assessment of hypoxia in advanced aortic atherosclerosis in rabbits where hypoxia has been found to be predominantly confined to the macrophage-rich regions within the atheromatous core, whereas the macrophages close to the lumen were hypoxia negative [47]. This was then related to hypoxia assessed by *ex vivo* tissue staining using pimonidazole, and immuno-staining for macrophages (RAM-11), new vessels (CD31) and hypoxia-inducible factor-1 α. ^{18}F-fluoromisonidazole (^{18}F-FMISO), a cell permeable 2-nitroimidazole derivative that is reduced *in vivo* by nitroreductases, regardless of the intracellular oxygen concentration, has been one of the leading radiotracers for imaging hypoxia [47]. In human studies, this imaging approach has been coupled with quantitative polymerase chain reaction (qPCR) and immune-staining of plaques tissues recovered by carotid endarterectomy to determine the gene expression of HIF-1α and cluster of differentiation 68 (CD68, a marker of inflammation). HIF-1α and CD68 expression were both found to be significantly correlated with F-FDG-uptake, indicating an association between the presence of hypoxia, inflammation and increased glucose metabolism *in vivo* [59].

Imaging plaque biomarkers such as CRP, interleukins 6, 10 and 18, soluble CD40 ligand, P- and E-selectin, NT-proBNP, fibrinogen and cystatin C show great potential in the prediction and improvement for vascular patients [60].

4.2. The development of a hypoxic environment within the atherosclerotic plaque

Hypoxia has been identified as a potential factor in the formation of vulnerable plaque, and it is clear that decreased oxygen plays a role in the development of plaque angiogenesis leading to plaque destabilization [61]. There have been a number of hypotheses of atherogenesis (plaque angiogenesis) proposing that an imbalance between the demand for and supply of oxygen in the arterial wall is a key factor in the development of atherosclerosis [2, 62].

During atherogenesis, the intima (the innermost layer of the artery wall) may thicken by the accumulation of cells and matrix, and the diffusion of oxygen can then become impaired. The vasa vasorum, forming the network of small blood vessels, are vulnerable to hypoxia especially at the site of arterial branching as they are end arteries and the blood flow is reduced in this region. It has been hypothesized that hypoxia within the vasa vasorum is due to reduced blood flow and consequent endothelial dysfunction, local inflammation and permeation of large particles such as microbes, LDL-lipoprotein and fatty acids which are transformed by macrophages into foam cells [63, 64], which may be an initiating factor in atherosclerosis [65]. Therefore, the micro-environment within the atherosclerotic plaque is thought to be an important determinant of whether a plaque progresses, and the likelihood of clinical complications. Recent reports provide substantial evidence that there are regions within the plaque in which hypoxia can be identified [46].

In addition to being a marker of hypoxia, HIF-1α may directly enhance atherogenesis through several mechanisms, including smooth muscle cell proliferation and migration, new vessel formation (angiogenesis) and altered lipid metabolism [66]. The effects of HIF-1α on macrophage biology and subsequent promotion of atherogenesis has been studied in mice. HIF-1α expression in macrophages affects their intrinsic inflammatory profile and promotes the development of atherosclerosis [67]. Hence, HIF-1α may play a key role in the progression of atherosclerosis by initiating and promoting the formation of foam cells, endothelial cell dysfunction, apoptosis, increasing inflammation and angiogenesis [68].

It has been also proposed that the state of hypoxia, present in the atherosclerotic plaques of mice deficient in apolipoprotein E (ApoE$^{-/-}$ mice), may promote lipid synthesis, and reduce cholesterol efflux through the ATP-binding cassette transporter (ABCA1) pathway: processes that are known to be mediated by HIF-1α [55]. Hypoxia has also been reported to increase the formation of lipid droplets in macrophages to promote the secretion of inflammatory mediators, and atherosclerotic lesion progression by exacerbating ATP depletion and lactate accumulation in this model of atherosclerosis [53].

Several HIF-responsive genes have been found to be upregulated in atherosclerosis, such as VEGF, endothelin-1 and matrix-metalloproteinase-2 [69]. Hypoxia has the potential to fundamentally change the function, metabolism and responses of many of the cell types found within the developing atherosclerotic plaque, and this may in turn determine whether the plaque evolves into a stable or unstable phenotype. It is likely that this is mediated through effects on angiogenesis, extracellular matrix elaboration and lipoprotein metabolism. The hypoxic milieu in the atherosclerotic plaque may therefore also have implications for the putative therapeutic interventions for atherosclerosis. However, most *in vitro* studies have been conducted under normoxic conditions. The effects observed under these conditions may not accurately reflect those extant within the plaque [69].

The role of HIF-1 in atherosclerosis is not univocal. Silencing of HIF-1α in macrophages reduces proinflammatory factors and increases macrophage apoptosis. Hyperlipidaemia impairs angiogenesis in an HIF-1b and nuclear factor (NF)-κB-dependent manner. Specific knockdown of HIF-1α in endothelial cells reduces atherosclerosis through reduced monocyte recruitment [26], whereas knockdown in antigen-presenting cells results in aggravation of atherosclerosis through T-cell polarization [70]. There is another non-lipid-driven mechanism by which alternative macrophages present in human atherosclerosis M(Hb) promote plaque neoangiogenesis and microvessel incompetence throughan HIF-1α/VEGF-A-dependent pathway [71].

HIF-1α has also been also implicated in the pathogenesis of in-stent restenosis following coronary revascularisation, stroke, peripheral artery disease, aortic aneurysm formation and pulmonary artery hypertension [72], and also appears to be involved in the calcification of blood vessels, which often accompanies atherosclerosis [73]. Despite being an intracellular transcription factor, HIF-1 could be possible released into the circulation from damaged cells, similar to other transcriptional factors such as NF-κB and p53 [73-75].

4.3. Other atherogenic mechanisms of hypoxia

Although plaque angiogenesis is a physiological response that facilitates the increased oxygen demand in the plaque, it can have adverse effects by facilitating intra-plaque haemorrhage (IPH) and the influx of inflammatory mediators. IPH as a result of immature plaque neovessels is associated with subsequent ischemic events. Inflammatory cell, endothelial cell and pericyte interactions can provide insight into the biological mechanisms of plaque angiogenesis [70].

The recruitment of T lymphocytes and proliferation and migration of smooth muscle and endothelial cells are essential for atherosclerotic plaque formation and development. During this process, a number of pro-inflammatory factors and cytokines, leukotrienes and chemokines are increased in expression, especially in lipid-loaded foam cells, such as IL8, tumour necrosis factor α (TNFα), interleukin (IL)-1,vascular cell adhesion molecule 1 (VCAM-1) and 15-lipoxygenase-2 (15-LOX-2). Moreover, macrophages are trapped in hypoxic areas of the lesion; however, the exact mechanisms have yet to be determined.

The majority of inflammatory cells contributing to early atherosclerosis probably enter the artery wall from the lumen [76, 77]. However, the vasa vasorum and associated microvessels may provide an alternate route by which leucocytes can enter the vascular wall [78]. As atherosclerosis progresses, angiogenic factors within the micro-environment of the plaque may stimulate new vessel formation. This combination of delicate new vessel network and inflammatory cells, that elaborate proteolytic enzymes, may contribute to intra-plaque haemorrhage and subsequent plaque rupture [79]. The involvement of vasa vasorum and intimal hyperplasia in the pathophysiology of atherosclerosis is supported by several experimental animal studies [80, 81].

Hypoxia may also induce macrophage migration inhibitory factor (MIF). MIF plays a critical role in the progression of atherosclerosis by several different mechanisms. These include the MIF-triggered arrest and chemotaxis of monocytes and T cells through its receptors CXCR2/4. Further, in vivo studies have shown that the blockade of MIF in mice with advanced atherosclerosis leads to plaque regression and reduced monocyte and T-cell content. Additionally, the neuronal signalling molecule Netrin-1 was recently shown to play an important role in macrophage retention in atherosclerotic plaques. Notably, netrin-1 expression has been shown to be regulated by hypoxia, but this may be tissue or disease specific [55].

Atherosclerotic lesion formation is associated with vessel wall thickening resulting in regional limited oxygen exchange. Vascular cells respond to hypoxic conditions with changes in cell metabolism, angiogenesis, apoptosis and inflammatory responses comparable to cells in tumours. Local hypoxic regions and hypoxic cells have been identified in human atherosclerotic lesions and in experimental models. Increased oxygen consumption by cells with a high metabolic activity, such as macrophages, further depletes the oxygen availability, creating a hypoxic environment in the atherosclerotic lesion. In macrophages, hypoxia not only affects the metabolism and lipid uptake but also results in an increased inflammatory response characterized by increased IL-1β and caspase-1 activation. Hypoxia also augments the thrombogenic potential of atherosclerotic plaques through upregulation of tissue factor.

The identification of specific inflammatory markers pertaining to the arterial wall in atherosclerosis may be useful for both diagnosis and treatment. These include macrophage inhibiting factor (MIF), leucocytes and P-selectin. Purinergic signalling is involved in the control of vascular tone and remodelling. Endothelial cells release purines and pyrimidines in response to changes in blood flow (evoking shear stress) and hypoxia. They then act on P2Y, P2X and P1 receptors on endothelial cells leading to release of EDRF mediated by nitric oxide and prostaglandins and EDHF, resulting in vasodilatation. The therapeutic potential of purinergic compounds for the treatment of vascular diseases, including hypertension, ischaemia, atherosclerosis, migraine and coronary artery and diabetic vascular disease as well as vasospasm is discussed [82]. Modern therapeutic modalities involving endothelial progenitor cells therapy, angiotensin II type-2 (AT2R) and ATP-activated purinergic receptor therapy are notable to mention. Future drugs may be designed to target three signalling mechanisms of AT2R which are (a) activation of protein phosphatases resulting in protein dephosphorylation, (b) activation of bradykinin/nitric oxide/ cyclic guanosine 3″,5″-monophosphate pathway by vasodilation and (c) stimulation of phospholipase A(2) and release of arachidonic acid. Drugs may also be designed to act on ATP-activated purinergic receptor channel type P2X7 molecules which acts on cardiovascular system. Better understanding of the vascular inflammatory processes and the cells involved in the formation of plaques may prove to be beneficial for future diagnosis, clinical treatment and planning innovative novel anti-atherosclerotic drugs [83].

Systemic hypoxia that is, for example, associated with obstructive sleep apnoea (OSA) also promotes atherosclerosis. The processes by which it may do this include effects on lipid metabolism and efflux, inflammation, altered macrophage polarization and glucose metabolism [84].

5. Conclusion

Hypoxia is involved in several pathophysiological processes, including embryogenesis, angiogenesis and atherogenesis. HIF-1 appears to be an important mediator controlling cellular response to hypoxia. It also appears to be related to atherosclerotic progression and rupture. A better understanding of the mechanism involved in these processes may provide some novel therapeutic approaches to the treatment of cardiovascular disease.

Author details

Lamia Heikal * and Gordon Ferns

*Address all correspondence to: l.heikal@bsms.ac.uk

Brighton and Sussex Medical School, University of Sussex, Brighton, United Kingdom

References

[1] Zimna A and Kurpisz M. Hypoxia-inducible factor-1 in physiological and pathophysi-ological angiogenesis: applications and therapies. BioMed Research International. 2015;**2015**:13DOI: 10.1155/2015/549412

[2] Bjornheden T, Levin M, Evaldsson M and Wiklund O. Evidence of hypoxic areas within the arterial wall in vivo. Arteriosclerosis, Thrombosis and Vascular Biology. 1999;**19** (4):870-6 (4PT).

[3] Michiels C, Deleener F, Arnould T, Dieu M and Remacle J. Hypoxia stimulates human endothelial cells to release smooth muscle cell mitogens–role of prostaglandins and BFGF. Experimental Cell Research. 1994;**213**(1):43–54. DOI: 10.1006/excr.1994.1171

[4] Humar R, Kiefer FN, Berns H, Resink TJ and Battegay EJ. Hypoxia enhances vascular cell proliferation and angiogenesis in vitro via rapamycin (mTOR) -dependent signaling. The FASEB Journal. 2002;**16**(8):771–780. DOI: 10.1096/fj.01-0658com

[5] Krock BL, Skuli N and Simon MC. Hypoxia-induced angiogenesis: good and evil. Genes & Cancer. 2011;**2**(12):1117–33. DOI: 10.1177/1947601911423654

[6] Chen L, Endler A and Shibasaki F. Hypoxia and angiogenesis: regulation of hypoxia-inducible factors via novel binding factors. Experimental and Molecular Medicine. 2009;**41**:849–857.

[7] Chan CK and Vanhoutte PM. Hypoxia, vascular smooth muscles and endothelium. Acta Pharmaceutica Sinica B. 2013;**3**(1):1–7. DOI: 10.1016/j.apsb.2012.12.007

[8] Singh RB, Mengi SA, Xu Y-J, Arneja AS and Dhalla NS. Pathogenesis of atherosclerosis: a multifactorial process. Experimental & Clinical Cardiology. 2002;**7**(1):40–53.

[9] Cines DB, Pollak ES, Buck CA, et al.. Endothelial cells in physiology and in the patho-physiology of vascular disorders. Blood. 1998;**91**(10):3527–3561.

[10] Semenza GL. Regulation of hypoxia-induced angiogenesis: a chaperone escorts VEGF to the dance. The Journal of Clinical Investigation. 2014;**108**(1):39–40. DOI: 10.1172/ JCI13374

[11] Goggins BJ, Chaney C, Radford-Smith GL, Horvat JC and Keely S. Hypoxia and integrin-mediated epithelial restitution during mucosal inflammation. Frontiers in Immunology. 2013;**4**DOI: 10.3389/fimmu.2013.00272

[12] Ziello JE, Jovin IS and Huang Y. Hypoxia-inducible factor (HIF)-1 regulatory pathway and its potential for therapeutic intervention in malignancy and ischemia. The Yale Journal of Biology and Medicine. 2007;**80**(2):51–60.

[13] Ahluwalia A and Tarnawski AS. Critical role of hypoxia sensor HIF-1 alpha in VEGF gene activation. Implications for angiogenesis and tissue injury healing. Current Medicinal Chemistry. 2012;**19**(1):90–97.

[14] Fandrey J. Oxygen-dependent and tissue-specific regulation of erythropoietin gene expression. American Journal of Physiology–Regulatory, Integrative and Comparative Physiology. 2004;**286**(6):R977–R988. DOI: 10.1152/ajpregu.00577.2003

[15] Heikal L, Ghezzi P, Mengozzi M, Stelmaszczuk B, Feelisch M and Ferns GAA. Erythropoietin and a nonerythropoietic peptide analog promote aortic endothelial cell repair under hypoxic conditions: role of nitric oxide. Hypoxia. 2016;**4**:121–133.

[16] Heikal L, Ghezzi P, Mengozzi M and Ferns G. Low oxygen tension primes aortic endothelial cells to the reparative effect of tissue-protective cytokines. Molecular Medicine. 2015;**21**:709–716. DOI: 10.2119/molmed.2015.00162

[17] Myllyharju J. Prolyl 4-hydroxylases, master regulators of the hypoxia response. Acta Physiologica. 2013;**208**(2):148–165. DOI: 10.1111/apha.12096

[18] Milkiewicz M, Pugh CW and Egginton S. Inhibition of endogenous HIF inactivation induces angiogenesis in ischaemic skeletal muscles of mice. The Journal of Physiology. 2004;**560**(1):21–26. DOI: 10.1113/jphysiol.2004.069757

[19] Provenzano R, Besarab A, Sun CH, et al. Oral hypoxia-inducible factor prolyl hydroxylase inhibitor roxadustat (FG-4592) for the treatment of anemia in patients with CKD. Clinical Journal of the American Society of Nephrology. 2016;**11**(6):982–991. DOI: 10.2215/cjn.06890615

[20] Jain MR, Joharapurkar AA, Pandya V, et al. Pharmacological characterization of ZYAN1, a novel prolyl hydroxylase inhibitor for the treatment of anemia. Drug Research. 2016;**66**(2):107–112. DOI: 10.1055/s-0035-1554630

[21] Beuck S, Schaenzer W and Thevis M. Hypoxia-inducible factor stabilizers and other small-molecule erythropoiesis-stimulating agents in current and preventive doping analysis. Drug Testing and Analysis. 2012;**4**(11):830–845. DOI: 10.1002/dta.390

[22] Yousaf F and Spinowitz B. Hypoxia-inducible factor stabilizers: a new avenue for reducing BP while helping hemoglobin?. Current Hypertension Reports. 2016;**18**(3)DOI: 10.1007/s11906-016-0629-6

[23] Forristal CE, Winkler IG, Nowlan B, Barbier V, Walkinshaw G and Levesque JP.. Pharmacologic stabilization of HIF-1α increases hematopoietic stem cell quiescence in vivo and accelerates blood recovery after severe irradiation. Blood. 2013;**121**(5):759–769. DOI: 10.1182/blood-2012-02-408419

[24] Maxwell PH and Eckardt KU. HIF prolyl hydroxylase inhibitors for the treatment of renal anaemia and beyond. Nature Reviews in Nephrology. 2016;**12**(3):157–168. DOI: 10.1038/nrneph.2015.193

[25] Kuschel A, Simon P and Tug S. Functional regulation of HIF-1a under normoxi-auis there more than post-translational regulation?. Journal of Cellular Physiology. 2012;**227**(2):514–524. DOI: 10.1002/jcp.22798

[26] Pajusola K, Kunnapuu J, Vuorikoski S, et al. Stabilized HIF-1 alpha is superior to VEGF for angiogenesis in skeletal muscle via adeno-associated virus gene transfer. Faseb Journal. 2005;**19**(8):1365. DOI: 10.1096/fj.05-3720fje

[27] Tsurumi Y, Takeshita S, Chen DF, et al. Direct intramuscular gene transfer of naked DNA encoding vascular endothelial growth factor augments collateral development and tissue perfusion. Circulation. 1996;**94**(12):3281–3290.

[28] Eckle T, Köhler D, Lehmann R, El Kasmi KC and Eltzschig HK. Hypoxia-inducible factor-1 is central to cardioprotection. A New Paradigm for Ischemic Preconditioning. 2008;**118**(2):166–175. DOI: 10.1161/circulationaha.107.758516

[29] Tekin D, Dursun AD and Xi L. Hypoxia inducible factor 1 (HIF-1) and cardioprotection. Acta Pharmacologica Sinica. 2010;**31**(9):1085–1094. DOI: 10.1038/aps.2010.132

[30] Zhao J, Du F, Shen G, Zheng F and Xu B. The role of hypoxia-inducible factor-2 in digestive system cancers. Cell Death Disease. 2015;**6**:e1600. DOI: 10.1038/cddis.2014.565

[31] Agnieszka L, Alicja J and Jozef D. HIF-1 and HIF-2 transcription factors - similar but not identical. Molecules and Cells. 2010;**29**(5):435–442.

[32] Carroll VA and Ashcroft M. Role of hypoxia-inducible factor (HIF)-1 alpha-versus HIF-2 alpha in the regulation of HIF target genes in response to hypoxia, insulin-like growth factor-1, or loss of von Hippel-Lindau function: implications for targeting the HIF pathway. Cancer Research. 2006;**66**(12):6264–6270. DOI: 10.1158/0008-5472.can-05-2519

[33] Eubank TD, Roda JM, Liu HW, O'Neil T and Marsh CB. Opposing roles for HIF-1 alpha and HIF-2 alpha in the regulation of angiogenesis by mononuclear phagocytes. Blood. 2011;**117**(1):323–332. DOI: 10.1182/blood-2010-01-261792

[34] Li QF, Wang XR, Yang YW and Lin H. Hypoxia upregulates hypoxia inducible factor (HIF)-3 alpha expression in lung epithelial cells: characterization and comparison with HIF-1 alpha. Cell Research. 2006;**16**(6):548–558. DOI: 10.1038/sj.cr.7310072

[35] Pugh CW and Ratcliffe PJ. Regulation of angiogenesis by hypoxia: role of the HIF system. Nature Medicine. 2003;**9**(6):677–684.

[36] Graham CH, Fitzpatrick TE and McCrae KR. Hypoxia stimulates urokinase receptor expression through a heme protein-dependent pathway. Blood. 1998;**91**(9):3300–3307.

[37] Phelan MW, Forman LW, Perrine SP and Faller DV. Hypoxia increases thrombospon-
     din-1 transcript and protein in cultured endothelial cells. Journal of Laboratory and
     Clinical Medicine. 1998;**132**(6):519–529. DOI: 10.1016/s0022-2143(98)90131-7

[38] Kuwabara K, Ogawa S, Matsumoto M, et al. Hypoxia-mediated induction of acidic/basic
     fibroblast growth factor and platelet derived growth factor in mononuclear phagocytes stim-
     ulates growth of hypoxic endothelial cells. Proceedings of the National Academy of Sciences
     of the United States of America. 1995;**92**(10):4606–4610. DOI: 10.1073/pnas.92.10.4606

[39] Wykoff CC, Pugh CW, Maxwell PH, Harris AL and Ratcliffe PJ. Identification of
     novel hypoxia dependent and independent target genes of the von Hippel-Lindau
     (VHL) tumour suppressor by mRNA differential expression profiling. Oncogene.
     2000;**19**(54):6297–6305. DOI: 10.1038/sj.onc.1204012

[40] Sakuda H, Nakashima Y, Kuriyama S and Sueishi K. Media conditioned by smooth mus-
     cle cells cultured in a variety of hypoxic environments stimulates in vitro angiogenesis-
     a relationship to transforming growth factor-beta-1. American Journal of Pathology.
     1992;**141**(6):1507–1516.

[41] Phillips PG, Birnby LM and Narendran A. Hypoxia induces capillary network forma-
     tion in cultured bovine pulmonary microvessel endothelial cells. American Journal of
     Physiology-Lung Cellular and Molecular Physiology. 1995;**268**(5):L789–L800.

[42] Norrby K. Mast cells and angiogenesis. Apmis. 2002;**110**(5):355–371. DOI:
     10.1034/j.1600-0463.2002.100501.x

[43] Goerlach A, Dimova EY, Petry A, et al. Reactive oxygen species, nutrition, hypoxia
     and diseases: Problems solved?. Redox Biology. 2015;**6**:372–385. DOI: 10.1016/j.
     redox.2015.08.016

[44] Kim YW and Byzova TV.. Oxidative stress in angiogenesis and vascular disease. Blood.
     2014;**123**(5):625–631. DOI: 10.1182/blood-2013-09-512749

[45] Semenza G L. Hypoxia-inducible factor 1 and cardiovascular disease. Annual Review of
     Physiology. 2014;**76**:39–56. DOI: 10.1146/annurev-physiol-021113-170322

[46] Lahoz C and Mostaza JM. Atherosclerosis as a systemic disease. Revista Espanola De
     Cardiologia. 2007;**60**(2):184–195. DOI: 10.1157/13099465

[47] Mateo J, Izquierdo-Garcia D, Badimon JJ, Fayad ZA and Fuster V. Noninvasive assess-
     ment of hypoxia in rabbit advanced atherosclerosis using (18)F-fluoromisonidazole
     PET imaging. Circulation. Cardiovascular imaging. 2014;**7**(2):312–320. DOI: 10.1161/
     CIRCIMAGING.113.001084

[48] Varani J and Ward PA. Mechanisms of endothelial cell injury in acute inflammation.
     Shock. 1994;**2**(5):311–319.

[49] Andrade PJ, Medeiros MM, Andrade AT, Lima AA. Coronary angioplasty versus CABG:
     review of randomised trials. Arquivos Brasileiros De Cardiologia. 2011;**97**(3):E60–E69.

[50] Solomon AJ, Gersh BJ. Management of chronic stable angina: medical therapy, percu- taneous transluminal coronary angioplasty and coronary artery bypass graft surgery- Lessons from randomized trials. Annals of Internal Medicine. 1998;**128**(3):216–223.

[51] Xiao W, Jia Z, Zhang Q, Wei C, Wang H and Wu Y. Inflammation and oxidative stress, rather than hypoxia, are predominant factors promoting angiogenesis in the initial phases of atherosclerosis. Molecular Medical Report. 2015;**12**(3):3315–3322. DOI: 10.3892/mmr.2015.3800

[52] Nie XY, Randolph GJ, Elvington A, et al. Imaging of hypoxia in mouse atherosclerotic plaques with Cu-64-ATSM. Nuclear Medicine and Biology. 2016;**43**(9):534–542. DOI: 10.1016/j.nucmedbio.2016.05.011

[53] Hulten LM and Levin M. The role of hypoxia in atherosclerosis. Current Opinion in Lipidology. 2009;**20**(5):409–414. DOI: 10.1097/MOL.0b013e3283307be8

[54] Van der Veken B, De Meyer GRY and Martinet W. Intraplaque neovascularization as a novel therapeutic target in advanced atherosclerosis. Expert Opinion on Therapeutic Targets. 2016;**20**(10):1247–1257. DOI: 10.1080/14728222.2016.1186650

[55] Parathath S, Yang Y, Mick S and Fisher EA. Hypoxia in murine atherosclerotic plaques and its adverse effects on macrophages. Trends in Cardiovascular Medicine. 2013;**23**(3):80–84. DOI: 10.1016/j.tcm.2012.09.004

[56] Bjornheden T, Evaldsson M and Wiklund O. A method for the assessment of hypoxia in the arterial wall, with potential application in vivo. Arteriosclerosis, Thrombosis and Vascular Biology. 1996;**16**(1):178–185.

[57] Webster L, Hodgkiss RJ and Wilson GD. Cell cycle distribution of hypoxia and progres- sion of hypoxic tumour cells in vivo. British Journal of Cancer. 1998;**77**(2):227–234.

[58] Buscombe JR. Exploring the nature of atheroma and cardiovascular inflammation in vivo using positron emission tomography (PET). British Journal of Radiology. 2015;**88**(1053) DOI: 10.1259/bjr.20140648

[59] Pedersen SF, Grabe M, Hag AMF, Hojgaard L, Sillesen H and Kjar A. (18)F-FDG imag- ing of human atherosclerotic carotid plaques reflects gene expression of the key hypoxia marker HIF-1alpha. American Journal of Nuclear Medicine and Molecular Imaging. 2013;**3**(5):384–92.

[60] van Lammeren GW, Moll FL, Borst GJD, de Kleijn DPV, de Vries JPPM and Pasterkamp G.. Atherosclerotic plaque biomarkers: beyond the horizon of the vulnerable plaque. Current Cardiology Reviews. 2011;**7**(1):22–27. DOI: 10.2174/157340311795677680

[61] Sluimer JC and Daemen MJ. Novel concepts in atherogenesis: angiogenesis and hypoxia in atherosclerosis. Journal of Pathology. 2009;**218**(1):7–29. DOI: 10.1002/path.2518

[62] Gainer JL. Hypoxia and atherosclerosis. Re-evaluation of the old hypothesis. Atherosclerosis. 1987;**68**(3):263–266. DOI: 10.1016/0021-9150(87)90206-1

[63] Jarvilehto M and Tuohimaa P. Vasa vasorum hypoxia: initiation of atherosclerosis. Medical Hypotheses. 2009;**73**(1):40–41. DOI: 10.1016/j.mehy.2008.11.046

[64] Barger AC, Beeuwkes R, Lainey LL and Silverman KJ. Hypothesis-vasa vasorum and neovascularisation of human coronary arteries- a possible role in the path-physiology of atherosclerosis. New England Journal of Medicine. 1984;**310**(3):175–177. DOI: 10.1056/nejm198401193100307

[65] Ferns G and Heikal L. Atherogenesis and hypoxia. Angiology. 2016; August 27:1-22. DOI: 10.1177/0003319716662423

[66] Lim CS, Kiriakidis S, Sandison A, Paleolog EM and Davies AH. Hypoxia-inducible factor pathway and diseases of the vascular wall. Journal of Vascular Surgery. 2013;**58**(1):219–230. DOI: 10.1016/j.jvs.2013.02.240

[67] Aarup A, Pedersen TX, Junker N, et al. Hypoxia-inducible factor-1α expression in macrophages promotes development of atherosclerosis. Arteriosclerosis, Thrombosis, and Vascular Biology. 2016; 36:1782-1790;DOI: 10.1161/atvbaha.116.307830

[68] Gao L, Chen Q, Zhou X and Fan L. The role of hypoxia-inducible factor 1 in atherosclerosis. Journal of Clinical Pathology. 2012;**65**(10):872–876. DOI: 10.1136/jclinpath-2012-200828

[69] Sluimer JC, Gasc J-M, van Wanroij JL, et al. Hypoxia, hypoxia-inducible transcription factor, and macrophages in human atherosclerotic plaques are correlated with intraplaque angiogenesis. Journal of the American College of Cardiology. 2008;**51**(13):1258–1265. DOI: 10.1016/j.jacc.2007.12.025

[70] de Vries MR and Quax PHA. Plaque angiogenesis and its relation to inflammation and atherosclerotic plaque destabilisation. Current Opinion in Lipidology. 2016;**27**(5):499–506.

[71] Finn AV, Akahori H, Guo L, et al. Alternative macrophages promote intraplaque angiogenesis and vascular permeability in human atherosclerosis. Journal of the American College of Cardiology. 2016;**67**(13):2241–2241.

[72] Kasivisvanathan V, Shalhoub J, Lim CS, Shepherd AC, Thapar A and Davies AH. Hypoxia-inducible factor-1 in arterial disease: a putative therapeutic target. Current Vascular Pharmacology. 2011;**9**(3):333–349.

[73] Li G, Lu W-h, Ai R, Yang J-h, Chen F and Tang Z. The relationship between serum hypoxia-inducible factor 1 alpha and coronary artery calcification in asymptomatic type 2 diabetic patients. Cardiovascular Diabetology. 2014;**13**DOI: 10.1186/1475-2840-13-52

[74] Ismail S, Mayah W, Battia HE, et al. Plasma nuclear factor kappa B and serum peroxiredoxin 3 in early diagnosis of hepatocellular carcinoma. Asian Pacific Journal of Cancer Prevention: APJCP. 2015;**16**(4):1657–63.

[75] Attallah AM, Abdel-Aziz MM, El-Sayed AM and Tabll AA. Detection of serum p53 protein in patients with different gastrointestinal cancers. Cancer Detection and Prevention. 2003;**27**(2):127–131. DOI: http://dx.doi.org/10.1016/S0361-090X(03)00024-2

[76] Faggiotto A, Ross R and Harker L. Studies of hypercholesterolemia in the non-human primate. 1. Changes that lead to fatty streak formation. Arteriosclerosis. 1984;**4**(4):323–340.

[77] Ross R. Mechanisms of disease - atherosclerosis - an inflammatory disease. New England Journal of Medicine. 1999;**340**(2):115–126.

[78] Rademakers T, Douma K, Hackeng TM, et al. Plaque-associated vasa vasorum in aged apolipoprotein E-deficient mice exhibit proatherogenic functional features In Vivo. Arteriosclerosis, Thrombosis and Vascular Biology. 2013;**33**(2):249–256. DOI: 10.1161/atvbaha.112.300087

[79] Moreno PR, Purushothaman KR, Zias E, Sanz J and Fuster V. Neovascularization in human atherosclerosis. Current Molecular Medicine. 2006;**6**(5):457–477. DOI: 10.2174/156652406778018635

[80] Barker SGE, Talbert A, Cottam S, Baskerville PA and Martin JF. Arterial intimal hyperplasia after occlusion of the adventitial vasa vasorum in the pig. Arteriosclerosis and Thrombosis. 1993;**13**(1):70–77.

[81] Khurana R, Zhuang Z, Bhardwaj S, et al. Angiogenesis-dependent and independent phases of intimal hyperplasia. Circulation. 2004;**110**(16):2436–2443. DOI: 10.1161/01.cir.0000145138.25577.f1

[82] Burnstock G. Purinergic signalling and endothelium. Current Vascular Pharmacology. 2016;**14**(2):130–145. DOI: 10.2174/1570161114666151202204948

[83] Thent ZC, Chakraborty C, Mahakkanukrauh P, Kosai N, Rajan R and S D. The molecular concept of atheromatous plaques. Current Drug Target. 2016; 17: 1–9.

[84] Marsch E, Sluimer JC and Daemen MJAP. Hypoxia in atherosclerosis and inflammation. Current Opinion in Lipidology. 2013;**24**(5):393–400. DOI: 10.1097/MOL.0b013e32836484a4

5

Platelet Lysate to Promote Angiogenic Cell Therapies

Scott T. Robinson and Luke P. Brewster

Abstract

Cellular therapies for patients with ischemic muscle have been limited by poor cell retention and survivability. Platelets are a robust source of growth factors and structural proteins, and extracts from this peripheral blood component may be manipulated to improve both cell retention and survivability in percutaneous delivery methods. Human platelet lysate is generated from pooled human platelets and contains a growth factor milieu that promotes robust human mesenchymal stem cell (MSC) proliferation without risk of xenogenic contamination. As such, platelet lysate is a practical alternative to animal serum for MSC culture and, with minor adjustments to the production process, can also be used as a scaffold for cell delivery. Human platelet lysate is a promising substrate that can provide nutritive delivery both in vitro and during cell implantation, potentially improving retention and survivability of MSCs that may improve angiogenic function for cell therapy in *treatment* of ischemic tissues.

Keywords: critical limb ischemia, mesenchymal stromal cells, platelet lysate, angiogenic cell therapy

1. Introduction

The legs are a site of ischemic muscle that are particularly attractive to application of angiogenic therapies. Decreased perfusion of the legs is known as peripheral arterial disease (PAD), and PAD is pandemic with extreme costs to society. In its most severe form, it is called critical limb ischemia (CLI). CLI patients do not have adequate perfusion to their resting nutritional needs resulting in rest pain or even tissue loss. While only 1–2% of PAD patients will develop CLI, CLI affects 1 million individuals annually [1]. Surgical revascularization of CLI patients can prevent major amputation. Current treatment for limb salvage includes endovascular therapy (angioplasty or stent placement) and surgical bypass. However, despite improvements in medical and surgical therapies, successful management of CLI is difficult with ~0.5

of patients with CLI dying or undergoing major amputation within 1 year [2]. Since many patients with CLI either fail revascularization therapy or are not candidates for these procedures, amputation is commonly performed. In addition to the impaired quality of life that results from lower limb amputation, historically mortality rates for this procedure have been reported to approach 40% [3]. New and innovative therapies are imperative to improve mortality and quality of life in patients with CLI and provide an alternative to limb amputation.

Cell therapy is a promising new treatment strategy for patient with CLI. The concept of cell therapy for treatment of critical limb ischemia coincided with the discovery of a circulating endothelial progenitor cell (EPC) in 1997, which described a population of circulating peripheral blood mononuclear cells that presumably arise from the bone marrow yet is also capable of displaying characteristics of a mature endothelium [4]. This discovery challenged the prevailing paradigm of postnatal neovascularization [5] in which blood vessel growth was the result of angiogenesis (the formation of new blood vessels from the existing endothelium through sprouting or intussusception) and arteriogenesis (the expansion of preexisting collateral vessels due to an increase in blood flow in response to changes in shear stress [6]). The work by Asahara et al. was significant for two reasons. First, it introduced the concept of postnatal vasculogenesis, suggesting that bone marrow-derived cells could contribute to the formation of new blood vessels in the adult similar to the process of vasculogenesis seen in embryogenesis, where primitive hemangioblasts give rise to de novo blood vessels in the developing fetus. Second, it pioneered the idea of cell therapy, through experiments in which the ischemic limbs of nude mice were injected with a population of human peripheral blood mononuclear cells enriched for CD34+ and Flk-1 (VEGFR-2), and found that the transplanted cells incorporated into the blood vessel endothelium at sites of neovascularization.

The notion that bone marrow-derived cells incorporate directly into native endothelium is controversial. Despite several initial reports suggesting differentiation of bone marrow cells into endothelial cells [7–9], several subsequent studies demonstrated that endogenous and transplanted bone marrow cells did not directly incorporate into the endothelium but instead support neovascularization through a paracrine mechanism [10–13]. Numerous stem and progenitor cell populations derived from the bone marrow, adipose tissue, and embryonic stem cells and induced pluripotent stem cells have been shown to enhance blood vessel growth in animal models of hind limb ischemia, suggesting a role for cell therapy in therapeutic neovascularization [4, 14–16]. Mesenchymal stromal cells (MSCs) are a potential cell source that can be easily isolated, rapidly expanded ex vivo, and have potent proangiogenic qualities [17] mediated through paracrine stimulation of endogenous tissues [18]. The use of MSCs for cell therapy is advantageous over other cell types because they can be derived from an autologous source, thereby avoiding the immunogenicity and loss of tolerance observed when allogeneic MSCs are exposed to an inflammatory environment [19, 20].

Despite numerous animal studies and small clinical pilot trials demonstrating the ability of MSCs to promote angiogenesis [17, 21, 22], the biology and clinical benefit of this approach has not yet been demonstrated in patients with CLI. Two major limitations have prevented the translation of MSC therapy from the laboratory to the clinical arena. First, the use of an autologous cell source in this demographic is complicated by the fact that progenitor cell populations are depleted or functionally impaired in patients with coronary artery disease [23], stroke [24], and diabetes mellitus [25–27] and who are smokers [28]; all risk factors or comorbidities are highly prevalent in patients with CLI. A second major limitation of stem cell therapy thus far has been maintaining a clinically significant cell number in target tissues, as direct intramuscular injection or intra-arterial infusion alone typically does not enable adequate cell delivery [29–31]. In order to fully realize the potential of cell therapy, these limitations must be addressed before successful clinical deployment of MSC therapy can be achieved.

As cell therapy is translated from preclinical animal studies to human clinical trials, strict cell culture techniques must be employed to ensure human safety. The vast majority of clinical trials to date have utilized fetal bovine serum (FBS) for ex vivo expansion and growth of MSCs. However, FBS has considerable xenogenic potential and transplanted autologous MSCs can be rapidly rejected after culture in FBS [32]. Therefore, new human-derived alternatives have been evaluated as possible cell culture supplements to ensure that growth and expansion of MSCs are complain with current good manufacturing processes (GMPs).

Platelets are small enucleated cell fragments derived from megakaryocytes in the bone marrow and play a critical role in initiating hemostasis by binding and adhering to extracellular matrix components after endothelial injury, which in turns leads to platelet activation. Activated platelets then subsequently aggregate and become crosslinked with fibrin through activation of the coagulation cascade, thereby generating a platelet plug capable of blocking the flow of the blood. Platelets normally represent 0.1–0.25% of the blood and typically circulate for 5–9 days. Platelets are also an abundant source of growth factors, accounting for the majority of growth factors found in serum [33, 34]. As a result, various platelet extracts have been used for regenerative medicine applications. Platelet lysate (PL) is one such supplement that has been utilized as a supplement for culture of MSCs and has been shown to be superior to FBS [35, 36]. We and several collaborators have performed extensive characterization of platelet lysate as a cell culture supplement for expansion of human MSCs suitable for cell therapy trials. More recently, we have modified the PL production process such that PL may be used to form a 3D scaffold for MSC growth and invasion. In this chapter, we elaborate on our experience with PL as it pertains to culture of MSCs as well as describe a novel scaffold for cell delivery derived from PL extract.

2. Platelet lysate

2.1. Soluble platelet lysate for expansion of human MSCs

2.1.1. Generation of fibrinogen-depleted platelet lysate

The platelet lysate supplement for cell culture used by our group and our collaborators is manufactured through the Emory Personal Immunotherapy Center (EPIC). The specific production strategy was initially optimized and described by Copland et al. The current protocol employed by EPIC emphasizes good manufacturing process (GMP) technique and results in a fibrinogen-depleted form of platelet lysate (dPL) that is a soluble media supplement for ex vivo expansion of human MSCs. EPIC has provided numerous research groups with dPL and has received FDA approved for use of dPL for human cell therapy trials using MSCs for treatment of Crohn's disease (NCT01659762) and graft vs. host disease following allogenic bone marrow transplantation (NCT02359929). The production process utilizes outdated plateletpheresis products obtained from the Emory University Hospital blood bank. For each lot of dPL, five plateletpheresis products are exposed to sequential freeze-thaw cycles to ensure adequate membrane fracturing. The platelet products are first stored at -20°C, then thawed at 4°C, and aliquoted into smaller volumes of 20–25 mL. The aliquots are then refrozen at -80°C and filtered through a 40 µm filter. The filtered PL is then centrifuged at 4000×g for 20 min at room temperature and refiltered in 40 µm filters. The PL is then mixed with CaCl$_2$ and heparin solution and stored at 4°C overnight to allow formation of a fibrin clot. Following this, the dPL samples are centrifuged again at 4000×g at room temperature, filtered at 0.2 µm, and then stored at -80°C [37]. These final aliquots are then thawed and immediately ready for use in cell culture.

The standard plateletpheresis process employed by the American Red Cross involves the addition of 10% v/v acid citrate dextrose (ACD) to platelet products, which serves as a calcium chelator to disrupt the coagulation cascade and prevent clot formation. In order to generate fibrin clot for depletion of the fibrinogen from the platelet lysate supplement, 20 mM CaCl$_2$ is added to the platelet lysate, which enables the protease-driven conversion of fibrinogen to fibrin, thus leading to spontaneous clot formation. The addition of heparin at a concentration of 2 U/mL also stabilizes clot formation and increases yield of the soluble fraction of the platelet lysate. Under these conditions, over 85% of the platelet lysate is recovered with a final fibrinogen concentration of less than 5 µg/mL (compared to a fibrinogen concentration of ~120 µg/mL in the unfractionated platelet lysate) [37].

The growth factor content of dPL has been well characterized and contains numerous abundant mitogens for cell culture. Specifically, dPL contains ample amounts of PDG-BB, TFG-β1, VEGF, EGF, and BDNF. These growth factors exist in levels significantly higher than standard serum and are preserved in both unfractionated and fibrinogen-depleted PL preparations. Furthermore, dPL is remarkably stable, with room temperature preparations of PL capable of maintaining consistent levels of PDGF-BB and EGF for up to 3 weeks [37]. The stability of dPL and low interlot variability are extremely desirable qualities in a cell culture supplement and therefore are well suited for ex vivo growth and expansion of human therapeutic cell lines.

2.1.2. Immunomodulatory effect of PL fibrinogen depletion on MSCs

The use of dPL as a cell culture supplement is advantageous because it not only decreases the risk of xenogenic contamination but dPL also induces a robust proliferative response in human MSCs. When compared to cells grown in FBS, low passage MSCs cultured in equivalent concentrations of dPL had significantly decreased doubling times and decreased cell volumes. Despite the increase in proliferation, cells grown in dPL maintained expression of typical MSC markers including CD44, CD90, CD73, HLA-I, and CD105 and lacked expression of CD45 and CD34 [37].

In addition to impacting proliferative capacity of MSCs, platelet lysate composition may also affect the immunomodulatory properties of MSCs. MSCs can have a profound immunosuppressive effect on various inflammatory processes. Exposure of MSCs to fibrinogen upregulates integrin and non-integrin fibrinogen-binding complexes. Furthermore, the analysis of the secretome of MSCs exposed to fibrinogen in vitro demonstrated a significant increase in pro-inflammatory cytokines IL-8, MCP-1, and IL-6 [37]. The impact of fibrinogen content in various PL formulations on T-cell activation and proliferation has also been examined. Recently, upregulation of indoleamine 2,3-dioxygenase (IDO) in MSCs has been shown to correlate with suppression of T-cell proliferation [38]. MSCs cultured in unfractionated PL had decreased IDO expression compared to cells cultured in FBS; however, the IDO response was restored when dPL was used as a culture supplement. This functional effect of MSCs on T-cell proliferation was also examined through a coculture assay where MSCs were cocultured with PBMCs exposed to CD3/CD8. T-cell proliferation was noted to be higher in the unfractionated PL compared to dPL and standard FBS. These data suggest that an increased fibrinogen content promotes a pro-inflammatory phenotype of MSCs in vitro, and conversely fibrinogen depletion of PL preserves the immunosuppressive properties of MSCs.

2.1.3. Ex vivo enhancement of MSCs with dPL

The ex vivo expansion for MSCs is essential for cell therapy, as a large number of cells are needed to achieve a desired therapeutic effect. Bone marrow aspirates and peripheral blood cultures provide a relatively low yield of MSCs, and this necessitates prolonged in vitro expansion in order to obtain an adequate number of cells for autologous cell therapy. An unfortunate consequence of this process is that prolonged culture leads to MSC senescence, loss of plasticity, and loss of self-renewal capacity. Typically, human MSCs grown in media supplemented with FBS begin to show signs of senescence after 10 passages, so either increasing proliferation at early passages or delaying the effect of senescence would improve the yield of MSCs for treatment of CLI.

The enriched milieu of growth factors contained within dPL can potentially overcome the senescence associated with long-term MSC culture. Griffith et al. demonstrated that proliferation in senescent MSCs (passage 13 or greater) could be reversed with culture in dPL. MSCs cultured in 5% dPL showed reduction in cell size and a decrease in doubling time while maintaining MSC markers and reducing β-gal production compared to control MSCs cultured in FBS. These effects were short-lived, however, and by passage 16, MSCs failed to proliferate adequately regardless of culture conditions. The transient increase in proliferative response was also evident in *late* passage MSCs (passages 10–11). Culturing in dPL led to a marked decrease in doubling time, but by passage 16, MSCs showed severe signs of senescence in both dPL and FBS treatment groups. Consistent with these results, no changes in telomerase activity were noted between groups [39]. This study clearly established that poor-quality MSCs could be rescued and restored to a robust proliferative state using dPL, even if the effect was only temporary.

2.1.4. Expansion of MSCs from patients with CLI

Expanding on the research of our collaborators, we have worked to exploit the benefits of dPL for cell therapy in patients with CLI. By generating patient-specific MSC cell lines from individuals with CLI, we were able to test the feasibility of expanding MSCs with dPL for future cell therapy trials. In our initial series, we isolated MSCs from bone marrow of amputated limbs of four patients with critical limb ischemia and four patients with critical limb ischemia and concomitant diabetes mellitus. This cohort of patients had no further surgical or endovascular revascularization options and therefore is representative of the population of patients who would benefit from new cell therapy strategies. Additionally, we obtained MSCs from four healthy donors through EPIC. All MSCs were initially plated in media containing FBS; however, at passage 4 they were transitioned to either media containing FBS or dPL. As demonstrated in previous studies, MSCs grown in dPL maintained a similar phenotype based on cell surface markers compared to cells grown in FBS (**Figure 1**), with no notable differences detected across all patient groups. Additionally, differentiation capacity was preserved in MSCs from all patient groups and culture conditions, with all cells differentiating toward osteogenic or adipogenic lineage under appropriate assay conditions [40].

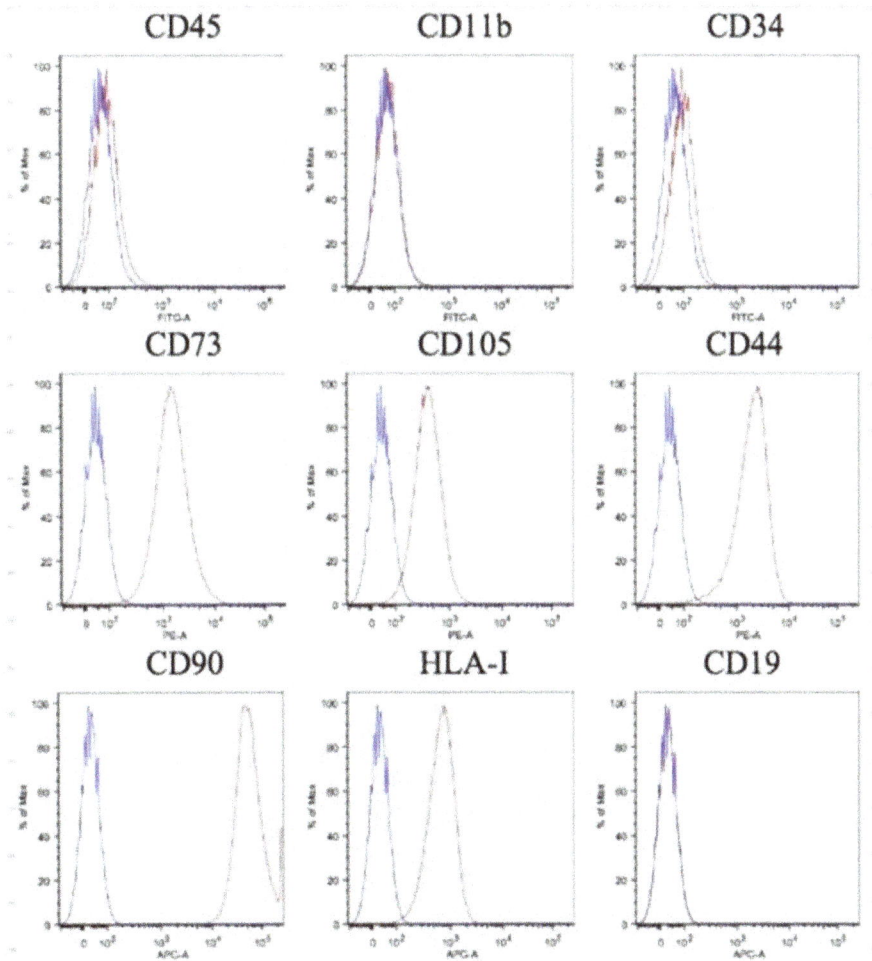

Figure 1. Representative flow cytometry of human MSCs cultured in dPL expresses typical MSC markers. Reprinted from Brewster et al. [40] with permission from Elsevier.

The proliferative response of MSCs from all patient groups and in culture conditions containing both FBS and dPL was examined by quantifying population doublings over multiple passages. For these experiments, a direct comparison of FBS and PL was performed, such that cells were cultured in either 5% FBS or 5% dPL. Cell counts were recorded at 7-day intervals, at which point MSCs were replated up to passage 11. We found that when all patient groups were analyzed together, the number of mean population doublings was increased in the dPL group at earlier passages, but by mid to late passage, the benefit of culturing cells in dPL had disappeared (**Figure 2**). When stratified according to disease state, cells cultured in dPL were non-inferior to cells cultured in FBS, and at early passage, cells cultured in dPL had increased number of population doublings across all groups. At early passage, there was also no difference when disease states were compared, suggesting that proliferative capacity of MSCs was preserved regardless of patient characteristics. From a practical standpoint, it should be noted that MSCs grown in dPL grew so rapidly at early passages that they quickly became confluent prior to subculturing, and thus proliferation was likely impaired by contact inhibition, so our experimental design may not have captured the full proliferative effect of dPL [40].

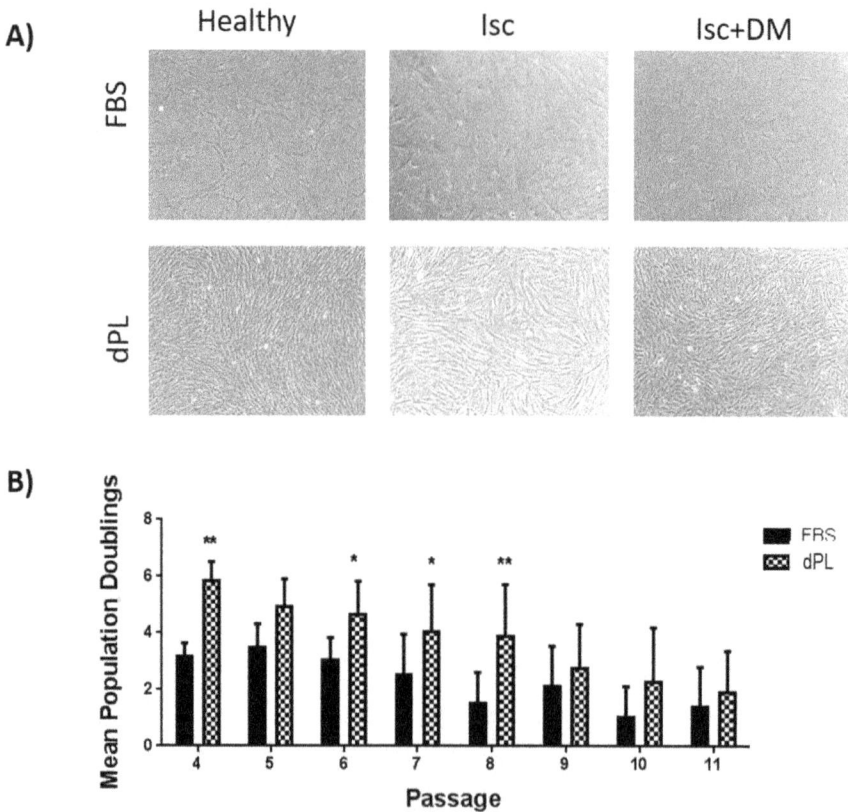

Figure 2. Cell culture with dPL leads to robust proliferation of human MSCs. In (A), MSCs from healthy controls are shown in comparison to MSCs isolated from the bone marrow of patients with CLI or CLI with concomitant diabetes mellitus. In (B), quantification of population doublings in MSCs across all patient groups was higher when grown in dPL than FBS at early passages, but by later passages, there was no difference between culture conditions. Reprinted from Brewster et al. [40] with permission from Elsevier.

We also characterized the functional capacity of MSCs across the different patient groups in vitro, in order to predict potential efficacy of MSCs for therapeutic angiogenesis in future human trials. A colony-forming unit (CFU) assay was performed on MSCs from each patient group. The number of CFUs in MSCS from patients with critical limb ischemia was similar to healthy control donors, suggesting that clonal capacity was independent of patient characteristics. A robust secretome analysis was also performed for all patient groups on MSCs that were cultured in either FBS or dPL. We specifically examined MSC production of bFGF, VEGF, HGF, and MCP-1. The secretome profiles were similar across all patient groups and culture conditions, with only minor differences noted. Furthermore, there were no obvious functional differences when conditioned media from the different treatment and patient groups were used to stimulate endothelial cell migration or proliferation. In order to assess the proangiogenic function of MSCs from patients with fibrinogen-rich platelet lysate (frPL), a coculture assay was used where MSCs from each patient mixed with a human endothelial cell line and embedded as cell pellets in 3D fibrin hydrogels. In this model the two cell types form sprouts which invade the fibrin hydrogel. Sprout length was quantified as a surrogate for angiogenic potential and was noted to be similar among all patient groups when MSCs were precultured in dPL. When MSCs were precultured in FBS, sprout length in the CLI group (without diabetes) was significantly lower than the CLI group with diabetes and the health controls. Despite any residual impairment within MSCs from patients with CLI that may result from epigenetic changes to the cells, the functional quality of MSCs from patients with CLI cultured with dPL appears to be equivalent of that healthy controls. These data support the use of dPL for expansion of MSCs and suggest that autologous cell therapy with MSCs for augmentation of neovascularization is a viable treatment strategy in patients with CLI.

Our study was the first in vitro testing of the proangiogenic characteristics of the bone marrow from amputated limbs in patients with CLI, but it is notably limited by the small sample size for each group. However, two important conclusions can be drawn from this study. First, we provide compelling data that, despite numerous reports that progenitor cell populations are impaired in patients with cardiovascular disease or associated risk factors, at least early-passage MSCs from patients with CLI are similar in quality to healthy controls when expanded ex vivo. Diabetes specifically has been shown to impair mesenchymal stem cell (MSC) function [41], at least partially due the effect of oxidative stress from Nox4 upregulation. Diabetes has also been shown to induce epigenetic changes in the promoter of IL-12 in bone marrow cells, such that cell fate is predisposed toward a pro-inflammatory phenotype. This raises the possibility that MSCs in patients with diabetes mellitus may have irreversible changes to the epigenetic signature. However, our study is consistent with other reports that demonstrate functional capacity of MSCs in patients with CLI is equivalent to healthy controls after short-term culture [42] and that ex vivo expansion in either FBS or PL may at least transiently overcome the epigenetic changes induced by patient comorbidities.

2.2. Platelet lysate as a scaffold for MSC delivery

2.2.1. Generation of fibrinogen-rich platelet lysate

Poor cell retention and viability at targeted sites of delivery have impaired advancement of cell therapies, as the number of functioning cells in the desired tissue appears to be critical for therapeutic efficacy [31, 43, 44]. Numerous biologic materials have been developed to promote cell retention and viability including encapsulation with alginate [45, 46], prefabrication of a tissue engineered patch [47, 48], and seeding of elongated fibrin strands [49]. While these approaches demonstrate that scaffold-mediated cell delivery improves the functional impact of cell therapy, the scaffold designs fail to incorporate any nutritive support for MSCs. In contrast to the fibrinogen-depleted form of platelet lysate used as a cell culture supplement for MSC growth, modifying the production process to retain clotting factors within platelet lysate (fibrinogen-rich platelet lysate or frPL) permits thrombin-induced self-assembly of a hydrogel with incorporated growth factors.

In order to generate platelet lysate that can spontaneously polymerize into 3D hydrogels, we modified the production process of dPL to maximize fibrinogen content of the platelet lysate. This was achieved by eliminating the step in which fibrin clot is formed and extracted from the solution. Our protocol again involves obtaining human platelets from Emory University blood bank in collaboration with EPIC. The platelets are then pooled and exposed to two sequential freeze-thaw cycles [freezing at -80°C for 48 h, then rapidly thawing at 37°C for 8 h] followed by centrifugation at 1500×g for 10 min. The rapid thawing phase is essential to prevent the formation of cryoprecipitate, which will deplete the solution of soluble clotting factors. The supernatant is then collected and stored at -20°C until ready for use. For hydrogel formation, the frPL is rapidly thawed at 37°C immediately prior to use and then centrifuged at 10,000×g for 10 min in 1.5 mL microcentrifuge tubes and sequentially filtered through 0.45 and 0.2 μm syringe tip filters.

Using this processing technique, we generated frPL with a fibrinogen concentration of 450 μg/mL which rapidly self-assembled into a 3D hydrogel with the addition of thrombin [50]. The hydrogel production process was refined for optimal durability and seeding with MSCs. For most applications, a 50% frPL hydrogel has preferential mechanical properties and provides appropriate MSC support. For hydrogel formation, an activating solution is prepared containing αMEM media with calcium chloride and thrombin so that the final concentrations are 5 mM and 2 U/mL, respectively, in a 50% PL gel. MSCs are then added to the activating solution at the desired cell density. The complete activating solution is then quickly mixed in a 1:1 ratio with frPL and cast in a cell culture plate and stored at 37°C for 1 h.

2.2.2. Structural composition of frPL

Microstructural analysis of [50] frPL indicates that fibrin is an essential component of frPL hydrogels. To evaluate the contribution to the frPL scaffold, frPL hydrogels and fibrin controls were loaded with 5% fluorescein isothiocyanate (FITC)-labeled fibrinogen and imaged with confocal microscopy to visualize the fibrin microstructure. The resulting images reveal an organized fibrin network within the frPL hydrogels that is more dense than control fibrin hydrogels but lacks clear elongated fibers (**Figure** 3). Additional imaging with scanning electron microscopy shows that the morphology of the frPL consists of thin, highly interconnected branched networks that are distinct from the fibrin hydrogels, which formed more distinct elongated fibrils (**Figure** 3) [50]. This was surprising since the 50% frPL contained only 225 μg/mL of fibrinogen, compared to the 1 mg/mL concentration of the fibrin-only controls. The proteolytic activity of thrombin rapidly initiates the polymerization for liquid frPL into a 3D scaffold. The conversion of fibrinogen to fibrin clearly plays an important role in hydrogel formation, but other structural components are also likely. At present, it is unclear which specific proteins contribute to the mesh network visualized with microscopy, although we speculate that there are additional clotting factors and retained membrane and cytoskeletal elements from platelets that incorporate into the scaffold.

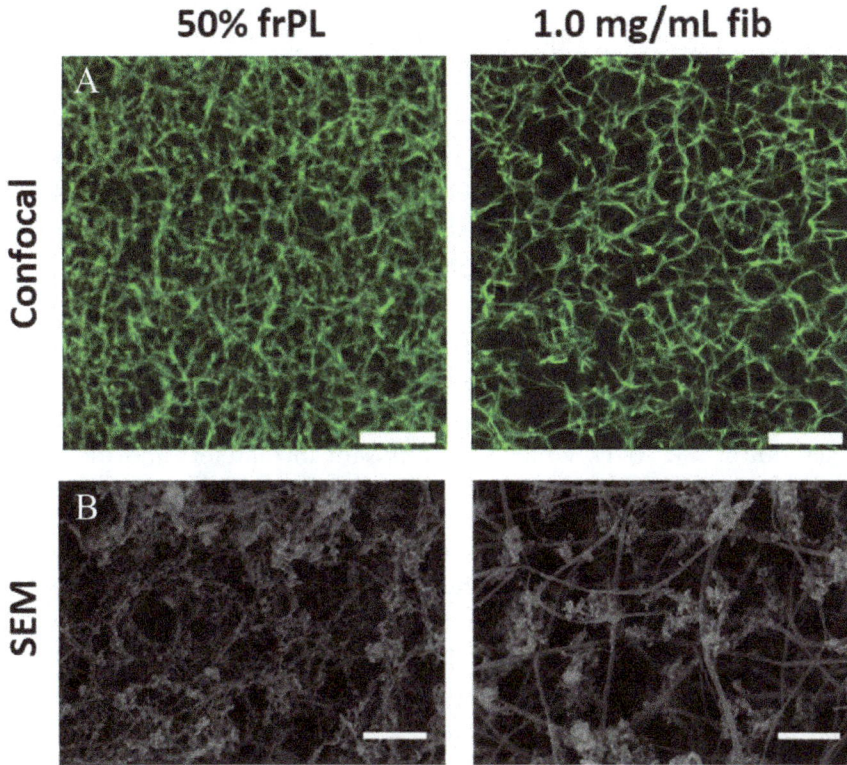

Figure 3. Microstructure of frPL and fibrin hydrogels is visualized in (A) with confocal microscopy after spiking with 5% FITC-labeled fibrinogen (scale bar equal to 20 μm) and (B) with scanning electron microscopy (SEM, scale bar equal to 1.0 μm). Reprinted from Robinson et al. [50], with permission from Elsevier.

The functional attributes of frPL hydrogels are also unique when compared to gels containing only fibrin. Mechanical testing on frPL revealed that these hydrogels behave as a viscoelastic solid with a storage and loss modulus equivalent to fibrin hydrogels with four times greater fibrin content [50]. The specific etiology of this property is unclear, but it may be the result of enhanced fibrin crosslinking due to the presence of additional components of the coagulation cascade, including Factor XIII. Additionally, numerous extracellular proteins (i.e., fibronectin, collagen), proteoglycans, and adhesion proteins such as Von Willebrand factor within the PL may reinforce the underlying fibrin network. Under experimental conditions, composite hydrogels containing additional elements such as collagen have improved mechanical strength over their homogenous control hydrogels without a change in total protein content [51, 52]. Therefore, the presence of these additional proteins may essentially act to form composite fibrin hydrogels with improved mechanical properties. The improved mechanical properties of frPL may also result from thrombin-induced polymerization of alternative macromolecules within the frPL that either alter fibrin binding sites or function as molecular crowders, thereby enhancing the viscoelastic behavior of the gel at relatively low fibrin concentrations [53, 54].

The microstructural differences between frPL and standard fibrin hydrogels extend beyond the microscopic appearance of the scaffold. Diffusion of FITC-labeled dextran molecules from 20 to 150 kDa that were embedded in hydrogels and diffusion of labeled dextran were significantly decreased. However, these differences between diffusion rates within hydrogels were due, at least in part, to the resistance of frPL hydrogels to proteolytic degradation [50]. This was supported by the fact that inclusion of aprotinin (a protease inhibitor) in culture media abrogated the differences between frPL and fibrin hydrogels. Additionally, frPL hydrogels containing 5% FITC-labeled fibrinogen retained labeled fibrin for up to 7 days, while fibrin-only gels rapidly degraded. Again, degradation rates were significantly decreased in fibrin gels with the addition of aprotinin, indicating that frPL is highly resistant to protease degradation compared to pure fibrin hydrogels [50]. Although the specific mechanism by which frPL hydrogels are stabilized has not been explored, it is likely due to the presence of serine protease inhibitors within frPL such as α2-antiplasmin or plasminogen activator inhibitor-1 (PAI-1), which are abundant in platelets and plasma and significantly impair fibrinolysis.

During hydrogel polymerization, the abundant growth factors present in soluble PL become entrapped within the frPL scaffold. We found that frPL hydrogels are enriched in PDGF-BB, which is released over 20 days in vitro, and ~45% of PDGF-BB persisted within the frPL gel at completion of that time course [50]. The retention of PDGF-BB in frPL hydrogels is superior to that seen in optimized formulations of fibrin-only hydrogels in vitro [55, 56], where greater than 90% of PDGF-BB is released after 7 days [57]. In addition to serving as a proangiogenic growth factor [58], PDGF-BB is also a critical mediator of MSC engraftment into tissue [59]; therefore, frPL can serve to both enhance engraftment of MSCs delivered within the scaffold and also exert a proangiogenic effect on native endothelial cells. The unique microstructure of frPL and resistance to degradation permit sustained release of these growth factors, such that the therapeutic window of MSCs embedded within the frPL scaffold is prolonged.

2.2.3. Impact of frPL on MSC function

The enriched milieu of growth factors and cytokines contained within frPL hydrogel has numerous beneficial effects on both MSCs and endothelial cells in vitro. Seeding of MSCs in frPL hydrogels leads to extensive proliferation of MSCs when quantified with MTS assay. In fact, cell number was higher in an frPL gel than fibrin-only gels when quantified over 7 days and also higher than in cells grown in a monolayer with dPL supplemented media. The frPL does not appear to have the same mitogenic effect on endothelial cells, as HUVECs grown in frPL hydrogels showed very little proliferative activity compared to controls [50].

The frPL hydrogel also has a significant impact on cell invasion. Sprout length from MSC/EC coculture pellets embedded in hydrogels was significantly longer than sprout length in fibrin controls (**Figure 4**) [50]. When MSCs or ECs alone were embedded in frPL, there was a notable difference in effect between the two different cell types. MSC sprouting appeared to be dependent on fibrin content, as sprout invasion was greater in low concentration fibrin hydrogels in addition to frPL. In contrast to its effect on MSCs, the frPL scaffold led to superior invasion of HUVECs compared to both high and low fibrin controls. Cells with the frPL scaffold receive both biochemical and biomechanical cues, which have a variable effect on different cell types. The frPL induces endothelial migration through biochemical signaling, but does not impact proliferation. On the other hand, growth factor signaling within the frPL causes substantial proliferation in MSCs, while the soft substrate of the scaffold provides mechanical cues to stimulate cell migration of MSCs. Based on this in vitro data, we can infer that frPL hydrogels embedded with MSCs have the ability to recruit remote endothelial cells, as demonstrated in the transwell migration assay. These data support the proposed clinical treatment strategy, whereby PL gel embedded with MSCs recruits host ECs for neovascularization following implantation in ischemic tissues.

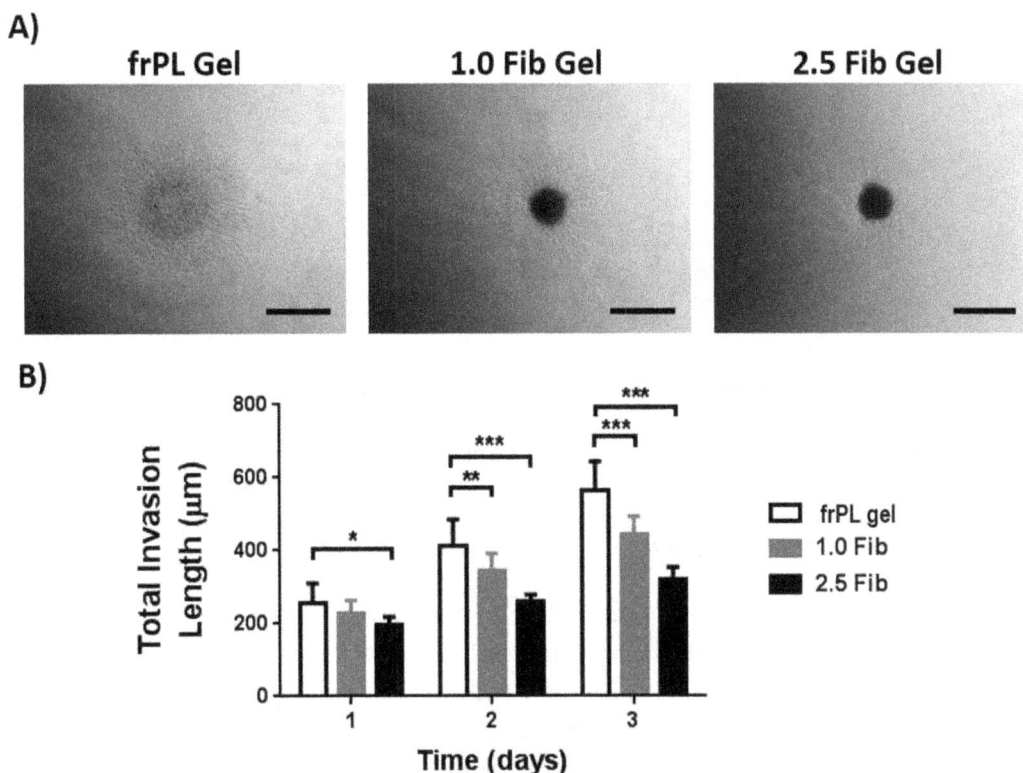

Figure 4. Cell sprouting of hydrogels. Human MSCs and HUVECs were mixed in a 1:1 ratio and embedded in frPL, 1.0 mg/mL fibrin, or 2.4 mg/mL fibrin hydrogels. Sprout length was assessed over 3 days in culture. Representative bright field images of each group at day 3 are shown in (A). Sprout length is quantified in (B). Reprinted from Robinson et al. [50], with permission from Elsevier.

Preliminary testing in a mouse model of hind limb ischemia supports this treatment strategy. Implantation of MSCs embedded in PL into ischemic limbs in a mouse model of HLI led to rapid neovascularization of ischemic tissues by 8 days when assessed with LDPI. Rapid and complete neovascularization of gastrocnemius muscle occurred in 8 days, which was increased significantly when compared to PL gel alone and MSCs alone (**Figure 5**) [50].

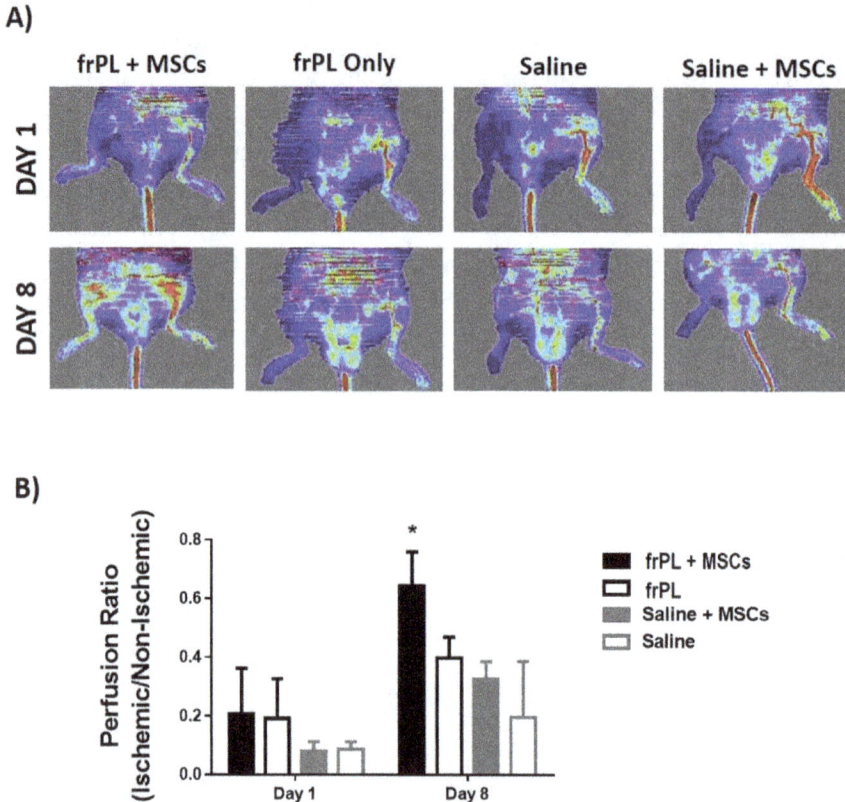

Figure 5. MSCs in saline or frPL were injected into the ischemic hind limb of mice, and perfusion with LDPI was assessed after 8 days. (A) Representative LDPI images are shown of the different groups. (B) Perfusion ratio of the ischemic to nonischemic limb is quantified for each group. Reprinted from Robinson et al. [50] with permission from Elsevier.

2.2.4. Encapsulation of MSCs with frPL

More recently, we have identified an additional novel application of frPL that results from its unique effect on MSCs. For most experiments hydrogels are cast in sterile, tissue culture treated polystyrene wells. In most cases the hydrogel will adhere to the walls and floor of the dish. However, when tissue culture plates are preincubated with a solution containing 2% albumin, hydrogels are no longer tethered to the plastic. When MSCs are embedded in fibrin gels, they exert a modest contractile effect on the scaffold that results in ~75% reduction in gel volume. However, when MSCs are embedded in an untethered frPL, hydrogel gel volume is reduced to 1–2% of the initial volume over 3 days (**Figure 6**). Cells were stained with CellTracker Red, and labeled fibrinogen was added to the frPL, and the reorganization of fibrin strands can clearly be seen with rounding of the cell bodies with loss of extending processes (**Figure 6**). Cell viability is preserved in cells encapsulated within frPL pellets. The pellets can be degraded and MSCs can be released with dispase treatment. Viability of MSCs within the frPL pellets is preserved for up to 3 days in vitro, as determined with a live/dead assay. The ability of frPL to form dense cell spheroids containing MSCs provides yet another practical application of platelet lysate. The frPL MSC spheroids could serve as an additional mechanism of cell delivery, by encapsulating MSCs in a thin fibrin shell.

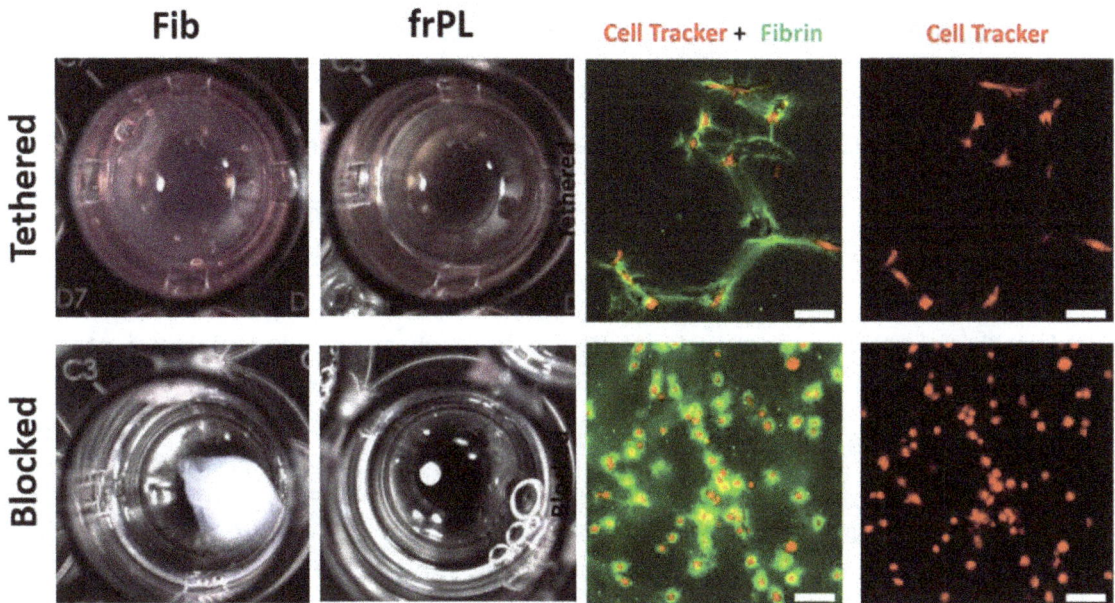

Figure 6. MSCs embedded in untethered frPL form cell spheroids. $2×10^5$ MSCs/mL were embedded in frPL or fibrin hydrogels in six well tissue culture dishes with (untethered) and without (tethered) preblocking the plate with 2% albumin solution. MSCs within the frPL formed dense spheroids. Hydrogels were labeled with 5% FITC-dextran and seeded with CellTracker Red-labeled MSCs in tethered and untethered culture conditions. Scale bars represent 20 μm (original figure).

3. Conclusion

Innovative strategies are needed for enhancing quality of MSCs in patients with CLI while also improving delivery and retention of MSCs for cell-based therapy. Here we discuss the dual use of human platelet lysate as both a cell culture supplement and a scaffold for cell delivery. When bereft of clotting factors, depleted form of platelet lysate (dPL) supplemented media enables rapid expansion of MSCs without diminishing their angiogenic activity. In contrast, with preservation of clotting factors, frPL forms a rapidly assembling hydrogel with desirable structural properties and biological activity on MSC and ECs. In both soluble and hydrogel form, PL augments the proangiogenic qualities of MSCs and is readily derived from human source materials that have been tested for safe delivery to patients. As a result of these unique traits, PL hydrogel is ideally suited to serve as a cell culture supplement for MSC growth and as a vector for delivery of MSCs to ischemic tissues.

Author details

Scott T. Robinson[1] and Luke P. Brewster[2, 3*]

*Address all correspondence to: lbrewst@emory.edu

1 Department of Surgery, University of Michigan School of Medicine, Ann Arbor, MI, USA

2 Department of Surgery, Emory University of Medicine, Atlanta, GA, USA

3 Atlanta VA Medical Center, Surgical and Research Services, Decatur, GA, USA

References

[1] Hirsch, A. T. et al. Peripheral arterial disease detection, awareness, and treatment in primary care. *JAMA* **286**, 1317–24 (2001).

[2] Norgren, L. et al. Inter-society consensus for the management of peripheral arterial disease (TASC II). *J. Vasc. Surg.* **45 Suppl S**, S5–67 (2007).

[3] Otteman, M. G. & Stahlgren, L. H. Evaluation of factors which influence mortality and morbidity following major lower extremity amputations for arteriosclerosis. *Surg. Gynecol. Obstet.* **120**, 1217–20 (1965).

[4] Asahara, T. et al. Isolation of putative progenitor endothelial cells for angiogenesis. *Science (80-.).* **275**, 964–966 (1997).

[5] Risau, W. Mechanisms of angiogenesis. *Nature* **386**, 671–4 (1997).

[6] Heil, M., Eitenmüller, I., Schmitz-Rixen, T. & Schaper, W. Arteriogenesis versus angiogenesis: similarities and differences. *J. Cell. Mol. Med.* **10**, 45–55 (2006).

[7] Asahara, T. et al. Bone marrow origin of endothelial progenitor cells responsible for postnatal vasculogenesis in physiological and pathological neovascularization. *Circ. Res.* **85**, 221 (1999).

[8] Takahashi, T. et al. Ischemia- and cytokine-induced mobilization of bone marrow-derived endothelial progenitor cells for neovascularization. *Nat. Med.* **5**, 434–8 (1999).

[9] Shi, Q. et al. Evidence for circulating bone marrow-derived endothelial cells. *Blood* **92**, 362 (1998).

[10] Rajantie, I. et al. Adult bone marrow-derived cells recruited during angiogenesis comprise precursors for periendothelial vascular mural cells. *Blood* **104**, 2084 (2004).

[11] Ziegelhoeffer, T. *et al.* Bone marrow-derived cells do not incorporate into the adult growing vasculature. *Circ. Res.* **94**, 230–8 (2004).

[12] O'Neill, T. J., Wamhoff, B. R., Owens, G. K. & Skalak, T. C. Mobilization of bone marrow-derived cells enhances the angiogenic response to hypoxia without transdifferentiation into endothelial cells. *Circ. Res.* **97**, 1027–35 (2005).

[13] Purhonen, S. *et al.* Bone marrow-derived circulating endothelial precursors do not contribute to vascular endothelium and are not needed for tumor growth. *Proc. Natl. Acad. Sci.* **105**, 6620 (2008).

[14] Planat-Benard, V. *et al.* Plasticity of human adipose lineage cells toward endothelial cells: physiological and therapeutic perspectives. *Circulation* **109**, 656–63 (2004).

[15] Cho, S. W. *et al.* Improvement of postnatal neovascularization by human embryonic stem cell derived endothelial-like cell transplantation in a mouse model of hindlimb ischemia. *Circulation* **116**, 2409–19 (2007).

[16] Lian, Q. *et al.* Functional mesenchymal stem cells derived from human induced pluripotent stem cells attenuate limb ischemia in mice. *Circulation* **121**, 1113–23 (2010).

[17] Al-Khaldi, A., Al-Sabti, H., Galipeau, J. & Lachapelle, K. Therapeutic angiogenesis using autologous bone marrow stromal cells: improved blood flow in a chronic limb ischemia model. *Ann. Thorac. Surg.* **75**, 204–209 (2003).

[18] Gnecchi, M., Zhang, Z., Ni, A. & Dzau, V. J. Paracrine mechanisms in adult stem cell signaling and therapy. *Circ. Res.* **103**, 1204–19 (2008).

[19] Eliopoulos, N., Stagg, J., Lejeune, L., Pommey, S. & Galipeau, J. Allogeneic marrow stromal cells are immune rejected by MHC class I- and class II-mismatched recipient mice. *Blood* **106**, 4057–65 (2005).

[20] Nauta, A. J. *et al.* Donor-derived mesenchymal stem cells are immunogenic in an allogeneic host and stimulate donor graft rejection in a nonmyeloablative setting. *Blood* **108**, 2114–20 (2006).

[21] Kinnaird, T. *et al.* Local delivery of marrow-derived stromal cells augments collateral perfusion through paracrine mechanisms. *Circulation* **109**, 1543–9 (2004).

[22] Moon, M. H. *et al.* Human adipose tissue-derived mesenchymal stem cells improve postnatal neovascularization in a mouse model of hindlimb ischemia. *Cell. Physiol. Biochem.* **17**, 279–90 (2006).

[23] Heeschen, C. *et al.* Profoundly reduced neovascularization capacity of bone marrow mononuclear cells derived from patients with chronic ischemic heart disease. *Circulation* **109**, 1615–22 (2004).

[24] Ghani, U. *et al.* Endothelial progenitor cells during cerebrovascular disease. *Stroke.* **36**, 151–3 (2005).

[25] Loomans, C. J. M. *et al.* Endothelial progenitor cell dysfunction: a novel concept in the pathogenesis of vascular complications of type 1 diabetes. *Diabetes* **53**, 195–9 (2004).

[26] Pistrosch, F. *et al.* PPARgamma-agonist rosiglitazone increases number and migratory activity of cultured endothelial progenitor cells. *Atherosclerosis* **183**, 163–7 (2005).

[27] Tepper, O. M. Human endothelial progenitor cells from type II diabetics exhibit impaired proliferation, adhesion, and incorporation into vascular structures. *Circulation* **106**, 2781–2786 (2002).

[28] Kondo, T. *et al.* Smoking cessation rapidly increases circulating progenitor cells in peripheral blood in chronic smokers. *Arterioscler. Thromb. Vasc. Biol.* **24**, 1442–7 (2004).

[29] Fan, W. *et al.* Adipose stromal cells amplify angiogenic signaling via the VEGF/mTOR/ Akt pathway in a murine hindlimb ischemia model: a 3D multimodality imaging study. *PLoS One* **7**, e45621 (2012).

[30] van der Bogt, K. E. A. *et al.* Comparison of different adult stem cell types for treatment of myocardial ischemia. *Circulation* **118**, S121–9 (2008).

[31] Sheikh, A. Y. *et al.* In vivo functional and transcriptional profiling of bone marrow stem cells after transplantation into ischemic myocardium. *Arterioscler. Thromb. Vasc. Biol.* **32**, 92–102 (2012).

[32] Spees, J. L. *et al.* Internalized antigens must be removed to prepare hypoimmunogenic mesenchymal stem cells for cell and gene therapy. *Mol. Ther.* **9**, 747–56 (2004).

[33] Sporn, M. B. & Roberts, A. B. Transforming growth factor-beta. Multiple actions and potential clinical applications. *JAMA* **262**, 938–41 (1989).

[34] Ross, R., Bowen-Pope, D. F. & Raines, E. W. Platelet-derived growth factor and its role in health and disease. *Philos. Trans. R. Soc. Lond. B. Biol. Sci.* **327**, 155–69 (1990).

[35] Bieback, K. *et al.* Human alternatives to fetal bovine serum for the expansion of mesenchymal stromal cells from bone marrow. *Stem Cells* **27**, 2331–41 (2009).

[36] Schallmoser, K. *et al.* Human platelet lysate can replace fetal bovine serum for clinical-scale expansion of functional mesenchymal stromal cells. *Transfusion* **47**, 1436–46 (2007).

[37] Copland, I. B., Garcia, M. A., Waller, E. K., Roback, J. D. & Galipeau, J. The effect of platelet lysate fibrinogen on the functionality of MSCs in immunotherapy. *Biomaterials* **34**, 7840–50 (2013).

[38] François, M., Romieu-Mourez, R., Li, M. & Galipeau, J. Human MSC suppression correlates with cytokine induction of indoleamine 2,3-dioxygenase and bystander M2 macrophage differentiation. *Mol. Ther.* **20**, 187–95 (2012).

[39] Griffiths, S., Baraniak, P. R., Copland, I. B., Nerem, R. M. & McDevitt, T. C. Human platelet lysate stimulates high-passage and senescent human multipotent mesenchymal stromal cell growth and rejuvenation in vitro. *Cytotherapy* **15**, 1469–83 (2013).

[40] Brewster, L. L. *et al.* Expansion and angiogenic potential of mesenchymal stem cells from patients with critical limb ischemia. *J. Vasc. Surg.* 2016 Feb 24. pii: S0741-5214(16)00222-6. doi: 10.1016/j.jvs.2015.02.061. [Epub ahead of print] PMID:26921003.

[41] Yan, J. *et al.* Type 2 diabetes restricts multipotency of mesenchymal stem cells and impairs their capacity to augment postischemic neovascularization in db/db mice. *J. Am. Heart Assoc.* **1**, e002238 (2012).

[42] Gremmels, H. *et al.* Neovascularization capacity of mesenchymal stromal cells from critical limb ischemia patients is equivalent to healthy controls. *Mol. Ther.* **22**, 1960–70 (2014).

[43] Swijnenburg, R. J. J. *et al.* Timing of bone marrow cell delivery has minimal effects on cell viability and cardiac recovery after myocardial infarction. *Circ. Cardiovasc. Imaging* **3**, 77–85 (2010).

[44] Hong, K. U. *et al.* C-Kit+ cardiac stem cells alleviate post-myocardial infarction left ventricular dysfunction despite poor engraftment and negligible retention in the recipient heart. *PLoS One* **9**, 1–7 (2014).

[45] Landázuri, N. & Levit, R. Alginate microencapsulation of human mesenchymal stem cells as a strategy to enhance paracrine-mediated vascular recovery after hindlimb ischaemia. *J Tissue Eng Regen Med.* 2016 Mar; 10(3):222–32. doi: 10.1002/term.1680. Epub 2012 Dec 21.

[46] Levit, R. D. *et al.* Cellular encapsulation enhances cardiac repair. *J. Am. Heart Assoc.* **2**, e000367 (2013).

[47] Simpson, D. L., Boyd, N. L., Kaushal, S., Stice, S. L. & Dudley, S. C. Use of human embryonic stem cell derived-mesenchymal cells for cardiac repair. *Biotechnol. Bioeng.* **109**, 274–83 (2012).

[48] Wei, H. J. *et al.* Bioengineered cardiac patch constructed from multilayered mesenchymal stem cells for myocardial repair. *Biomaterials* **29**, 3547–3556 (2008).

[49] Guyette, J. P. *et al.* A novel suture-based method for efficient transplantation of stem cells. *J. Biomed. Mater. Res.–Part A* **101 A**, 809–818 (2013).

[50] Robinson, S. T. *et al.* A novel platelet lysate hydrogel for endothelial cell and mesenchymal stem cell-directed neovascularization. *Acta Biomater.* **36**, 86–98 (2016).

[51] Rowe, S. L. & Stegemann, J. P. Microstructure and mechanics of collagen-fibrin matrices polymerized using ancrod snake venom enzyme. *J. Biomech. Eng.* **131**, 61012 (2009).

[52] Rowe, S. L. & Stegemann, J. P. Interpenetrating collagen-fibrin composite matrices with varying protein contents and ratios. *Biomacromolecules* **7**, 2942–8 (2006).

[53] Stabenfeldt, S. E., Gourley, M., Krishnan, L., Hoying, J. B. & Barker, T. H. Engineering fibrin polymers through engagement of alternative polymerization mechanisms. *Biomaterials* **33**, 535–44 (2012).

[54] Barker, T. H., Fuller, G. M., Klinger, M. M., Feldman, D. S. & Hagood, J. S. Modification of fibrinogen with poly(ethylene glycol) and its effects on fibrin clot characteristics. *J. Biomed. Mater. Res.* **56**, 529–35 (2001).

[55] Thomopoulos, S. & Zaegel, M. PDGF-BB released in tendon repair using a novel delivery system promotes cell proliferation and collagen remodeling. *J Orthopaedic Res.* 1358–1368 (2007). doi:10.1002/jor

[56] Sakiyama-Elbert, S. & Das, R. Controlled-release kinetics and biologic activity of platelet-derived growth factor-BB for use in flexor tendon repair. *J Hand Sur.* **33**, 1548–1557 (2008).

[57] Greisler, H. P. *et al.* Enhanced endothelialization of expanded polytetrafluoroethylene grafts by fibroblast growth factor type 1 pretreatment. *Surgery* **112**, 244-54–5 (1992).

[58] B-receptors, P. *et al.* PDGF-BB modulates endothelial proliferation and angiogenesis in vitro. **125**, 917–928 (1994).

[59] Lin, R.-Z. *et al.* Human endothelial colony-forming cells serve as trophic mediators for mesenchymal stem cell engraftment via paracrine signaling. *Proc. Natl. Acad. Sci. U. S. A.* **111**, 10137–42 (2014).

6

Corneal Angiogenesis: Etiologies, Complications, and Management

Sepehr Feizi

Abstract

A large subset of corneal pathologies involves the formation of new blood vessels, leading to compromised visual acuity. Additionally, neovascularization of the cornea worsens the prognosis of subsequent penetrating keratoplasty, keeping the patient in a vicious circle of poor prognosis. Ocular angiogenesis results from the upregulation of proangiogenic and downregulation of antiangiogenic factors. There is a tremendous need for developing effective measures to prevent and/or treat corneal neovascularization. Topical steroid medication, cautery, argon and yellow dye laser, and fine needle diathermy have all been advocated with varying degrees of success. The process of corneal neovascularization is primarily mediated by the vascular endothelial growth factor family of proteins, and current therapies are aimed at disrupting the various steps in this pathway. This article aims to review the clinical causes and presentations of corneal neovascularization caused by different etiologies. Moreover, this chapter reviews different complications caused by corneal neovascularization and summarizes the most relevant treatments available so far.

Keywords: cornea, angiogenesis, etiologies, complications, management

1. Introduction

A normal cornea is necessary to protect the eye against structural damage to the deeper ocular components as well as to provide a proper anterior refractive surface. Optimal vision and corneal clarity entail an avascular cornea, and maintaining the stromal avascularity is an important feature of the corneal pathophysiology. Corneal vascularization, which is a sign of corneal disease processes than a diagnosis, results from an imbalance between angiogenic and antiangiogenic factors [1]. The angiogenic factors stimulate the proliferation and migration of vascular endothelial cells, resulting in the formation of a capillary tube [2, 3]. Corneal neovascularization is part of the natural healing processes, which are triggered by exposure of the cornea to trauma or pathogens, and is not necessarily 'harmful.' In the long-term and under certain circumstances, however, corneal neovascularization can surpass a threshold, invading the cornea, reducing visual acuity, and, in case of lamellar keratoplasty or penetrating kerato-plasty, endangering corneal graft survival [4–7]. These complications have prompted clinicians to devise means to shut vessels. Topical steroid medication, cautery, argon and yellow dye laser, and fine needle diathermy (FND) have all been advocated with varying degrees of success. The advent of anti-vascular endothelial growth factor (VEGF) antibodies has resulted in a surge of interest in using these agents to treat corneal neovascularization. These approaches, however, have a limited clinical efficacy and can result in a multitude of undesirable complications. This chapter aims to review the causes, pathogenesis, and clinical presentations of corneal neovascu-larization caused by different etiologies, such as contact lens–induced keratitis, corneal ulcers, and herpes simplex stromal keratitis. Moreover, it reviews different complications caused by corneal neovascularization and summarizes the most relevant treatments available so far.

2. Etiologies

Corneal vascularization occurs as a nonspecific response to different clinical insults. Diseases associated with corneal neovascularization include corneal graft rejection, inflammatory dis-orders, chemical burns, contact lens–related hypoxia, stromal ulceration, infectious keratitis, limbal stem cell deficiency, and congenital disease (**Table 1**) [8–10].

Categories	Cause
Infectious keratitis	Parasitic
	Viral
	Bacterial
	Fungal
Hypoxia	Contact lens wearing
Conjunctival/corneal degeneration	Pterygium
Inflammatory disorder	Stevens-Johnson syndrome
	Mucous membrane pemphigoid
	Corneal graft rejection
	Rosacea
	Atopic conjunctivitis
Ocular surface neoplasia	Conjunctival or corneal intraepithelial neoplasia
	Conjunctival or corneal squamous cell carcinoma
	Papilloma
Loss of limbal barrier function	Congenital (e.g., aniridia)
	Thermal burn, chemical burn, or other injury

Table 1. Causes of corneal neovascularization.

Hypoxia related to contact lens wear is a common cause where corneal neovascularization is usually superficial and involves only the corneal periphery [11, 12]. However, if contact lens wear is not discontinued, deep stromal and central corneal invasion can take place.

Infections can result in corneal neovascularization with the patterns of response being different. Herpes simplex virus (HSV) keratitis is likely to cause extensive vascularization and lipid keratopathy, while, in Acanthamoeba keratitis, vascularization tends to develop late in the course of the disease (**Figure 1**). The continued presence of HSV-DNA and HSV-immune complexes

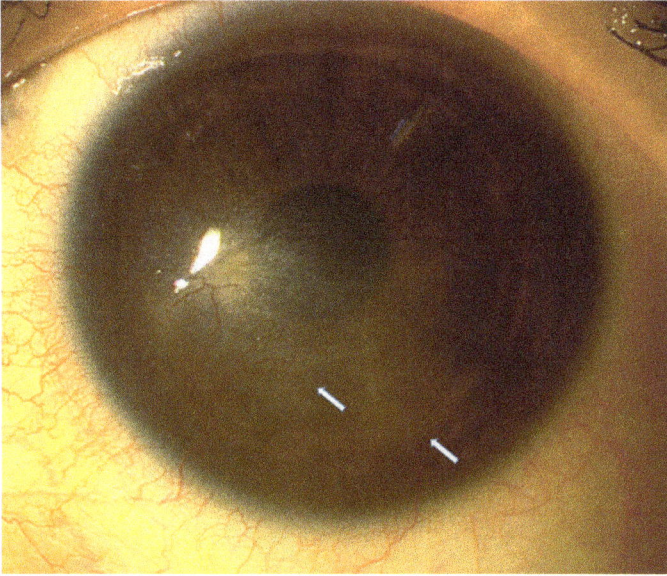

Figure 1. Acanthamoeba keratitis. Corneal opacity and vascularization (arrows) developed four months after corneal ulcer caused by Acanthamoeba in a contact lens wearer.

contributes to inflammation and angiogenesis in HSV stromal keratitis through increased levels of matrix metalloproteinase (MMP)-9 and vascular endothelial growth factor (VEGF) [13, 14]. There is a close link between extent (i.e., superficial or stromal) and location (i.e., central or peripheral) of infections, and the location and extent of corneal neovascularization.

Limbal stem cell deficiency (LSCD) occurs in a variety of ocular pathologies both congenital (e.g., aniridia) and acquired (e.g., contact lens use, drugs, chemical burns, etc.), which lead to partial or total loss of limbal stem cells [15, 16]. Chemical (acidic and alkaline) substances can penetrate and damage the cornea and anterior chamber, with alkali burns being more severe [17]. Conjunctivalization of the cornea with massive neovascularization may develop, leading to severe reductions in corneal clarity and visual acuity through the pannus formation on the cornea and an unstable and irregular epithelium [17, 18]. Deep vascularization may develop in the late healing phase following severe chemical burns (**Figure 2**).

Degenerative conditions such as pterygium are associated with corneal neovascularization that usually is accompanied with a fibrovascular pannus located on, rather than in, the corneal stroma. Long-standing irritation of the ocular surface such as in vernal keratoconjunctivitis can lead to aggressive corneal neovascularization (**Figure 3**).

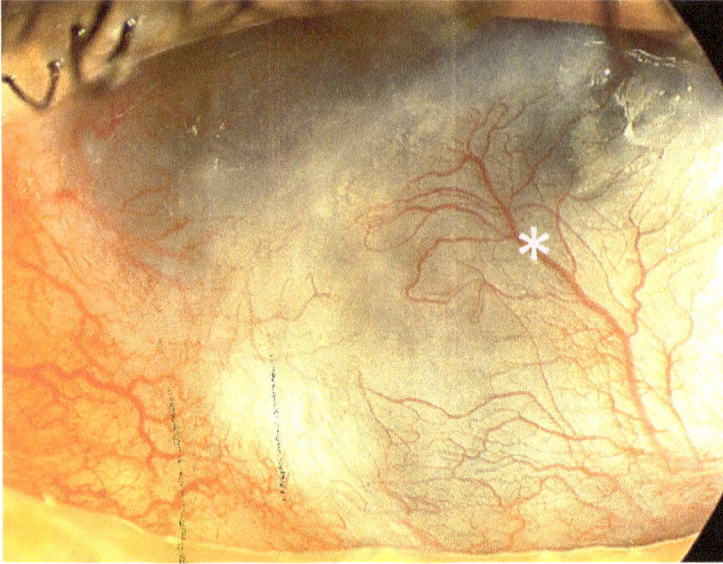

Figure 2. Limbal stem cell deficiency after alkali burn. The Figure demonstrates invasion of conjunctival vessels into the cornea (conjunctivalization) along with corneal stromal opacification and vascularization (asterisk).

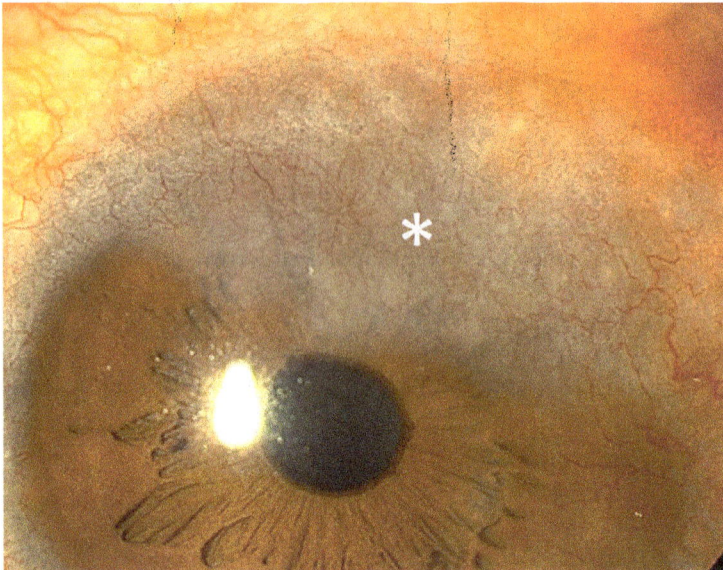

Figure 3. Corneal vascularization (asterisk) in a patient with vernal keratoconjunctivitis.

Ocular surface neoplasia, including papilloma and conjunctival/corneal intraepithelial neoplasia, can cause corneal neovascularization as part of the tumor angiogenic response. Initially, the vessels can be limited to the tumor but eventually invade the entire cornea. Other specific etiologies of corneal neovascularization include persistent corneal edema as in chronic hydrops of keratoconus and bullous keratopathy as well as corneal allograft rejection. Less common causes of corneal neovascularization are corneal foreign bodies and exposure to chemical toxins including mustard gas, radiation, or sun [19–21]. Intrastromal corneal ring implants, loose sutures, suture knots, and broken sutures seem to provide a stimulus for corneal vascularization

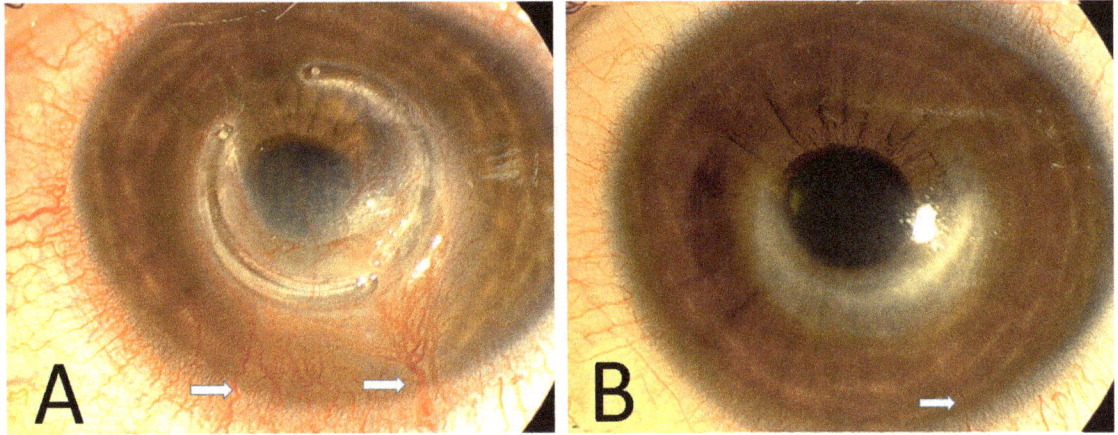

Figure 4. Intrastromal corneal ring segment implants complicated by corneal neovascularization. (A) Active young vessels (arrows) emanating from the limbus invade to the site of segment implantation. (B) The vessels have regressed after intrastromal corneal ring segment implants were removed. Partially regressed vessels are present in the inferior cornea (arrow).

(**Figure 4**). The mucus that collects around loose and broken sutures can trap polymorphonuclear cells and microbes inciting localized inflammation/infection, thus attracting vessels.

3. Pathogenesis

The upstream molecular pathway mechanisms resulting in corneal neovascularization differ in the different underlying pathologies. Nonetheless, core molecular pathways governing the processes of corneal hemangiogenesis seem to be shared among various conditions leading to the active stage of corneal neovascularization. The normally avascular cornea may vascularize in circumstances in which a disequilibrium between angiogenic and antiangiogenic stimuli results in a surplus of proangiogenic factors, such as VEGF, basic fibroblast growth factor (bFGF), interleukin-1 (IL-1), and MMP, and a deficiency in antiangiogenic agents, such as endostatin, angiostatin, and pigment epithelium-derived factor (PEDF) [22].

The so-called VEGF family consists of VEGF-A, VEGF-B, VEGF-C, VEGF-D, and placental growth factor [23]. VEGF-A is the most important member of this family, especially relating to pathologic hemangiogenesis through VEGF receptor (VEGFR)-2. VEGF-C and VEGF-D can stimulate lymphangiogenesis through VEGFR-2 and VEGFR-3, respectively [24, 25]. Macrophages, activated by injury or inflammation, can also produce VEGF-A, VEGF-C, and VEGF-D in corneal stroma [26]. VEGF-A sustains various steps of hemangiogenesis including vascular endothelial cell proliferation and migration, capillary lumen formation, and proteolytic activity [1]. The importance of VEGF-A in corneal neovascularization was exhibited experimentally on animal studies by inhibiting angiogenesis following stromal application of an anti-VEGF-A antibody [27].

Platelet-derived growth factors (PDGFs) are involved in cell division, growth, tissue remodeling, and angiogenesis. Receptors, such as PDGFR-a and PDGFR-b, and ligands, such as PDGF-A and PDGF-B, can be found in cornea and are associated with corneal neovascularization [28, 29]. Improved understanding of the molecular mechanisms of vascularization has enabled identification of specific factors that suppress angiogenesis to maintain the avascularity of the cornea. Because several molecules are involved in corneal neovascularization, a multipronged approach is desirable.

4. Clinical presentations

Corneal neovascularization which arises from the limbus, conjunctiva, and iris can lead to a reduction in the clarity of the cornea and visual acuity because of edema, scarring, intracorneal lipid and protein deposition, and persistent inflammation. Additionally, there is a robust association between the presence of corneal neovascularization and corneal graft rejection with the risk increasing as more quadrants are affected by vessels (**Figure 5**) [4–7]. The presence of corneal neovascularization can also cause intraoperative bleeding, which can be associated with hyphema.

Abnormal vessels may invade the cornea at different planes depending on the location and nature of the inflammatory stimulus. Corneal neovascularization has three clinical patterns, based on the depth of involvement. The first type, superficial vascularization, results from ocular surface disease (**Figure 6**). The second type is stromal vessels, which results from alkaline injury or stromal keratitis (**Figure 7**). The third is deep vessels overlying Descemet's membrane, which can be associated with interstitial keratitis or HSV keratitis, or after deep anterior lamellar keratoplasty (**Figure 8**) [1, 8, 9, 22]. Mixed patterns are often observed clini-

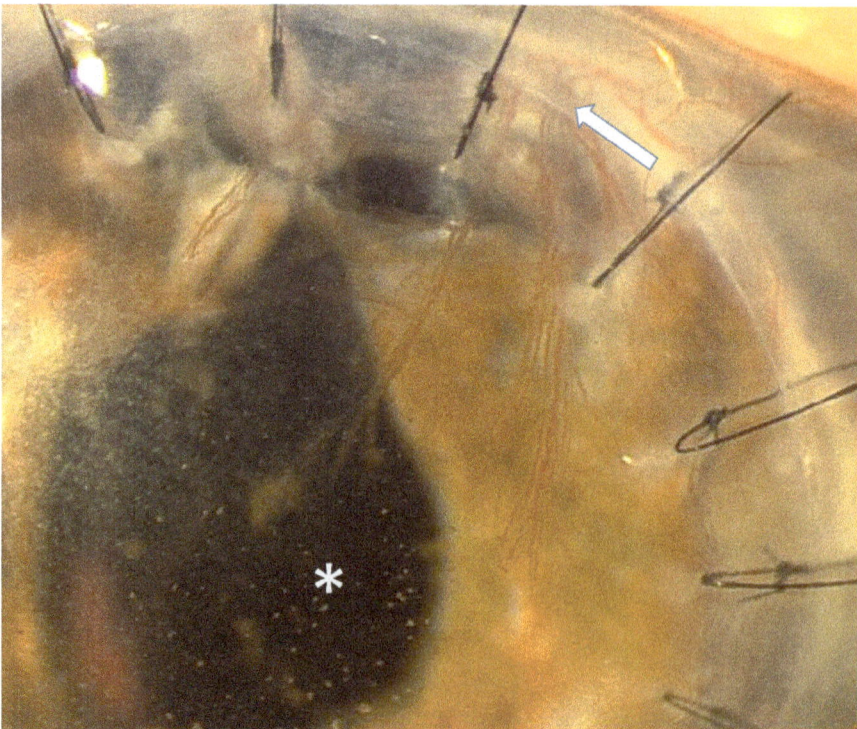

Figure 5. Endothelial corneal graft rejection in a high-risk graft. Active old corneal vessels (arrow) arising from the limbus sharply dip into a deep suture track and continue to the graft in an eye that underwent penetrating keratoplasty. The presence of keratic precipitates (asterisk) indicates an episode of endothelial graft rejection.

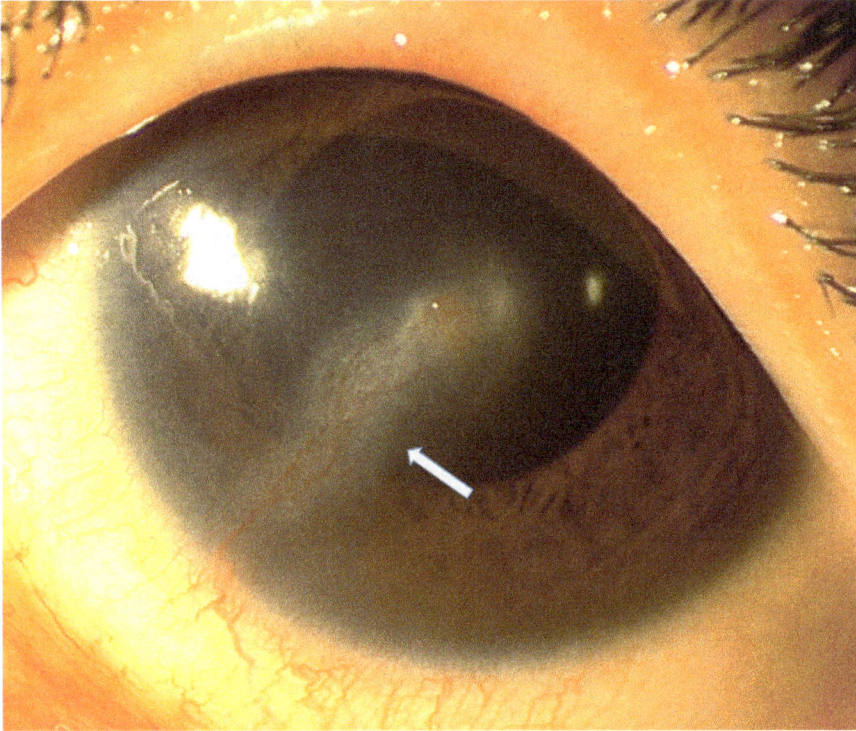

Figure 6. Phlyctenular keratitis. Superficial corneal vascularization (arrow) is evident in an eye with severe blepharitis. Adjacent stroma shows edema and infiltration.

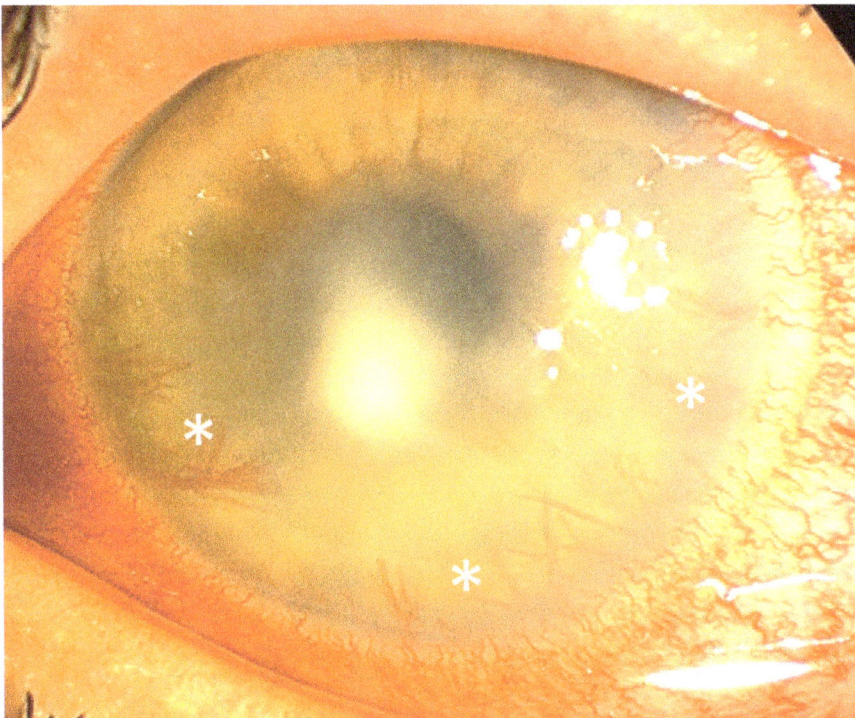

Figure 7. Deep stromal vascularization in an eye with recurrent herpes simplex stromal keratitis. Active young, bright red, brush-like vessels (asterisks) invade in to the corneal stroma.

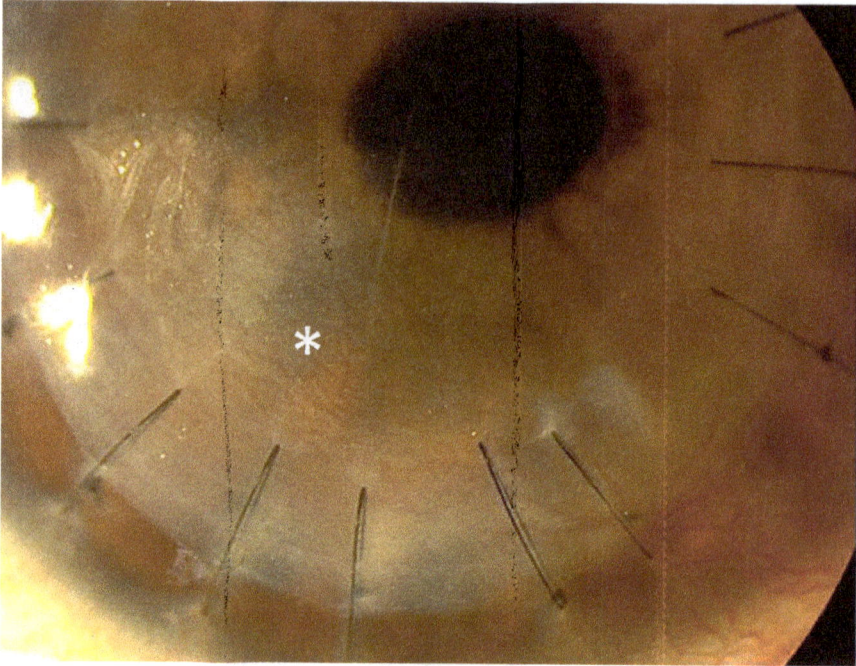

Figure 8. Partially regressed vessels with lipid keratopathy (asterisk) at the donor-recipient interface in a patient who underwent deep anterior lamellar keratoplasty (DALK). Vessels arising from the limbus sharply dip into a deep suture track and continue to the deep lamellar plane created by the DALK procedure, before fanning out. The vessels are dull red with a slow circulation, and some parts of the complex are less visible or have undergone attrition.

cally. The level of vascularization is chiefly related to the level of pathology rather than to the etiology. Superficial corneal pathology results in superficial vascularization, and deep pathology results in deep vessels. Often when the disease process extends through the thickness of the cornea, superficial and deep vessels are seen in the same cornea.

A detailed clinical evaluation of corneal neovascularization, including extension (the number of quadrants involved) and depth, is crucial for treatment planning. In addition to the extent and level of corneal vascularization, the state of vessel activity is also important [30]. Clinically, corneal vascularization can be classified as active young, active old, mature, partially regressed, and regressed. This often corresponds with the stage of activity or chronicity of the disease. Active young vessels are freshly formed vessels that are full of blood, appear bright red in color, have minimal surrounding fibrous tissue sheathing, and are actively progressing in the cornea with a well-defined arborizing network of fine (capillary) vessels (**Figures 4A** and **7**). The corneal stroma surrounding the vessels shows signs of leakage and edema. Active old vessels appear less bright and maintain a brisk circulation (**Figure 5**). This represents the stage when the vessels have reached and surrounded or covered the offending lesion in the cornea. Their progression ceases but consolidation continues. Mature vessels are relatively large vessels, with minimal arborization and regressed or absent capillary networks, seen to persist in scar tissue or in the corneal stroma after the corneal pathology has healed. These vessels contain blood and maintain a circulation (**Figure 9**). Partially regressed vessels are seen when the corneal pathology has abated in response to therapy or the arrival

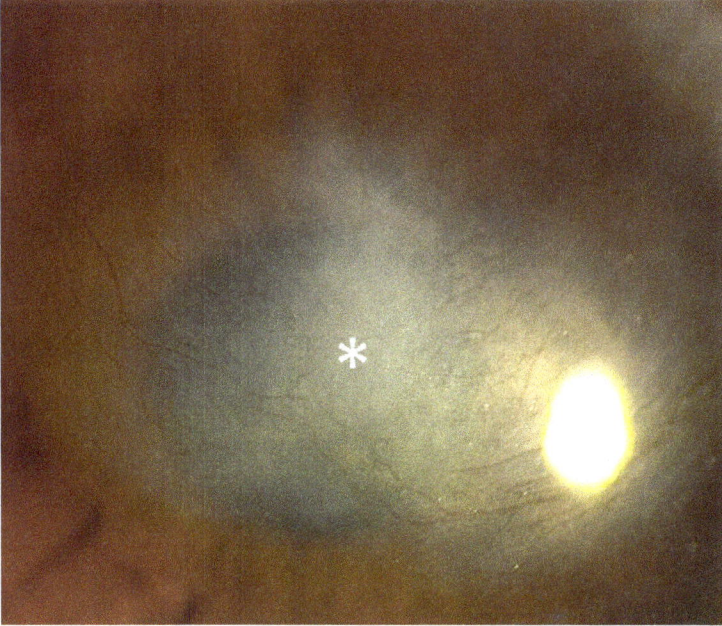

Figure 9. Mature vessels in the corneal stroma after the improvement of corneal ulcer (asterisk). The vessels are relatively large, with minimal arborization and regressed or absent capillary networks. These vessels which persist in scar tissue contain blood and maintain a circulation.

of corneal vessels. The circulation in the vascular complex is relatively slow, the vessels are less engorged, and some parts of the complex have become less visible or undergo attrition (**Figures 4B** and **8**). Regressed (ghost) vessels present as fine white lines mirroring the morphology of the original vessels. These do not have an active circulation, and the cornea where they are located is not edematous. Although clinically undetectable, lymphangiogenesis almost always accompanies hemangiogenesis in the cornea [31].

5. Paraclinical evaluation of corneal vascularization

Accurate evaluation and documentation of corneal neovascularization are essential to monitor the effect of any treatment modality employed. Case note entries can be used to assess the extent of corneal vascularization, and the depth of penetration and the centripetal progression of vessels, which allows a semiquantitative measurement of corneal neovascularization. It is neither time efficient nor practical, however, to manually trace the corneal vessels in each follow-up examination. Furthermore, the reproducibility is questionable, and the opportunity for variability and human error is very high.

The need to measure corneal neovascularization motivated researchers to explore measurement tools. An ideal measurement tool should allow rapid, reproducible, accurate, and objective measurement of corneal neovascularization. Digitized photographs with good contrast can be analyzed, based on the grayscale values, to evaluate the progression of vascularization [32]. Corneal vessels can be quantified on the basis of contrast enhancement, density threshold identification for the blood vessels, and pixel measurement [33]. A more novel automatic approach on the basis of gray filter sampling and threshold analyses of digital photographs using an image analysis software has also been investigated [34, 35]. Despite the recent progress in the graphic editing software, automated methods have some limitations. First, the optimization and validation of any automated quantitative tool are questionable [36–38]. Second, it does not allow sufficient appreciation of details on vessel extent, localization, leakage, origin, and differentiation of the afferent and efferent systems. This information is of importance for guidance of clinical judgment and treatment [39].

Corneal angiography, using fluorescein and indocyanine green, provides excellent details of the neovascular complexes, thus enabling an enhanced clinical assessment and decision-making even in patients with complex corneal neovascularization [39]. The required technological equipment for corneal angiography is readily available in most ophthalmologic centers, as angiography is widely used to diagnose vascular disorders of the retina of various origin. It is a relatively inexpensive and safe diagnostic intervention, and serious adverse events like anaphylaxis to the intravenous dye are extremely rare [40, 41].

Fluorescein angiography gives an indication of the vessel maturity and leakage activity, whereas indocyanine green angiography allows better depiction of capillaries and deeper corneal neovascularization, particularly in the presence of vessel obscuration because of corneal haze and scarring [39]. It is possible to calculate the area of corneal neovascularization, the time to first detection of fluorescein dye leakage, corneal neovascular vessel diameter, and vascular tortuosity and activity. These parameters reliably quantify changes in corneal neovascularization over time [39]. Therefore, it allows monitoring of the natural course and treatment success [42].

6. Treatments

The treatment for corneal neovascularization aims at the occlusion of afferent corneal blood vessels to reduce exudative lipid keratopathy, and stromal edema and inflammation or as a preoperative conditioning intervention before keratoplasty to increase chances of graft survival [17, 43]. Current treatments for corneal neovascularization consist of topical nonsteroid anti-inflammatory and corticosteroid medications [44], photodynamic therapy [45], laser photocoagulation [46, 47], fine needle diathermy [48], and limbal, conjunctival, and amniotic membrane transplantation (AMT) [49]. More recently, manipulation of VEGF activity and manipulation of proangiogenic mediators like interleukin have been under investigation [50,51]. Unfortunately, all of these approaches have a limited clinical efficacy, especially when the vessels are large because large vessels are difficult to occlude and easily recanalized. In addition, a multitude of undesirable side effects can occur after the treatment of corneal neovascularization. The following section reviews the available treatment approaches for corneal neovascularization and their limitations.

6.1. Corticosteroid therapy

Inflammation is a potent driver for corneal neovascularization. When inflammation settles, spontaneous regression of corneal neovascularization can occur and lead to gradual resolution of lipid keratopathy if present. Topical and periocular steroids have been popular and can effectively reduce inflammation and consequently corneal neovascularization in various disease conditions. However, the risks of superinfection, glaucoma, and cataract associated with the long-term use of corticosteroids have been a limiting factor [44]. Additionally, steroids have only limited antiangiogenic effects [52]. Cyclosporine A and nonsteroidal anti-inflammatory agents were reported to be largely ineffective in controlling or limiting corneal angiogenesis [53].

6.2. Laser photocoagulation

Photocoagulation of vessels has been shown to be an effective method to obliterate corneal vascularization [46, 47]. The argon laser [46] and the 577 nm yellow dye lasers [47] have been used effectively for treating vascularization in lipid keratopathy and graft rejection. Laser obliteration of corneal efferent vessels is comparatively easy as they are wider and have a relatively slower blood flow. Conversely, the afferent vessels are narrower and deeper, have a rapid blood flow, and are more difficult to obliterate. Consequently, reopening of the afferent vessels takes place in a high proportion of patients. In such cases, the procedure can be repeated more than once. Laser photocoagulation may not be effective in cases with extensive corneal neovascularization [46]. Other drawbacks include damage to iris and accidental suture lysis, which has a significant implication for grafts with running sutures. Furthermore, the expense of this equipment and the lack of availability in most centers make the treatment inaccessible to most surgeons.

6.3. Fine needle diathermy

Fine needle diathermy (FND) is an inexpensive and useful procedure that can serve as an adjunct or alternative to laser photocoagulation for the management of established corneal vessels. FND is simple and inexpensive and can be performed under topical anesthesia by any ophthalmologist. It can be applied at any depth to obliterate both afferent and efferent vessels with equal efficacy. However, it may have to be repeated to obtain the desired result [48]. Corneal microperforation is a potentially serious adverse event that can occur during passage of the needle. This is particularly so when the vascularized cornea is thin [48]. Other adverse events, such as striae, whitening, and intracorneal hemorrhages, are reversible [48]. Transient opacification of the cornea is observed in the stroma immediately surrounding the needle in all patients and persists for 24–48 h, with complete resolution. Intracorneal hemorrhage occurring intraoperatively or immediately postoperatively is the commonest adverse event. Though dramatic in appearance, intracorneal hemorrhages all resolve over a week or two. Sometimes, crystalline deposits can develop in the site of hemorrhage [48].

6.4. Corneal anti-angiogenesis target therapies

The advent of anti-VEGF agents has introduced a new dimension to the management of corneal vessels [54]. Active young vessels which usually indicate an underlying ongoing pathology continuing to induce further vascularization are probably best treated with anti-VEGF drops or subconjunctival injections. There is a growing list of therapeutic agents that target corneal angiogenesis (**Table 2**). Currently, only limited experience using anti-VEGFs on the cornea and only in an off-label setting is available [54].

Targets	Mechanisms	Therapeutics
Vascular endothelial growth factor	Anti–VEGF-A antibodies	Bevacizumab
		Ranibizumab
	Soluble or modified VEGF receptors	VEGFR-2-Fc
		sVEGFR-3 overexpression gene therapy
		VEGFR-1 morpholino
		Recombinant dimeric
		sVEGFR-1 overexpression gene therapy
		VEGFR intraceptor gene therapy (Flt23k, Flt24k)
		Aflibercept/VEGF-Trap(R1R2)
	VEGF-A aptamer	Pegaptanib
Pigment epithelium-derived factor	PEDF direct effect	PEDF
		PEDF gene therapy
		PEDF-derived peptide
Angiostatin	Angiostatin direct effect	Angiostatin pump
Platelet-derived growth factor	Multitargeted receptor tyrosine kinase inhibitor	Sunitinib
	PDGF receptor inhibitor	AG 1296
12-Hydroxyeicosatrienoic acid	siRNA for cytochrome P450 mono-oxygenase	CYP4B1 siRNA gene therapy
Hypoxia-inducible factors	shRNA for hypoxia-inducible factors	HIF-1a shRNA gene therapy (HIF-1a RNAi-A)
Decorin	Decorin direct effect	Decorin gene therapy
Vascular adhesion protein	VAP-1/SSAO inhibitor	U-V002
		LJP1207
Cannabinoid receptor CB1	CB1 antagonist	Rimonabant
Vasohibin-1	Vasohibin-1 directly effect	Vasohibin-1 gene therapy

HIF-1a: hypoxia-inducible factor 1a, CYP: cytochrome P450 mono-oxygenase, PDGF: platelet-derived growth factor, SSAO: semicarbazide-sensitive amine oxidase, PEDF: pigment epithelium-derived factor, VAP-1: vascular adhesive protein-1, sVEGFR: soluble form of vascular endothelial growth factor receptor, VEGF: vascular endothelial growth factor, VEGFR: vascular endothelial growth factor receptor.

Table 2. Corneal antiangiogenesis target therapies.

6.4.1. Anti-VEGF antibody

Inhibition of VEGF activity by a specific neutralizing anti-VEGF antibody is one possible strategy for treating corneal angiogenesis. VEGF inhibitors such as pegaptanib sodium (Macugen™, OSI/Eyetech), off-label bevacizumab (Avastin™, Genentech), and ranibizumab (Lucentis™, Genentech) are currently used for the treatment of different retinal pathologies including wet-type age-related macular degeneration [55]. Both animal models and clinical trials have demonstrated that these agents are effective in reducing corneal neovascularization. Both ranibizumab and bevacizumab use the same mechanisms and nonspecifically inhibit the VEGF-A isoforms [56]. Nevertheless, differently from ranibizumab and bevacizumab, pegaptanib specifically binds to VEGF-A165 and does not inhibit all of the VEGF isoforms. Subconjunctival ranibizumab, pegaptanib sodium, and bevacizumab are effective with no epitheliopathy in reducing corneal angiogenesis. Repeated subconjunctival injections with higher doses and concentrations and combination therapy with other antiangiogenic agents may be valid options to improve the effectiveness of treatments [57].

Treating corneal new vessel with the anti-VEGF antibody has some limitations. In contrast to superficial and active vascularization, in which clear regression is observed, anti-VEGF agents have a lower effect on deep vascularization. The effect of the anti-VEGF antibodies depends on the time of the treatment after the onset of neovascularization. In contrast to newly formed vessels, stable vessels are less affected by VEGF blockade [58]. The vessels mature in chronic neovascularization, and pericytes are recruited to the area around the region of corneal neovascularization [59]. Such coverage may reduce the influence of anti-VEGF agents on the regression of newly formed immature vessels. Anti-VEGF therapy is only a symptomatic treatment of corneal neovascularization that does not cure the underlying pathology, making it necessary to repeat the treatment to maintain its positive effect over a span of time [27].

Bevacizumab, which is FDA approved for intravenous administration in the treatment of various cancers, is a full-length, humanized murine monoclonal antibody with a molecular weight of 149 kD. Bevacizumab recognizes all isoforms of VEGF and is in widespread use, off-label, as an intravitreal injection to treat different retinal diseases [60]. Additionally, studies have demonstrated that topical, subconjunctival, and intraocular application of bevacizumab can partially reduce corneal angiogenesis and inflammatory response, resulting in an increase in corneal transparency [61, 62]. Bevacizumab can inhibit macrophage migration to the corneal stroma in early but not late treatment. Macrophages are known to trigger neovascularization in ischemic or inflamed corneas [63]. There is a concern about the interference of the topical form but not subconjunctival form of bevacizumab with nerve regeneration and delayed wound healing [54, 64, 65].

Ranibizumab, which has VEGF-binding characteristics similar to bevacizumab, is a recombinant humanized monoclonal antibody fragment that binds and inhibits all VEGF-A isoforms. Bevacizumab and ranibizumab are related to each other, but ranibizumab is the Fab fragment from the same antibody used to create bevacizumab. Therefore, ranibizumab has a molecular weight of 48 kD, making it approximately one-third the size of bevacizumab and theoretically allowing a better corneal penetration. In addition, it has been affinity matured to optimize the VEGF-A binding potential. These characteristics may enable ranibizumab to reduce corneal angiogenesis more effectively than bevacizumab [66]. Subconjunctival ranibizumab significantly reduces VEGF levels not only in the bulbar conjunctiva and cornea but also in the iris and aqueous humor [67]. Clinically, stable corneal neovascularization can be effectively treated by topical ranibizumab 1% as evidenced by a significant reduction in vessel caliber and neovascular area with no significant change in invasion area. These findings suggest that the main outcome of ranibizumab treatment for stable corneal neovascularization is to induce the narrowing of vessels more than a reduction in their length.

6.4.2. Pigment epithelium-derived factor

PEDF is a glycoprotein with neurotrophic, antitumorigenic, and antiangiogenic functions. PEDF can inhibit FGF, VEGF, and interlukin-8 (IL-8/CXCL8)-mediated angiogenesis by inducing the cells' apoptosis and reducing endothelial cell migration simultaneously [68, 69]. It is also found to play an important role in the antiangiogenic effect of AMT [70]. Topical PEDF or PEDF-derived (P5-2 and P5-3) peptides can downregulate VEGF expression and inhibit corneal neovascularization in a chemical-induced corneal model [71].

6.4.3. Tyrosine kinase inhibitors

Anti-VEGF antibodies block the effect of VEGF before it attaches to the endothelial receptors. Tyrosine kinase with immunoglobulin and epidermal growth factor homology domain 2 (TIE2) that is predominantly or exclusively expressed in endothelial cells is an important regulator of angiogenesis. Tyrosine kinase inhibitors inhibit the activity of VEGF by blocking tyrosine kinase in the intracellular part of the VEGF cell membrane receptor. This may offer a different opportunity for the management of the angiogenesis process in corneal diseases. Regorafenib is a multikinase inhibitor that targets various kinases, including PDGF β, VEGFR1, VEGFR2, and VEGFR3, mutant oncogenic kinases, TIE2, and the FGF receptor, which are involved in neovascularization. The inhibitory effects of topical regorafenib are comparable to those of topical bevacizumab and dexamethasone [72]. Sunitinib is a multitargeted receptor tyrosine kinase inhibitor that blocks both VEGF and PDGF. Topically administered sunitinib can reduce corneal neovascularization more effectively than bevacizumab [73].

Trastuzumab is a monoclonal antibody that interferes with the HER2/ neu receptor. Lapatinib is a dual tyrosine kinase inhibitor, which interrupts the epidermal growth factor receptor (EGFR) and HER2/ neu pathways. Lapatinib used in the form of lapatinib ditosylate is an orally active drug for solid tumors such as breast cancer. In recent studies, both substances were compared for the treatment of experimental corneal angiogenesis. The results suggested that systemically administered lapatinib is more effective than systemically administered trastuzumab in preventing corneal angiogenesis [74].

7. Conclusion

Corneal neovascularization is a common clinical feature in different corneal diseases including ocular traumatic or chemical injury, autoimmune diseases, chronic contact lens wear, infectious keratitis, and keratoplasties. Although corneal neovascularization can serve a beneficial role in arresting stromal melts, wound healing, and the clearing of infections, its disadvantages are numerous and it frequently results in edema, tissue scarring, persistent inflammation, and lipid deposition that may significantly reduce vision. Furthermore, it plays a major role in corneal graft rejection by breaching corneal immune privilege. VEGF, which plays a crucial role in angiogenesis and the pathologic neovascularization associated with a variety of eye diseases, is the most important target for antiangiogenic therapies. Experience indicates that anti-VEGFs are effective in occluding actively growing corneal neovascularization but not established vessels. Surgical procedures, including laser photo-coagulation or fine needle diathermy, are useful particularly to obliterate large, established corneal vessels.

Author details

Sepehr Feizi

Address all correspondence to: sepehrfeizi@yahoo.com

Ophthalmic Research Center and Department of Ophthalmology, Labbafinejad Medical Center, Shahid Beheshti University of Medical Sciences, Tehran, Iran

References

[1] Chang JH, Gabison EE, Kato T, Azar DT. Corneal neovascularization. Curr Opin Ophthalmol 2001;12(4):242–249.

[2] Strömblad S, Cheresh DA. Integrins, angiogenesis and vascular cell survival. Chem Biol 1996;3(11):881–885.

[3] Lee HS, Chung SK. The effect of subconjunctival suramin on corneal neovascularization in rabbits. Cornea 2010;29(1):86–92.

[4] Bachmann B, Taylor RS, Cursiefen C. Corneal neovascularization as a risk factor for graft failure and rejection after keratoplasty: an evidence-based meta-analysis. Ophthalmology 2010;117(7):1300–1305.

[5] Huang PT. Penetrating keratoplasty in infants and children. J AAPOS 2007;11(1):5–6.

[6] Panda A, Vanathi M, Kumar A, Dash Y, Priya S. Corneal graft rejection. Surv Ophthalmol 2007;52(4):375–396.

[7] Sellami D, Abid S, Bouaouaja G, Ben Amor S, Kammoun B, Masmoudi M, Dabbeche K, Boumoud H, Ben Zina Z, Feki J. Epidemiology and risk factors for corneal graft rejection. Transplant Proc 2007;39(8):2609–2611.

[8] Menzel-Severing J. Emerging techniques to treat corneal neovascularisation. Eye (Lond) 2012;26(1):2–12.

[9]   Tshionyi M, Shay E, Lunde E, Lin A, Han KY, Jain S, Chang JH, Azar DT. Hemangiogenesis and lymphangiogenesis in corneal pathology. Cornea 2012;31(1):74–80.

[10] Beebe DC. Maintaining transparency: a review of the developmental physiology and pathophysiology of two avascular tissues. Semin Cell Dev Biol 2008;19(2):125–133.

[11] Madigan MC, Penfold PL, Holden BA, Billson FA. Ultrastructural features of contact lens-induced deep corneal neovascularization and associated stromal leukocytes. Cornea 1990;9(2):144–1451.

[12] Wong AL, Weissman BA, Mondino BJ. Bilateral corneal neovascularization and opacification associated with unmonitored contact lens wear. Am J Ophthalmol 2003;136(5):957–958.

[13] Remeijer L, Duan R, van Dun JM, Wefers Bettink MA, Osterhaus AD, Verjans GM. Prevalence and clinical consequences of herpes simplex virus type 1 DNA in human cornea tissues. J Infect Dis 2009;200(1):11–19.

[14] Hayashi K, Hooper LC, Detrick B, Hooks JJ. HSV immune complex (HSV-IgG: IC) and HSV-DNA elicit the production of angiogenic factor VEGF and MMP-9. Arch Virol 2009;154(2):219–226.

[15] Dua HS, Azuara-Blanco A. Limbal stem cells of the corneal epithelium. Surv Ophthalmol 2000;44(5):415–425.

[16] Kokotas H, Petersen MB. Clinical and molecular aspects of aniridia. Clin Genet 2010;77(5):409–420.

[17] Lee P, Wang CC, Adamis AP. Ocular neovascularization: an epidemiologic review. Surv Ophthalmol 1998;43(3):245–269.

[18] Mochimaru H, Usui T, Yaguchi T, Nagahama Y, Hasegawa G, Usui Y, Shimmura S, Tsubota K, Amano S, Kawakami Y, Ishida S. Suppression of alkali burn-induced corneal neovascularization by dendritic cell vaccination targeting VEGF receptor 2. Invest Ophthalmol Vis Sci 2008;49(5):2172–2177.

[19] Applegate LA, Ley RD. DNA damage is involved in the induction of opacification and neovascularization of the cornea by ultraviolet radiation. Exp Eye Res 1991;52(4):493–497.

[20] Cogan DG. Corneal vascularization. Invest Ophthalmol Vis Sci 1962;1:253–261.

[21] Javadi MA, Jafarinasab MR, Feizi S, Karimian F, Negahban K. Management of mustard gas-induced limbal stem cell deficiency and keratitis. Ophthalmology 2011;118(7):1272–1281.

[22] Chang JH, Garg NK, Lunde E, Han KY, Jain S, Azar DT. Corneal neovascularization: an anti-VEGF therapy review. Surv Ophthalmol 2012;57(5):415–429.

[23] Neufeld G, Cohen T, Gengrinovitch S, Poltorak Z. Vascular endothelial growth factor (VEGF) and its receptors. FASEB J 1999;13(1):9–22.

[24] Goldman J, Rutkowski JM, Shields JD, Pasquier MC, Cui Y, Schmökel HG, Willey S, Hicklin DJ, Pytowski B, Swartz MA. Cooperative and redundant roles of VEGFR-2 and VEGFR-3 signaling in adult lymphangiogenesis. FASEB J 2007;21(4):1003–1012.

[25] Shibuya M. Vascular endothelial growth factor (VEGF) and its receptor (VEGFR) signaling in angiogenesis: a crucial target for anti- and pro-angiogenic therapies. Genes Cancer 2011;2(12):1097–1105.

[26] Cursiefen C, Chen L, Borges LP, Jackson D, Cao J, Radziejewski C, D'Amore PA, Dana MR, Wiegand SJ, Streilein JW. VEGF-A stimulates lymphangiogenesis and hemangiogenesis in inflammatory neovascularization via macrophage recruitment. J Clin Invest 2004;113(7):1040–1050.

[27] Krizova D, Vokrojova M, Liehneova K, Studeny P. Treatment of corneal neovascularization using Anti-VEGF bevacizumab. J Ophthalmol. 2014;2014:178132. doi:10.1155/2014/178132.

[28] Kim WJ, Mohan RR, Mohan RR, Wilson SE. Effect of PDGF, IL-1alpha, and BMP2/4 on corneal fibroblast chemotaxis: expression of the platelet-derived growth factor system in the cornea. Invest Ophthalmol Vis Sci 1999;40(7):1364–1372.

[29] Hoppenreijs VP, Pels E, Vrensen GF, Felten PC, Treffers WF. Platelet-derived growth factor: receptor expression in corneas and effects on corneal cells. Invest Ophthalmol Vis Sci 1993;34(3):637–649.

[30] Pillai CT, Dua HS, Hossain P. Fine needle diathermy occlusion of corneal vessels. Invest Ophthalmol Vis Sci 2000;41(8):2148–2153.

[31] Cursiefen C, Chen L, Dana MR, Streilein JW. Corneal lymphangiogenesis: evidence, mechanisms, and implications for corneal transplant immunology. Cornea 2003;22(3):273–281.

[32] Proia AD, Chandler DB, Haynes WL, Smith CF, Suvarnamani C, Erkel FH, Klintworth GK. Quantitation of corneal neovascularization using computerized image analysis. Lab Invest 1988;58(4):473–479.

[33] Conrad TJ, Chandler DB, Corless JM, Klintworth GK. In vivo measurement of corneal angiogenesis with video data acquisition and computerized image analysis. Lab Invest 1994;70(3):426–434.

[34] Bock F, König Y, Kruse F, Baier M, Cursiefen C. Bevacizumab (Avastin) eye drops inhibit corneal neovascularization. Graefes Arch Clin Exp Ophthalmol 2008;246(2):281–284.

[35] Cursiefen C, Bock F, Horn FK, Kruse FE, Seitz B, Borderie V, Früh B, Thiel MA, Wilhelm F, Geudelin B, Descohand I, Steuhl KP, Hahn A, Meller D. GS-101 antisense oligonucleotide eye drops inhibit corneal neovascularization: interim results of a randomized phase II trial. Ophthalmology 2009;116(9):1630–1637.

[36] Wu PC, Liu CC, Chen CH, Kou HK, Shen SC, Lu CY, Chou WY, Sung MT, Yang LC. Inhibition of experimental angiogenesis of cornea by somatostatin. Graefes Arch Clin Exp Ophthalmol 2003;241(1):63–69.

[37] You IC, Kang IS, Lee SH, Yoon KC. Therapeutic effect of subconjunctival injection of bevacizumab in the treatment of corneal neovascularization. Acta Ophthalmol 2009;87(6):653–658.

[38] Jhanji V, Liu H, Law K, Lee VY, Huang SF, Pang CP, Yam GH. Isoliquiritigenin from licorice root suppressed neovascularisation in experimental ocular angiogenesis models. Br J Ophthalmol 2011;95(9):1309–1315.

[39] Kirwan RP, Zheng Y, Tey A, Anijeet D, Sueke H, Kaye SB. Quantifying changes in corneal neovascularization using fluorescein and indocyanine green angiography. Am J Ophthalmol 2012;154(5):850–858.

[40] Kwan AS, Barry C, McAllister IL, Constable I. Fluorescein angiography and adverse drug reactions revisited: the Lions Eye experience. Clin Experiment Ophthalmol 2006;34(1):33–38.

[41] Hope-Ross M, Yannuzzi LA, Gragoudas ES, Guyer DR, Slakter JS, Sorenson JA, Krupsky S, Orlock DA, Puliafito CA. Adverse reactions due to indocyanine green. Ophthalmology 1994;101(3):529–533.

[42] Steger B, Romano V, Kaye SB. Corneal indocyanine green angiography to guide medical and surgical management of corneal neovascularization. Cornea 2016;35(1):41–45.

[43] Romano V, Spiteri N, Kaye SB. Angiographic-guided treatment of corneal neovascularization. JAMA Ophthalmol 2015;133(3):e143544.

[44] Al-Torbak A, Al-Amri A, Wagoner MD. Deep corneal neovascularization after implantation with intrastromal corneal ring segments. Am J Ophthalmol 2005;140(5):926–927.

[45] Brooks BJ, Ambati BK, Marcus DM, Ratanasit A. Photodynamic therapy for corneal neovascularisation and lipid degeneration. Br J Ophthalmol 2004;88(6):840.

[46] Baer JC, Foster CS. Corneal laser photocoagulation for treatment of neovascularization. Efficacy of 577 nm yellow dye laser. Ophthalmology 1992;99(2):173–179.

[47] L'sEsperance FA Jr. Clinical photocoagulation with organic dye laser. A preliminary communication. Arch Ophthalmol 1985;103(9):1312–1316.

[48] Faraj LA, Elalfy MS, Said DG, Dua HS. Fine needle diathermy occlusion of corneal vessels. Br J Ophthalmol 2014;98(9):1287–1290.

[49] Liang L, Li W, Ling S, Sheha H, Qiu W, Li C, Liu Z. Amniotic membrane extraction solution for ocular chemical burns. Clin Exp Ophthalmol 2009;37(9):855–863.

[50] Oliveira HB, Sakimoto T, Javier JA, Azar DT, Wiegand SJ, Jain S, Chang JH. VEGF Trap(R1R2) suppresses experimental corneal angiogenesis. Eur J Ophthalmol 2010;20(1):48–54.

[51] Hos D1, Bock F, Dietrich T, Onderka J, Kruse FE, Thierauch KH, Cursiefen C. Inflammatory corneal (lymph) angiogenesis is blocked by VEGFR-tyrosine kinase inhibitor ZK 261991, resulting in improved graft survival after corneal transplantation. Invest Ophthalmol Vis Sci 2008;49(5):1836–1842.

[52] Cursiefen C, Wenkel H, Martus P, Langenbucher A, Nguyen NX, Seitz B, Küchle M, Naumann GO. Impact of short-term versus long-term topical steroids on corneal neovascularization after non-high-risk keratoplasty. Graefes Arch Clin Exp Ophthalmol 2001;239(7):514–521.

[53] Ey RC, Hughes WF, Bloome MA, Tallman CB. Prevention of corneal vascularization. Am J Ophthalmol 1968;66(6):1118–1131.

[54] Dastjerdi MH, Al-Arfaj KM, Nallasamy N, Hamrah P, Jurkunas UV, Pineda R 2nd, Pavan-Langston D, Dana R. Topical bevacizumab in the treatment of corneal neovascularization: results of a prospective, open-label, noncomparative study. Arch Ophthalmol 2009;127(4):381–389.

[55] Heier JS, Antoszyk AN, Pavan PR, Leff SR, Rosenfeld PJ, Ciulla TA, Dreyer RF, Gentile RC, Sy JP, Hantsbarger G, Shams N. Ranibizumab for treatment of neovascular age-related macular degeneration: a phase I/ II multicenter, controlled, multidose study. Ophthalmology 2006;113(4):633.e1–4.

[56] Bhisitkul RB. Vascular endothelial growth factor biology: clinical implications for ocular treatments. Br J Ophthalmol 2006;90(12):1542–1547.

[57] Akar EE, Oner V, Küçükerdönmez C, Aydın Akova Y. Comparison of subconjunctivally injected bevacizumab, ranibizumab, and pegaptanib for inhibition of corneal neovascularization in a rat model. Int J Ophthalmol 2013;6(2):136–140.

[58] Ferrari G, Dastjerdi MH, Okanobo A, Cheng SF, Amparo F, Nallasamy N, Dana R. Topical ranibizumab as a treatment of corneal neovascularization. Cornea 2013;32(7):992–997.

[59] Cursiefen C, Hofmann-Rummelt C, Küchle M, Schlötzer-Schrehardt U. Pericyte recruitment in human corneal angiogenesis: an ultrastructural study with clinicopathological correlation. Br J Ophthalmol 2003;87(1):101–106.

[60] Keating AM, Jacobs DS. Anti-VEGF treatment of corneal neovascularization. Ocul Surf 2011;9(4):227–237.

[61] Avisar I, Weinberger D, Kremer I. Effect of subconjunctival and intraocular bevacizumab injections on corneal neovascularization in a mouse model. Curr Eye Res 2010;35(2):108–115.

[62] Lee SH, Leem HS, Jeong SM, Lee K. Bevacizumab accelerates corneal wound healing by inhibiting TGF-beta2 expression in alkali-burned mouse cornea. BMB Rep 2009;42(12):800–805.

[63] Chen WL, Chen YM, Chu HS, Lin CT, Chow LP, Chen CT, Hu FR. Mechanisms control-ling the effects of bevacizumab (avastin) on the inhibition of early but not late formed cor-neal neovascularization. PLoS One 2014;9(4):e94205. doi:10.1371/journal.pone.0094205.

[64] Kim TI, Chung JL, Hong JP, Min K, Seo KY, Kim EK. Bevacizumab application delays epithelial healing in rabbit cornea. Invest Ophthalmol Vis Sci 2009;50(10):4653–4659.

[65] Koenig Y, Bock F, Horn F, Kruse F, Straub K, Cursiefen C. Short- and long-term safety profile and efficacy of topical bevacizumab (Avastin) eye drops against corneal neovas-cularization. Graefes Arch Clin Exp Ophthalmol 2009;247(10):1375–1382.

[66] Stevenson W, Cheng SF, Dastjerdi MH, Ferrari G, Dana R. Corneal neovasculariza-tion and the utility of topical VEGF inhibition: ranibizumab (Lucentis) vs bevacizumab (Avastin). Ocul Surf 2012;10(2):67–83.

[67] Liarakos VS, Papaconstantinou D, Vergados I, Douvali M, Theodossiadis PG. The effect of subconjunctival ranibizumab on corneal and anterior segment neovascularization: study on an animal model. Eur J Ophthalmol 2014;24(3):299–308.

[68] Duh EJ, Yang HS, Suzuma I, Miyagi M, Youngman E, Mori K, Katai M, Yan L, Suzuma K, West K, Davarya S, Tong P, Gehlbach P, Pearlman J, Crabb JW, Aiello LP, Campochiaro PA, Zack DJ. Pigment epithelium-derived factor suppresses ischemia-induced retinal neovascularization and VEGF-induced migration and growth. Invest Ophthalmol Vis Sci 2002;43(3):821–829.

[69] Mori K, Gehlbach P, Ando A, McVey D, Wei L, Campochiaro PA. Regression of ocular neovascularization in response to increased expression of pigment epithelium-derived factor. Invest Ophthalmol Vis Sci 2002;43(7):2428–2434.

[70] Shao C, Sima J, Zhang SX, Jin J, Reinach P, Wang Z, Ma JX. Suppression of corneal neo-vascularization by PEDF release from human amniotic membranes. Invest Ophthalmol Vis Sci 2004;45(6):1758–1762.

[71] Jin J, Ma JX, Guan M, Yao K. Inhibition of chemical cautery-induced corneal neo-vascularization by topical pigment epithelium-derived factor eyedrops. Cornea 2010;29(9):1055–1061.

[72] Onder HI, Erdurmus M, Bucak YY, Simavli H, Oktay M, Kukner AS. Inhibitory effects of regorafenib, a multiple tyrosine kinase inhibitor, on corneal neovascularization. Int J Ophthalmol 2014;7(2):220–225.

[73] Pérez-Santonja JJ1, Campos-Mollo E, Lledó-Riquelme M, Javaloy J, Alió JL. Inhibition of corneal neovascularization by topical bevacizumab (Anti-VEGF) and sunitinib (Anti-VEGF and Anti-PDGF) in an animal model. Am J Ophthalmol 2010;150(4):519–528.

[74] Kaya MK, Demir T, Bulut H, Akpolat N, Turgut B. Effects of lapatinib and trastuzumab on vascular endothelial growth factor in experimental corneal neovascularization. Clin Exp Ophthalmol 2015;43(5):449–457.

7

Coronary Collateral Growth: Clinical Perspectives and Recent Insights

Bhamini Patel, Peter Hopmann, Mansee Desai,

Kanithra Sekaran, Kathleen Graham, Liya Yin and

William Chilian

Abstract

This chapter summarizes recent research on the coronary collateral circulation. The chapter is focused on clinical perspectives and importance of a well-developed coronary collateral circulation, the mechanisms of growth induced by chemical factors and a role for stem cells in the process. Some discussion is devoted to the role of shear stress and mechanical signaling, but because this topic has been reviewed so extensively in the recent past, there is only small mention of its role in the growth of the coronary collateral circulation.

Keywords: arteriogenesis, coronary collateral, ischemic heart disease

1. Introduction

Although arteriogenesis has been studied for approximately a hundred years, there are still fundamental unanswered questions about the causes of collateral vessel growth, and whether different factors control growth at varying points in the maturation process. One line of investigation, spurred by the myriad contributions of Schaper and his colleagues have focused on mechanical shear stress being the main factor that stimulates collateral growth [1–4]. Although this hypothesis is well-founded on a large body of experimental data, it does not explain other observations that show collateral growth in the absence of altered shear stress [5, 6]. Accordingly investigators have proposed that ischemia (via cytokine, chemokine, and growth factor expression), and the consequential inflammation, is the cause of collateral growth, but assessing it has proven to be difficult due to the unclear lines between ischemic regions, nor-mal circulation, and collateral growth. The hypotheses regarding the causative factor(s) for collateral growth are not mutually exclusive as there are likely many mechanisms that are the principal driver, which vary at various points of the process. For example, even if one maintains that ischemia is the initiating mechanism for collateral growth, it is likely that other stimuli continue the growth of the vessel after the ischemic stimulus has waned. To provide perspective for this chapter, we refer to **Figure 1**, which summarizes four factors that exert important effects in this adaptive process. The bulk of this chapter will focus on the collateral growth from a clinical perspective, the role of stem cells, and chemical factors involved in this process. We will not extensively review the role that shear stress in coronary collateral growth as this has been reviewed ample times in the past. We also will not review the genetic aspects because the bulk of this information has been derived from studies of collateral growth in vascular beds other than the heart, e.g., skeletal muscle and brain [7, 8], although there is some preliminary information about genetic links to collateral growth in patients [9]. **Figure 1** also shows the anatomical structure of a collateral; namely, an arterial-arterial anastomosis that connect large coronary perfusion territories. Collateral growth, also known as arteriogenesis, in the heart involves the abluminal expansion of a preexisting arterial-arterial anastomosis [10]. The degree of expansion is profound—the caliber of collateral vessels can increase over an order of magnitude [10]. This degree of expansion would greatly reduce vascular resistance of these vessels, thereby increasing flow in the area of risk. This increase in flow is the reason why the collateral circulation exerts beneficial effects through the reduction in infarct size (fol-lowing a coronary occlusive event) and reduction in the incidence of sudden cardiac death.

We also would like to point out an obvious distinction between the growth of collateral ves-sels (arteriogenesis) and angiogenesis. These processes are often confused as the same, but

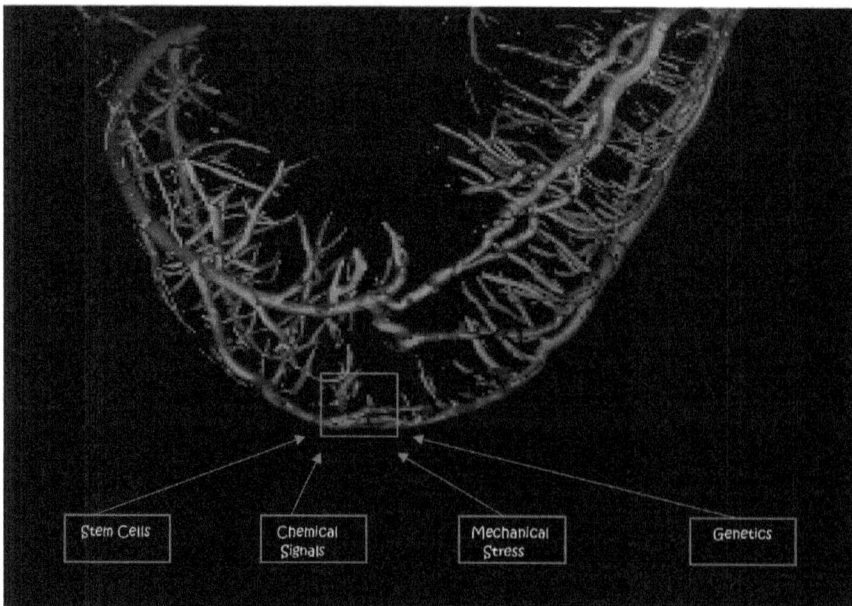

Figure 1. An image of the human coronary circulation depicting large collateral vessels that connect perfusion territories of major arteries and some factors that regulate their development.

they are distinct and have distinguishing characteristics. In *A Brief Etymology of the Collateral Circulation*, Faber et al. describe angiogenesis as the formation of capillaries from preexisting capillaries [11]. In contrast to angiogenesis, arteriogenesis is more the remodeling of preexisting vessels through the "anatomic increase in lumen area and wall thickness." The causes of arteriogenesis are more physical, specially, mechanical shear stress and ischemic conditions, while angiogenesis is caused by chemical conditions such as hypoxia [11].

2. Clinical perspective

Heart disease is extremely prevalent in the United States, where it accounts for every one in four deaths and almost 735,000 Americans suffer a heart attack each year (Centers for Disease Control, USA). However, there are numerous differences between these individuals in terms of response to treatment, future adverse events, and long-term survival rates. One explanation for these differences involves the presence of good collateral growth in certain individuals. A 5-year study called Osaka Acute Coronary Insufficiency Study (OACIS) assessed both acute and long-term survival in patients and came to three important conclusions: (1) patients with a Rentrop collateral score (RCS) of one or two showed the most promising 5-year survival rates, (2) RCS of three was associated with a worse 5-year survival rate, (3) RCS of three was associated with the best survival rates in a specific subgroup of patients with single vessel disease without previous myocardial infarction (MI) [12]. These first two conclusions can be explained due to the fact a higher baseline RCS can be indicative of a worse background of clinical characteristics such as previous MI or angina pectoris resulting in increased mortality rates, whereas an RCS of one or two was developed in the acute setting negating any adverse effects of chronic ischemia [12]. The third conclusion states RCS of three is more beneficial in the setting of single vessel occlusion and without previous MI, which would liken it to individuals who have RCS of one or two, but without any previous adverse events. In this subgroup, patients are having increased collateral flow, but without the chronic angina pectoris or previous MI improving survival rates [12]. This information leads to an important conclusion where the increased number of collaterals does not equate to decreased mortality rates, but rather is dependent upon a multitude of factors.

2.1. Methods

The literature is replete with the salubrious effects of a well-developed coronary collateral circulation and the potential benefit of a therapeutic process aimed at stimulating coronary collateral growth [13–19]. One patient study focused on coronary collateral growth in patients that had stable coronary artery disease. Specifically, the Möbius-Winkler et al. study looked at the impact of exercise on coronary collateral growth [20]. The patients were put into groups of usual care, moderate intensity exercise, and high-intensity exercise. The main findings of this study were that moderate and high-intensity exercise increased the coronary collateral blood flow. Scientists in this study postulated the cause of the coronary collateral growth. They questioned whether ischemia triggers collateral growth, since a percutaneous coronary intervention was performed before the study began; however, there is a large body of literature suggesting the PCI procedures may not completely resolve myocardial ischemia. The authors further speculated that the cause could be this increased blood flow and could have been from either increasing work done by preexisting blood vessels or an "improvement in endothelial function of small intramyocardial vessels." There was a CFI increase of 39% in the group of patients that did high-intensity exercise and a 41% CFI increase in the group that did moderate intensity exercise, which emphasized that exercise increased the coronary collateral blood flow in patients with coronary artery disease [20].

There has been much discussion for stimulating arteriogenesis in patients in order to give them proper blood perfusion to ischemic areas. Collaterals have been found to give patients many benefits over individuals who do not have collaterals, with a long-term mortality reduction, reduced myocardial infarct size, a greater postinfarction ejection fraction, and a reduced risk for rupture of the papillary muscle, myocardial free wall, or interventricular septum [21]. A reduction in infarct size was noted by the decreased peak creatinine levels as the number of collaterals increased depicting a cardioprotective effect [12]. Additionally, specific benefits have been noted between the presence of collaterals and sudden cardiac death and myocardial infarction.

There are three prevalent assessment methods of collateral growth circulation: the Rentrop score, collateral flow index (CFI), and intracoronary electrocardiogram. The Rentrop score can be most easily assessed when using coronary angiography as a visual assessment method. Circulation is then categorized into four different grades: Grade 0, Grade 1, Grade 2, and Grade 3. These categories range from no filling of the coronary collaterals to complete filling of collaterals, respectively. Although successful, the Rentrop method has some limitations due to being easily influenced by blood pressure changes and the force of injections during imaging procedures. Currently, the method considered to be the most accurate is the collateral flow index measurement. This method centers around utilizing a Doppler sensor tipped guide wire to quantify flow velocity in an occluded vessel compared with a normal vessel. Briefly mentioned was the intracoronary electrocardiogram, which is regarded as "simpler, cheaper, and very accurate" [22].

2.2. Benefits of coronary collaterals

Although many in the preclinical models have been employed in the study of coronary collateral growth, there is a relative paucity of clinical studies that have attempted to elucidate mechanisms of growth. One of the first studies done was in 1971 and was published in the *New England Journal of Medicine* [23]. This study only had three successful trials that demonstrated collaterals alleviating cardiovascular mortality. The inconsistency, according to Meier et al., could be rooted in the method by which they measured coronary collateral growth. The 1971 study "qualified" collaterals visually using coronary angiography, but Meier et al. postulates that had a better measurement method such as CFI been used, results could have been more promising [22].

One successful clinical study was performed by Seiler et al., which found that there is a direct correlation between collateral function and atherosclerotic lesions [24]. Patients with chronic total coronary occlusions had higher CFI values than those patients who did not have this condition. A CFI shift was quantified that patients with coronary occlusions had a CFI of 0.365 ± 0.190 versus 0.180 ± 0.105 of that of patients without occlusions. This study directly demonstrated that "collateral function is a direct indicator of CAD severity." The clinical importance of these findings suggests that human coronary collaterals can act as a "marker of poor outcome" in diseases such as acute coronary syndromes.

Sudden cardiac death (SCD) has several causes including electrical instability of the heart, specifically QRS complex variabilities can be used as markers for SCD and at times even trigger SCD [25]. The Oregon Sudden Unexpected Death Study (Ore-SUDS) has shown that prolongation of the QRS complex is associated with a large increase of SCD due to both known and unknown causes; therefore, methods to reduce this adverse event in the presence of myocardial ischemia can reduce mortality [26]. Additionally, fragmented QRS (fQRS), which are various RSR patterns in two continuous leads, have a well-established relationship with cardiac fibrosis caused by previous myocardial infarction or ischemia [27]. fQRS patterns have also been associated with increased morbidity and mortality, SCD, and repeat cardiovascular (CV) events and were found more often in individuals with poor collateral growth [27]. The presence of a well-developed collateral network has been shown to reduce QRS prolongation in left coronary artery occlusion and occurrence of fQRS in patients with chronic total occlusion [25, 27]. With this information, it can be concluded that with an increased number of coronary collaterals, patients can avoid QRS complex abnormalities thereby decreasing the chances of sudden cardiac death.

Additionally, the presence of collaterals has shown an increased time from symptom-onset-to-perfusion (>6 hours in good collateral versus poor collateral). This enables patients to increase the amount of time before onset of detrimental cardiac damage [28]. During an acute MI, the presence of a well-developed collateral circulation was seen in infarcted tissue that did not undergo cell necrosis, proving that increased collaterals will increase the chances of myocardial viability [29–31].

Overall, the presence of a well-developed collateral circulation in conjunction with healthy baseline characteristics (absence of repeat MI or angina pectoris) will be protective in patients who may suffer SCD, MI, or bouts of ischemia. Working to induce this collateral growth in patients both mechanically and chemically will prove to be very beneficial in decreasing mortality rates of patients with heart disease and perhaps ameliorate the possibility of recurrent cardiac events.

3. Mechanical factors involved in coronary collateral growth

The precise stimulation of arteriogenesis is yet to be found; however, both mechanical and chemical influences are required to induce the formation of collaterals in the heart. Mechanical shear stress occurs due to increased pressure gradients that form when an occlusion is present [32]. A stenotic artery will increase the pressure prior to the occlusion while decreasing the pressure distal to the occlusion. The increased pressure above the occlusion will cause an increase in blood flow into capillary beds prior to the occlusion increasing the shear stress [32]. The increased movement of blood into pre-existing collaterals and the resultant increased shear stress leads to several changes in the capillary endothelium. The first of which includes an increase in MCP-1 that serves to attract more monocytes to the proliferative site in order to transform them into the subsequent macrophages. The macrophages play a vital role in releasing cytokines and growth factors required for arteriogenesis. TNF-α, released by macrophages, helps form the inflammatory environment required for the growth of collaterals [33]. Another major factor includes basic fibroblast growth factor (bFGF), which helps with the actual development of collaterals [32]. A more in depth analysis on chemical inducers will be discussed later on in this chapter.

Although mechanical shear stress is thought to be a major contributor to arteriogenesis, it cannot be the sole solution due to the inability of fluid shear stress to completely replace the conducting artery. Fluid shear stress (FSS) has been found to only reach 35–40% of the maximal conductance possessed by the original stenotic artery [34]. An explanation for this phenomenon can be found in the relationships: FSS and blood flow velocity and FSS and cube of the vessel radius. FSS and blood flow velocity have a proportional relationship, while FSS is inversely related to the cube of the vessel radius [34]. The increase in blood flow velocity in the pre-existing collaterals leads to an increase in FSS. Since the shear stress causes growth in the collaterals (meaning an increase in the vessel radius), the FSS begins to decline preventing full recovery of the stenotic artery [34]. This indicates the need for both mechanical and chemical effectors for the production of proper coronary collaterals.

4. Chemical factors involved in coronary collateral growth

In addition to mechanical mechanisms of arteriogenesis, there are several chemical mediators involved in regulation of the process. Many of these chemical factors modulate the functions of the various cell types involved in arteriogenesis, including induction of cell proliferation, chemotaxis, and cellular remodeling. In this section, we will outline the various chemical mediators that are currently known to play a role in arteriogenesis.

4.1. Vascular endothelial growth factor (VEGF)

Vascular endothelial growth factor (VEGF) is known to play a major role in development of new vasculature. Under hypoxic conditions, VEGF production and release stimulates new capillary formation (angiogenesis) via endothelial cell sprouting, proliferation, and migration [35]. Alternatively, under different conditions, it can instead stimulate growth of new arteries, formation of collateral vessels, and modulation of lumen expansion—these actions are collectively referred to as arteriogenesis [35].

In VEGF signaling, there are three primary cell-surface receptors to which it binds: two tyrosine kinase receptors VEGFR-1 and VEGFR-2 and a nonkinase receptor neuropilin-1 (NRP-1) [35–37]. There are multiple isoforms of VEGF, with VEGF-A playing the major role in endothelial cell function via binding to VEGFR-2 [35]. VEGFR-2 is also involved in signaling pathways that lead to arteriogenesis via stimulation of proliferation, migration, survival, and lumenization of endothelial cells [35].

The first of these signaling cascades is activation of phosphatidylinositol 3-kinase (PI3K)/Akt that inhibits apoptosis in endothelial cells thus promoting cell survival [35]. The cascade is initiated by binding of VEGF-A to VEGFR-2 (Flk-1), which initiates receptor internalization via clathrin-coated pits followed by receptor autophosphorylation [35]. Active VEGFR-2 then phosphorylates PI3K, which goes on to phosphorylate the serine/threonine kinase Akt, which will go on to phosphorylate targets to inhibit apoptosis [38].

The second signal cascade is phosphorylation of profilin-1, indirectly via Src/FAK as well as directly via VEGFR-2, which stimulates migration of endothelial cells [35, 37]. Like the previous mechanism, this cascade is initiated by binding of VEGF-A to VEGFR-2. Activated VEGFR-2 then goes on to phosphorylate profilin-1 as well as Src kinase, which also phosphorylates profilin-1 [37]. Phosphorylated profilin-1 then goes on to catalyze the exchange of ADP for ATP on G-actin that stimulates polymerization of actin and resultant remodeling of the endothelial cell cytoskeleton [37]. This remodeling results in formation of actin-rich filopodia extending in the direction of the concentration gradient of VEGF, thus stimulating endothelial cell migration [37].

The third signal cascade is activation of the Raf-MEK-ERK signal cascade, which stimulates proliferation of endothelial cells, network formation, and increase in lumen size via phosphorylation of ERK1/2 [35]. While the exact mechanism of ERK1/2 action on cell proliferation and motility is not yet well understood, it has been suggested that a major component of this signaling cascade is downregulation of Rho-Kinase activity [39].

Finally, it is important to note that VEGF has been shown to be a critical factor in the process of coronary collateral growth. In a study of collateral growth following myocardial infarction in rats, it was observed that when the endogenous functions of VEGF were blocked by anti-VEGF neutralizing antibody, the result was a complete lack of collateral growth and subsequently no increase in coronary flow in the anti-VEGF group [40]. Additionally, upon treatment with dipyridamole (a potent vasodilator), it was observed that the increased coronary flow seen in the control group was in fact due to collateral growth, as there was no observed increase in coronary flow in the anti-VEGF group after the dipyridamole [40]. This study solidifies the importance of VEGF in the process of angiogenesis, particularly as it relates to coronary collateral growth.

4.2. bFGF and PDGF

In addition to VEGF, other growth factors are known to play a role in arteriogenesis—notably basic fibroblast growth factor (bFGF) and platelet-derived growth factor (PDGF) [41]. Basic FGF and PDGF are known to induce mitosis in both endothelial and smooth muscle cells and also exert other mitogenic effects such as promoting cell migration and differentiation [41, 42]. Basic FGF stimulates these mitogenic effects via binding to FGF receptors (FGFRs) expressed on cell surfaces [43]. These FGFRs are a part of the tyrosine kinase receptor family, and following binding of bFGF dimerize are autophosphorylated to become activated [43]. Activated FGFRs, notably FGFR-2 (FGFR-1 is thought to be a regulator of bFGF concentration available to bind FGFR-2), then continue the signal cascade by activation of cytoplasmic mitogen-activated protein kinase (MAPK), which then is translocated to the nucleus to initiate transcription promoting the aforementioned mitogenic effects [43]. PDGF, on the other hand, is known to activate multiple other downstream targets including PI3K, phospholipase C (PLC), as well as MAPK to mediate its mitogenic effects [44].

4.3. MCP-1 and macrophages

In addition to endothelial cells, macrophages are also heavily involved in arteriogenesis, but in order to do so must be directed to the correct location [36]. The primary molecule that has been studied as part of this mechanism is monocyte chemotactic protein 1 (MCP-1) [36]. Secretion of MCP-1 is initiated by activation of endothelial cell MAP-kinase-protein-kinase-2 (MK2) by elevation of fluid shear stress [45]. Released MCP-1 subsequently activates monocyte MK2, initiating migration to the correct location [45]. In the last step of the cycle, release of inflammatory cytokines by recruited monocytes cause increased secretion of MCP-1 from the endothelium, resulting in further monocyte recruitment [45]. Of similarly significant importance to MCP-1 are two adhesive molecules, intracellular adhesion molecule-1 (ICAM-1), and vascular cell adhesion molecule-1 (VCAM-1), which serve to bind the surface of migrating monocytes allowing them to roll along the luminal surface of the vasculature [36].

Once the macrophages have reached their destination, the correct phenotype must be expressed to stimulate new vessel growth [36]. There are two primary phenotypes of monocyte macrophages: M1 macrophages that secrete inflammatory molecules and help fight pathogens and M2 macrophages that play a role in vascular growth and wound healing [36]. These two phenotypes are induced by different cytokines, with interferon-γ causing a shift toward the M1 phenotype, while IL-4, IL-13, and several other factors such as IL-10 and IL-33 causing M2 differentiation. In histological analysis of hypoxia-induced arteriogenesis, the number of M2 macrophages was shown to increase indicating their essential role in development of new vasculature [36].

4.4. NO and eNOS

Nitric oxide (NO) is a potent vasodilator that is produced via the activity of endothelial nitric oxide synthase (eNOS). eNOS has been shown to function in stimulating production of new vasculature, and its expression is also known to be upregulated in response to elevated fluid shear stresses—a principal mechanical stimulus of arteriogenesis [46]. While the exact effects of NO and eNOS on arteriogenesis are still controversial, it has been shown that one contribution of elevated NO due to increased expression of eNOS is a reduction of vascular endothelial cadherin (VE-cadherin), resulting in increased vascular permeability and indirect promotion of macrophage invasion [46]. Additionally, eNOS activity and pharmacological inhibition of eNOS were shown to play a role in mediating vascular remodeling during collateral growth [47, 48].

4.5. Catestatin

Catestatin is a neuroendocrine peptide derived from a specific cleavage of the larger protein human chromogranin A (CgA) [49]. It functions in many different processes within the body including secretion of histamine from mast cells, defense against microbes, vasodilation, and attraction of monocytes. It has also been observed that catestatin acts in a pro-angiogenic capacity, involved in inducing proliferation and migration of endothelial cells as well as formation of capillary tubes [49, 50]. This is accomplished through stimulating release of bFGF, which in turn will activate MAPK via binding to FGFR-1 as previously discussed [49, 50]. It has also been shown that catestatin activates other signal cascades such as PI3K/Akt, serving an anti-apoptotic role to promote cell survival [50]. Finally, catestatin influences effects in both endothelial progenitor cells (EPCs) and vascular smooth muscle cells (VSMCs) in addition to its direct effects on endothelial cells, inducing chemotaxis to incorporate these cell types into formation of new vasculature [50].

4.6. Neuregulins

Neuregulins (NRG) are another class of molecules produced by endothelial cells. These growth factor ligands bind to erbB receptors expressed on the surface of endothelial cells—this action has been shown to induce angiogenesis [51]. NRG involvement in angiogenesis and arteriogenesis is tied to regulation of $\alpha_v\beta_3$ integrin, thus playing a role in cell migration, proliferation, and differentiation mechanisms as shown in a NRG-erbB knockout mouse model. The mechanism by which this occurs involves another proangiogenic protein, Cyr61, the expression of which is upregulated by NRG-erbB signaling, in addition to mediation via induction of VEGF release and subsequent activation of the ERK signaling cascade [51]. ErbB receptors have also been found to be expressed on EPCs, playing a role in increasing cell survival, and on certain types of VSMCs, though the role NRG-erbB signaling plays here is not well known [51].

4.7. Early growth response 1 (Egr-1)

Early growth response 1 (Egr-1) is a transcription factor of the zinc-finger family that has been shown to be upregulated during arteriogenesis [52]. It plays a major role in modulating the levels of other growth factors that are involved in the process of collateral growth, including playing a role in the recruitment and proliferation of leukocytes [52, 53]. Specific genes that are upregulated by Egr-1 include PDGF and transforming growth factor β (TGF-β), which then indirectly upregulates other factors involved in collateral growth such as VEGF and metalloproteinases [53]. Interestingly, despite the fact that most of these factors have been primarily shown to affect angiogenesis, it has been observed that Egr-1 primarily affects the growth of arterioles rather than capillaries, indicating its primary role in regulation of arteriogenesis [53].

Much like the other factors mentioned here, Egr-1 production is stimulated primarily by elevations in fluid shear stress, in this case by activating the Egr-1 gene promoter [54]. It has been suggested that this is mediated by the Ras-MEK-ERK1/2 signal cascade in which shear stress leads to activation of MEK1, which proceeds to activate ERK1/2 of the MAPK family, and finally ERK1/2 activate the protein Elk-1 that induces transcription of Egr-1 [54]. Interestingly, this pathway can be activated by very low levels of shear stress due to the sensitivity of ERK1/2 [54].

There are many varying chemical mediators of arteriogenesis, many of which share similar signaling pathways leading to their involvement. While some of these mediators have been studied extensively and are relatively well understood, there are others whose mechanisms have not yet been elucidated and require more investigation. There are likely even more chemical mediators involved that have not yet been studied. Going forward, more research will be extremely valuable in understanding the overall chemical mechanism behind collateral vessel growth and how to apply this knowledge to a clinical setting.

5. Role of Stem Cells in Coronary Collateral Growth

In addition to the aforementioned chemical mediators that mitigate the consequences of vascular occlusive diseases by stimulating collateral growth, in recent years, stem cell-based therapy has been implicated as a possible avenue for vascular regeneration. Stem cells have the unique potential of developing into many different cell types in the body. Under certain physiologic and experimental conditions, they can be manipulated to grow into specific tissues and organ cells with exclusive functionality. This revolutionary discovery for stem cells has demonstrated a clinical potential to create new networks of blood-perfused vessels and treat human patients with cardiovascular and vascular diseases [55]. The current theory is that stem cells may release a series of angiogenic factors, such as VEGF and bFGF, which mobilize vascular endothelial cells through a paracrine effect [56]. In this section, we will summarize the current state of regenerative approaches using stem cells to stimulate coronary collateral growth.

A 2012 study programmed endothelial cells to develop into induced vascular progenitor cells (iVPCs) and assessed their ability to induce coronary collateral growth in a rat model in efforts to increase blood flow to the collateral-dependent region of risk [57]. iVPCs are also known to be less tumorigenic compared with induced pluripotent cells (iPSCs) and are more likely to commit to a line of vascular differentiation (they will not turn into cardiomyocytes) [57]. When the iVPCs were transplanted into myocardium, they formed blood vessels and improved blood flow markedly better than did natural endothelial cells, mesenchymal stem cells, or iPSCs [57]. However, while results showed that partial programming of the endothelial cells was promising enough to sprout new blood vessels in the myocardium, one big challenge persists: how to maintain the partial programmed state of the cells until they get to their intended destination [57].

In addition, current literature posits that bone marrow-derived stem cells and endothelial progenitor cells in arteriogenesis do not physically deposit onto the walls of newly generated arteries but rather play the role of supporting cells [58]. The therapeutic induction of collateral growth from already established arteries improves any blood flow deficiencies caused by blockage in major arteries. Transplanted bone marrow-derived cells act as "cytokine factors" and secrete specific growth factors that mediate their effects through paracrine activity [59]. As Dr. Matthias Heil of the Netherlands puts it, "bone marrow stem cells provide the software and not the hardware in vascular growth" [59]. His group's study on the hindlimb ischemic model with mice revealed that GFP-tagged bone marrow was not localized to endothelial and smooth cell markers, but around burgeoning collaterals that were secreting chemokines and growth factors [59]. Hence, therapeutic arteriogenesis functions to boost the body's natural angiogenic ability by stimulating the release of pro-angiogenic factors rather than actually providing the buildings block for a new artery. A caveat to this is if the processes in the heart are different from those in the peripheral circulation.

While there is a continued debate on whether bone marrow-derived multipotent stromal cells (MSCs) exert their effect via transdifferentiation or through paracrine activity, there is unequivocal evidence showing that MSCs must first travel to ischemic tissue to achieve a therapeutic benefit [60]. MSCs localize to injured tissues by adhering to endothelial cells and migrating across the cell wall. Homing of MSCs to injured tissues is optimized by an expression of ligands on endothelial cells [60]. A 2009 study showed the importance of epidermal growth factor (EGF) and heparin-binding epidermal growth factor-like growth factor (HB-EGF) in inducing increased expression of these ligands [60]. Specifically, phosphorylation of the EGF-R leads to higher expression of ligands, VCAM-1, and ICAM-1 that enhanced MSC adherence and ultimately stimulated coronary collateral growth in rats that had undergone repetitive instances of myocardial ischemia [60]. Coronary collateral growth was assessed with the ratio of collateral dependent flow (CZ) to normal zone flow (NZ). Exposure of both MSCs and coronary endothelial cells (CECs) to a 100 ng/mL dose of EGF for 16 hours maximally increased expression of adhesion molecules compared with samples untreated with EGF [60]. The CZ/NZ ratio increased in rats whose MSCs were treated with EGF and showed improved cardiac function and decreased left ventricular remodeling compared to rats without EGF treatment of MSCs [60].

Another 2009 study involving a rat model of repetitive myocardial ischemia showed that granulocyte-colony stimulating factor (G-CSF), a glycoprotein responsible for hematopoietic cell proliferation and differentiation of neutrophil granulocytes, also stimulates coronary collateral growth [61]. G-CSF mounts a series of defenses against infectious agents, one of which is promotion of neutrophils to release reactive oxygen species (ROS) [61]. This generation of ROS was studied both *in vivo* and *in vitro* and was shown to directly act on injured cardiomyocytes. Cardiomyocytes under the influence of G-CSF-induced ROS generate angiogenic factors that lead to vascular growth and tube formation in levels comparative to cardiomyocytes induced by VEGF [61]. To the surprise of researchers, this study also demonstrated that G-CSF can promote coronary collateral growth without the impetus of repetitive ischemia and hence this cytokine can act as a surrogate for ischemia [61].

Majority of the recent clinical trials in humans purport that stem cell-based therapy adequately facilitates angiogenesis in patients suffering from peripheral arterial disease and promotes wound healing [55]. Specifically, bone marrow-derived stem cell transplantation has shown to improve ischemic symptoms, such as claudication, ischemic rest pain, and has augmented wound healing in ulcer-related conditions [55]. Nonetheless, these studies have been limited by a lack of care standardization, absence of a control group, small sample sizes, dissimilar inclusion criteria, and inconsistencies in methods of outcome assessment [55]. In other cases, the absence of follow-up procedures has prevented elucidation of long-term effects of treating peripheral artery disease with stem cells [55]. While the central issues of public safety and treatment efficacy linger over the field, progress, albeit limited, has been made in the arena of coronary collateral growth.

6. Summary

The process of coronary collateral growth is being better understood year by year. The role that the many chemical factors, mechanical factors, and stem cells play in the process is still incompletely understood. The study of these factors in "normal" preclinical models may be an oversimplification, because under conditions with risk factors for coronary disease, there may be shifts in the normal control mechanisms. We advocate that future studies incorporate models of cardiovascular disease and aging to better understand the mechanisms by which this adaptive process is abrogated in the majority of patients with ischemic heart disease.

Author details

Bhamini Patel, Peter Hopmann, Mansee Desai, Kanithra Sekaran, Kathleen Graham, Liya Yin and William Chilian*

*Address all correspondence to: wchilian@neomed.edu

Department of Integrative Medical Science, Northeast Ohio Medical University, Rootstown, Ohio, USA

References

[1] Cai W, Schaper W. Mechanisms of arteriogenesis. Acta Biochim Biophys Sin (Shanghai). 2008;40(8):681–692.

[2] Heil M, Schaper W. Influence of mechanical, cellular, and molecular factors on collateral artery growth (arteriogenesis). Circ Res. 2004;95(5):449–458.

[3] Pipp F, Boehm S, Cai WJ, Adili F, Ziegler B, Karanovic G, et al. Elevated fluid shear stress enhances postocclusive collateral artery growth and gene expression in the pig hind limb. Arterioscler Thromb Vasc Biol. 2004;24(9):1664–1668.

[4] Buschmann I, Schaper W. Arteriogenesis versus angiogenesis: two mechanisms of vessel growth. News Physiol Sci. 1999;14:121–125.

[5] Schaper W, De Brabander M, Lewi P. DNA synthesis and mitoses in coronary collateral vessels of the dog. Circ Res. 1971;28(6):671–679.

[6] Chilian WM, Mass HJ, Williams SE, Layne SM, Smith EE, Scheel KW. Microvascular occlusions promote coronary collateral growth. Am J Physiol. 1990;258(4 Pt 2):H1103–H1111.

[7] Chalothorn D, Clayton JA, Zhang H, Pomp D, Faber JE. Collateral density, remodeling and VEGF-A expression differ widely between mouse strains. Physiol Genom. 2007.

[8] Clayton JA, Chalothorn D, Faber JE. Vascular endothelial growth factor-A specifies formation of native collaterals and regulates collateral growth in ischemia. Circ Res. 2008;103(9):1027–1036.

[9] Gulec S, Karabulut H, Ozdemir AO, Ozdol C, Turhan S, Altin T, et al. Glu298Asp polymorphism of the eNOS gene is associated with coronary collateral development. Atherosclerosis. 2008;198(2):354–359.

[10] Schaper W, Gorge G, Winkler B, Schaper J. The collateral circulation of the heart. Prog Cardiovasc Dis. 1988;31(1):57–77.

[11] Faber JE, Chilian WM, Deindl E, van Royen N, Simons M. A brief etymology of the collateral circulation. Arterioscler Thromb Vasc Biol. 2014;34(9):1854–1859.

[12] Hara M, Sakata Y, Nakatani D, Suna S, Nishino M, Sato H, et al. Impact of coronary collaterals on in-hospital and 5-year mortality after ST-elevation myocardial infarction in the contemporary percutaneous coronary intervention era: a prospective observational study. BMJ Open. 2016;6(7):e011105.

[13] Fujita M, Sasayama S. Alleviation of myocardial ischemia by the development of coronary collateral circulation. Jpn Circ J. 1989;53(9):1164–1169.

[14] Fujita M, Sasayama S. Reappraisal of functional importance of coronary collateral circulation. Cardiology. 2010;117(4):246–252.

[15] Fujita M, Sasayama S. Coronary collateral growth and its therapeutic application to coronary artery disease. Circ J. 2010;74(7):1283–1289.

[16] Baklanov D, Simons M. Arteriogenesis: lessons learned from clinical trials. Endothelium. 2003;10(4–5):217–223.

[17] Bokeriia LA, Golukhova EZ, Eremeeva MV, Kiselev SL, Aslanidi IP, Vakhromeeva MN, et al. [New approaches to the treatment of ischemic heart disease: therapeutic angiogenesis in combination with surgical revascularization of the myocardium]. Ter Arkh. 2004;76(6):25–30.

[18] Emanueli C, Madeddu P. Angiogenesis gene therapy to rescue ischaemic tissues: achievements and future directions. Br J Pharmacol. 2001;133(7):951–958.

[19] Fujita M, Sasayama S, Asanoi H, Nakajima H, Sakai O, Ohno A. Improvement of treadmill capacity and collateral circulation as a result of exercise with heparin pretreatment in patients with effort angina. Circulation. 1988;77(5):1022–1029.

[20] Mobius-Winkler S, Uhlemann M, Adams V, Sandri M, Erbs S, Lenk K, et al. Coronary collateral growth induced by physical exercise: results of the impact of intensive exercise training on coronary collateral circulation in patients with stable coronary artery disease (EXCITE) trial. Circulation. 2016;133(15):1438–1448; discussion 48.

[21] Meier P, Gloekler S, Zbinden R, Beckh S, de Marchi SF, Zbinden S, et al. Beneficial effect of recruitable collaterals: a 10-year follow-up study in patients with stable coronary artery disease undergoing quantitative collateral measurements. Circulation. 2007;116(9):975–983.

[22] Meier P, Schirmer SH, Lansky AJ, Timmis A, Pitt B, Seiler C. The collateral circulation of the heart. BMC Med. 2013;11:143.

[23] Helfant RH, Vokonas PS, Gorlin R. Functional importance of the human coronary collateral circulation. N Engl J Med. 1971;284(23):1277–1281.

[24]   Seiler C, Stoller M, Pitt B, Meier P. The human coronary collateral circulation: development and clinical importance. Eur Heart J. 2013;34(34):2674–2682.

[25]   Meier P, Gloekler S, de Marchi SF, Zbinden R, Delacretaz E, Seiler C. An indicator of sudden cardiac death during brief coronary occlusion: electrocardiogram QT time and the role of collaterals. Eur Heart J. 2010;31(10):1197–1204.

[26]   Chugh SS, Reinier K, Singh T, Uy-Evanado A, Socoteanu C, Peters D, et al. Determinants of prolonged QT interval and their contribution to sudden death risk in coronary artery disease: the Oregon Sudden Unexpected Death Study. Circulation. 2009;119(5):663–670.

[27]   Erdogan T, Kocaman SA, Cetin M, Canga A, Durakoglugil ME, Cicek Y, et al. Relationship of fragmented QRS complexes with inadequate coronary collaterals in patients with chronic total occlusion. J Cardiovasc Med (Hagerstown). 2012;13(8):499–504.

[28]   Desch S, de Waha S, Eitel I, Koch A, Gutberlet M, Schuler G, et al. Effect of coronary collaterals on long-term prognosis in patients undergoing primary angioplasty for acute ST-elevation myocardial infarction. Am J Cardiol. 2010;106(5):605–611.

[29]   Seiler C, Meier P. Historical aspects and relevance of the human coronary collateral circulation. Curr Cardiol Rev. 2014;10(1):2–16.

[30]   van der Hoeven NW, Teunissen PF, Werner GS, Delewi R, Schirmer SH, Traupe T, et al. Clinical parameters associated with collateral development in patients with chronic total coronary occlusion. Heart. 2013;99(15):1100–1105.

[31]   Meier P, Hemingway H, Lansky AJ, Knapp G, Pitt B, Seiler C. The impact of the coronary collateral circulation on mortality: a meta-analysis. Eur Heart J. 2012;33(5):614–621.

[32]   Fujita M, Tambara K. Recent insights into human coronary collateral development. Heart. 2004;90(3):246–250.

[33]   Van Royen N, Piek JJ, Buschmann I, Hoefer I, Voskuil M, Schaper W. Stimulation of arteriogenesis; a new concept for the treatment of arterial occlusive disease. Cardiovasc Res. 2001;49(3):543–553.

[34]   Schaper W, Scholz D. Factors regulating arteriogenesis. Arterioscler Thromb Vasc Biol. 2003;23(7):1143–1151.

[35]   Kofler NM, Simons M. Angiogenesis versus arteriogenesis: neuropilin 1 modulation of VEGF signaling. F1000Prime Rep. 2015;7:26.

[36]   Hollander MR, Horrevoets AJ, van Royen N. Cellular and pharmacological targets to induce coronary arteriogenesis. Curr Cardiol Rev. 2014;10(1):29–37.

[37]   Simons M, Schwartz MA. Profilin phosphorylation as a VEGFR effector in angiogenesis. Nat Cell Biol. 2012;14(10):985–987.

[38]   Gerber HP, McMurtrey A, Kowalski J, Yan M, Keyt BA, Dixit V, et al. Vascular endothelial growth factor regulates endothelial cell survival through the phosphatidylinositol 3'-kinase/Akt signal transduction pathway. Requirement for Flk-1/KDR activation. J Biol Chem. 1998;273(46):30336–30343.

[39] Mavria G, Vercoulen Y, Yeo M, Paterson H, Karasarides M, Marais R, et al. ERK-MAPK signaling opposes Rho-kinase to promote endothelial cell survival and sprouting during angiogenesis. Cancer Cell. 2006;9(1):33–44.

[40] Toyota E, Warltier DC, Brock T, Ritman E, Kolz C, O'Malley P, et al. Vascular endothelial growth factor is required for coronary collateral growth in the rat. Circulation. 2005;112(14):2108–2113.

[41] Van Royen N, Piek JJ, Schaper W, Bode C, Buschmann I. Arteriogenesis: mechanisms and modulation of collateral artery development. J Nucl Cardiol. 2001;8(6):687–693.

[42] Wu S, Wu X, Zhu W, Cai WJ, Schaper J, Schaper W. Immunohistochemical study of the growth factors, aFGF, bFGF, PDGF-AB, VEGF-A and its receptor (Flk-1) during arteriogenesis. Mol Cell Biochem. 2010;343(1–2):223–229.

[43] Mason IJ. The ins and outs of fibroblast growth factors. Cell. 1994;78(4):547–552.

[44] Tsioumpekou M, Papadopoulos N, Burovic F, Heldin CH, Lennartsson J. Platelet-derived growth factor (PDGF)-induced activation of Erk5 MAP-kinase is dependent on Mekk2, Mek1/2, PKC and PI3-kinase, and affects BMP signaling. Cell Signal. 2016;28(9):1422–1431.

[45] Limbourg A, von Felden J, Jagavelu K, Krishnasamy K, Napp LC, Kapopara PR, et al. MAP-kinase activated protein kinase 2 links endothelial activation and monocyte/macrophage recruitment in arteriogenesis. PLoS One. 2015;10(10):e0138542.

[46] Yang B, Cai B, Deng P, Wu X, Guan Y, Zhang B, et al. Nitric oxide increases arterial endothelial permeability through mediating VE-cadherin expression during arteriogenesis. PLoS One. 2015;10(7):e0127931.

[47] Dai X, Faber JE. Endothelial nitric oxide synthase deficiency causes collateral vessel rarefaction and impairs activation of a cell cycle gene network during arteriogenesis. Circ Res. 2010;106(12):1870–1881.

[48] Matsunaga TDCW, Moniz M, Tessmmer J, Weihrauch D, Chilian WM. Role of nitric oxide and vascular endothelial growth factor in coronary collateral growth. Circulation. 2000;102:3098–3103.

[49] Xu W, Yu H, Li W, Gao W, Guo L, Wang G. Plasma catestatin: a useful biomarker for coronary collateral development with chronic myocardial ischemia. PLoS One. 2016;11(6):e0149062.

[50] Theurl M, Schgoer W, Albrecht K, Jeschke J, Egger M, Beer AG, et al. The neuropeptide catestatin acts as a novel angiogenic cytokine via a basic fibroblast growth factor-dependent mechanism. Circ Res. 2010;107(11):1326–1335.

[51] Hedhli N, Dobrucki LW, Kalinowski A, Zhuang ZW, Wu X, Russell RR, 3rd, et al. Endothelial-derived neuregulin is an important mediator of ischaemia-induced angiogenesis and arteriogenesis. Cardiovasc Res. 2012;93(3):516–524.

[52] Pagel JI, Ziegelhoeffer T, Heil M, Fischer S, Fernandez B, Schaper W, et al. Role of early growth response 1 in arteriogenesis: impact on vascular cell proliferation and leukocyte recruitment in vivo. Thromb Haemost. 2012;107(3):562–574.

[53] Sarateanu CS, Retuerto MA, Beckmann JT, McGregor L, Carbray J, Patejunas G, et al. An Egr-1 master switch for arteriogenesis: studies in Egr-1 homozygous negative and wild-type animals. J Thorac Cardiovasc Surg. 2006;131(1):138–145.

[54] Schwachtgen JL, Houston P, Campbell C, Sukhatme V, Braddock M. Fluid shear stress activation of egr-1 transcription in cultured human endothelial and epithelial cells is mediated via the extracellular signal-related kinase 1/2 mitogen-activated protein kinase pathway. J Clin Invest. 1998;101(11):2540–2549.

[55] Lee KB, Kim DI. Clinical application of stem cells for therapeutic angiogenesis in patients with peripheral arterial disease. Int J Stem Cells. 2009;2(1):11–17.

[56] Deindl E, Schaper W. The art of arteriogenesis. Cell Biochem Biophys. 2005;43(1):1–15.

[57] Yin L, Ohanyan V, Pung YF, Delucia A, Bailey E, Enrick M, et al. Induction of vascular progenitor cells from endothelial cells stimulates coronary collateral growth. Circ Res. 2012;110(2):241–252.

[58] Ziegelhoeffer T, Fernandez B, Kostin S, Heil M, Voswinckel R, Helisch A, et al. Bone marrow-derived cells do not incorporate into the adult growing vasculature. Circ Res. 2004;94(2):230–238.

[59] Heil M, Ziegelhoeffer T, Mees B, Schaper W. A different outlook on the role of bone marrow stem cells in vascular growth: bone marrow delivers software not hardware. Circ Res. 2004;94(5):573–574.

[60] Belmadani S, Matrougui K, Kolz C, Pung YF, Palen D, Prockop DJ, et al. Amplification of coronary arteriogenic capacity of multipotent stromal cells by epidermal growth factor. Arterioscler Thromb Vasc Biol. 2009;29(6):802–808.

[61] Carrao AC, Chilian WM, Yun J, Kolz C, Rocic P, Lehmann K, et al. Stimulation of coronary collateral growth by granulocyte stimulating factor: role of reactive oxygen species. Arterioscler Thromb Vasc Biol. 2009;29(11):1817–1822.

8

TGF-β Activation and Signaling in Angiogenesis

Paola A. Guerrero and Joseph H. McCarty

Abstract

The transforming growth factor-β (TGF-β) signaling pathway regulates various cellular processes during tissue and organ development and homeostasis. Deregulation of the expression and/or functions of TGF-β ligands, receptors or their intracellular signaling components leads to multiple diseases including vascular pathologies, autoimmune disorders, fibrosis and cancer. In vascular development, physiology and disease TGF-β signaling can have angiogenic and angiostatic properties, depending on expression levels and the tissue context. The objective of this chapter is to analyze the mechanisms that contribute to the activation and signaling of TGF-β in developmental, physiological and pathological angiogenesis, with a particular emphasis on the importance of TGF-β signaling in the mammalian central nervous system (CNS).

Keywords: TGF-β, vasculogenesis, angiogenesis, VEGF

1. Introduction

Discovery of TGF-βs was the result of independent efforts by several laboratories [1–4] during characterization of a secreted factor from fibroblasts transformed by the Moloney sarcoma virus (MSV). The TGF-β superfamily is now known to be composed of more than 30 chemokines such as TGF-β1-β3, activins, anti-Müllerian hormone (AMH), bone morphogenetic proteins (BMPs), growth and differentiation factors (GDFs) and NODAL that can signal via canonical and noncanonical receptors and intracellular effector proteins [5].

The best characterized member of the TGF-β family, TGF-β1, is initially produced from a single gene as a large precursor known as pre- and pro-TGF-βs which undergo two proteolytic cleavage events. The first signal peptide is cleaved in the rough endoplasmic reticulum. Furin, a proprotein convertase, subsequently cleaves the protein into two fragments [6]. The carboxy terminus corresponds to the functionally active cytokine and the large amino terminus is latency-associated protein (LAP), also referred to as the prodomain. Regardless of this processing by furin, the mature and LAP domains remain associated by noncovalent bonds to form the small latent complex (SLC). This complex subsequently covalently interacts with a second gene product, the latent TGF-β binding protein (LTBP), and is incorporated into a larger latent complex (LLC) that associates with the extracellular matrix (ECM) [6]. Three-dimensional crystal structure of porcine latent TGF-β1 shows a conformation that resembles a ring-like shape [7]. Two domains were defined in the structure: (i) an arm domain that contains an integrin-binding Arg-Gly-Asp (RGD) peptide motif and (ii) a "straitjacket" domain where the mature TGF-β is encased. At the opposite end of the arm domain, LTBP binds the prodomain forming the "ring head" [7] (**Figure 1**).

After secretion, the LLC complex interacts with various ECM proteins, such as fibronectin and fibrillin, and is maintained in an inactivated form [8]. TGF-β is activated by different mechanisms, including interactions with integrins, alterations in pH and extracellular proteases. αv integrin, which forms heterodimers with five different β integrin subunits (β1, β3, β5, β6 and β8), that bind to LAP-TGF-β1 and LAP-TGFβ-3 [9, 10]. However, only αvβ6 and αvβ8 have been shown to activate the latent TGF-β complex [11]. Activation by both αvβ6 and αvβ8 integrins requires the RGD motif in LAP. Activation by αvB6 requires an intact cytoplasmic domain [12, 13] and the presence of other ECM proteins [14]. Activation by αvβ8, however,

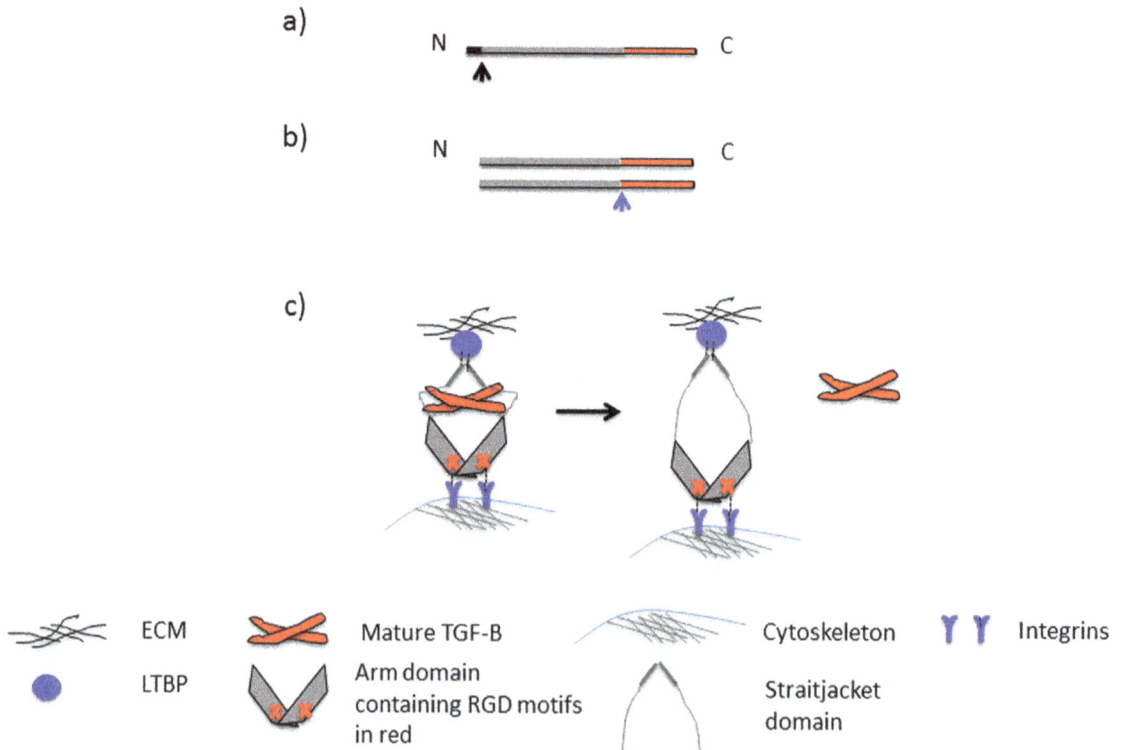

Figure 1. TGF-β processing and activation. **(a)**TGF-β precursor undergoes proteolysis at its N-terminus (black arrow head) which results in the removal of its signal peptide. **(b)**In a second proteolytic cleavage event by furin (blue arrow head), the precursor is separated into a large LAP or prodomain (gray) and the mature TGF-β (red) and **(c)**Schematic view of the closed ring structure (left) and unfastened straitjacket (right) conformation corresponding to the inactive LAP-TGF-β and mature TGF-β, respectively.

does not require the integrin cytoplasmic domain, but it is reported to require the presence of metalloproteinases (MMPs) on the cell surface or in the ECM [9]. Additionally, in T cells, αvβ6 and αvβ8 can activate LAP-TGF-β in cooperation with the glycoprotein-A repetitions predominant protein (GARP) [15, 16].

TGF-β is also activated by proteases. Aspartyl (e.g., cathepsin D) [17], cysteine (e.g., calpain) [18] and serine proteases (e.g., plasmin and kallikreins) and metalloproteases have shown to stimulate the release of chemokine from the latent complex, although most of these studies have been performed *in vitro* [19]. Moreover, TGF-β has been reported to be activated by other nonprotease mechanisms such as neuropilin1 (Nrp1), thrombospondin (TSP-1), F-spondin, pregnancy-specific beta-1-glycoprotein 1 (PSG1) and deglycosylation. Likewise, there are chemical and physical settings that activate TGF-β, for example, heat, ultraviolet radiation, physical shear, detergents and reactive oxygen species [8].

Three-dimensional structural studies of the LLC reveal that the RGD motifs are readily available for integrin engagement. Hydrophobic side chains, which have been identified near the RGD motif, likely enhance integrin binding [7]. In the presence of αvβ6, LLC can bind one or two integrin monomers. However, this binding does not induce required conformational changes to promote the complete activation of TGF-β, which is in agreement with prior mutational studies [12, 13, 20]. Furthermore, in accord with previous studies, the crystal structure of latent TGF-β predicts that pulling forces, emanating from the integrin C-terminal cytoplasmic tail that interacts with the cytoskeleton and binding RGD via the N-terminal extracellular region, are counteracted by associations with the ECM. Therefore, in the latent TGF-β, the straitjacket domain is maintained in a closed conformation until tensile forces are applied from both ends of the structure, resulting in loosening of the straitjacket domain and the release of the mature TGF-β. This study also showed that an additional feature of the prodomain is to prevent access to activating receptors [7].

2. TGF-β signaling pathways

Signaling is regulated by three major receptors: TGF-β receptor type I (TβRI), type II (TβRII) and type III (TβRIII). In general, TGF-β binds TβRIII, which facilitates its delivery to TβRII, a constitutively active kinase, leading to the subsequent phosphorylation and activation of TβRI. In humans, there are seven TβRIs, also known as activin receptor-like kinases (ALK), and five TβRIIs [5]. In most cells, ALK-5 forms a heterodimer with TβRII bound to TGF-β, which activates the ALK-5 kinase domain via phosphorylation of its GS domain. This receptor activation propagates intracellular signaling through 'canonical' effector proteins mothers against decapentaplegic homolog 2/SMAD family member 2 (Smad2) and Smad3, which are transcription factors. Once phosphorylated, these Smad proteins form a complex with Smad4 leading to nuclear translocation and initiation of genes transcription. In most normal cells, TGF-β-mediated activation of Smads leads to inhibition of cell growth. More specifically, the Smad2/3-4 complex partners with foxhead box O (FOXO) factors to activate p21Cip1 (*CDKN1A*), which inhibits cyclin-dependent kinase 1(CDK1), resulting in cell cycle arrest. Similarly, TGF-β can also activate p15Inkab (*CDKN2B*), the CDK4 inhibitor, through the SMAD2-3/4-FOXO1 axis (**Figure 2**) [5].

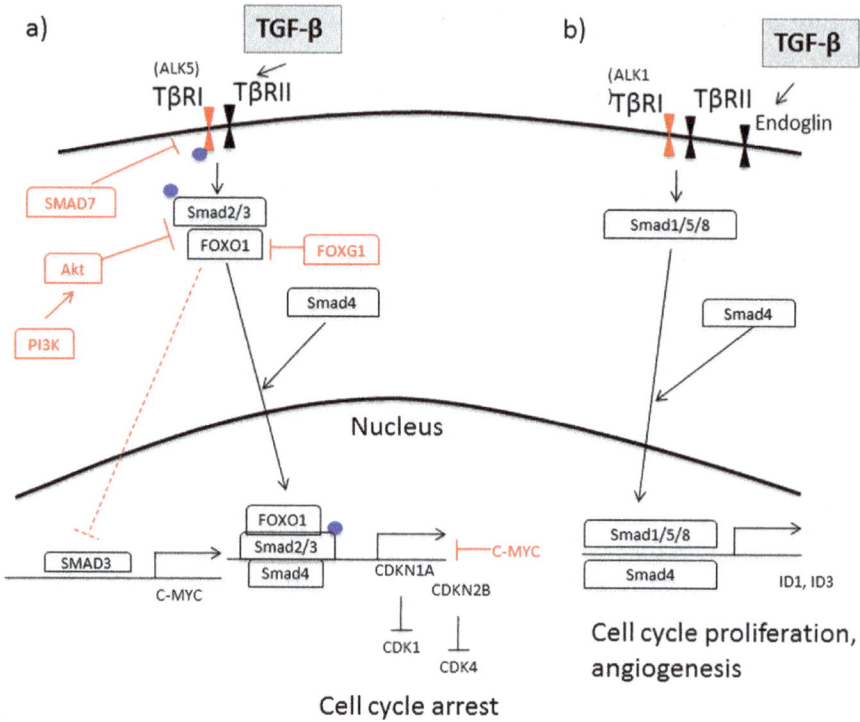

Figure 2. TGF-β canonical pathway. **(a)**In normal cells and early stages of cancer TGF-β promotes cell cycle arrest. Repressors of the pathway are shown in red. Blue dots represent protein phosphorylation and **(b)**in endothelial cells, an alternative pathway promotes cell proliferation.

Likewise, TGF-β acts as a cytostatic factor by decreasing c-Myc expression and downregulating the inhibitor of DNA-binding protein (ID) 1 and ID3 transcription factors. ID1 and ID3 are involved in differentiation, cell cycle progression and self-renewal of stem cells [21, 22]. TGF-β elicits c- Flk-1myc repression by promoting SMAD3 binding to a repressing Smad-binding element (RSBE) at the c-myc promoter [23]. c-Myc can be recruited to the promoters of *CDKN1A* and *CDKN2B* by the Myc-interacting zinc-finger (MIZ-1). This blocks CDK expression and results in apoptosis [24]. Additionally, in endothelial cells (ECs), TGF-β can target a second receptor type 1, ALK-1, which signals through Smad1/5/8 and stimulates angiogenic factors, such as interleukin 1 receptor-like 1 and ID1 (**Figure 2**) [25].

Several proteins are known to antagonize canonical TGF-β signaling. For example, (i) PI3K activates AKT which phosphorylates the SMADs-FOXO complex and inhibits its translocation to the nucleus [21], (ii) foxhead box G1 (FOXG1) inhibits the SMADs-FOXO complex [21], (iii) SMAD7 can trigger TβRI for proteosomal degradation by recruiting SMAD-specific E3 ubiquitin protein ligase (SMURF1) and SMURF2 [26], (iv) SMAD6 blocks SMAD1 through SMAD4 binding, (v) Erk proteins phosphorylate SMADs and inhibit their nuclear translocation, (vi) BAMBI, a pseudoreceptor, dimerizes with TβRI leading to its inactivation, (vii) FKBP12 binds to TβRI and impedes its phosphorylation, activation and signaling [27] and (viii) protein arginine N-methyltransferase 1 (PRMT1) methylates SMAD6 and allows BMP signaling through SMADs1/5 [28–30].

3. Vasculogenesis

During embryogenesis, the development of the vascular system is divided into three stages, vasculogenesis, angiogenesis and arteriogenesis. Vasculogenesis occurs in embryonic organs as well as extraembryonic tissues such as the placenta, yolk sac and allantois [31]. The earliest discernible structures in vasculogenesis, the blood islands, are formed in the mouse yolk sac by embryonic day (E) 6.5–7. This structure contains precursor cells or hemangioblasts, which differentiate to EC and hematopoietic cells [32]. At E8.5, cells located toward the periphery of the blood island, or angioblasts, differentiate into EC, while cells located toward the central region give rise to hematopoietic precursor cells. Next, lumenization takes place; tight junctions and basement membranes develop, and pericytes are recruited to blood vessels and promote maturation [33].

Several growth factors have been identified to regulate vasculogenesis, such as vascular endothelial growth factor (VEGF), fibroblast growth factor (FGF), the hedgehog family, neuropilins, integrins, fibronectin and TGF-βs. FGF-2 has been reported to participate in the generation of the angioblast in quail/chick chimeras and in vessel formation [34].

Hedgehog signaling has been shown to be crucial in the initial steps of vasculogenesis. It promotes differentiation of the primitive endoderm into both, endothelial and hematopoietic lineage [35]. For instance, blocking Indian hedgehog (Ihh) causes signaling repression from the visceral ectoderm and consequently abrogation of vasculogenesis and hematopoiesis in anterior epiblast [35]. Deletion of *Ihh* in mouse caused 50% lethality at midgestation with the remaining 50% dying at birth. Defects in blood vessel formation have been proposed as the cause for the lethality, which has been supported by experiments showing: (i) deletion of Sonic hedgehog (*Shh*) in mice resulted in a reduction in vascularization in lung [36], (ii) overexpression of *Shh* resulted in an increase in vascularization in neuroectoderm [37], (iii) depletion of *Shh* in zebrafish caused defective vasculature [38] and (iv) depletion of *Ihh* from stem cell-derived embroid bodies inhibited blood island differentiation [39].

VEGF signaling is crucial in vasculogenesis. Genetic studies have shown that deletion of *Flt-1* (VEGFR1), *Flk-1/KDR* (VEGFR2) and one or both alleles of *VEGF* cause embryonic lethality. VEGFR1 mutants exhibit aberrant central localization of the angioblasts in the blood island, instead of their normal localization toward the periphery [40]. These results implied that the growth of ECs was not inhibited in this region and led to the idea that VEGR1 hampers signaling from VEGF by ligand sequestration [33]. In addition, VEGFR2 mutants die around E9. In these embryos, both vasculogenesis and hematopoiesis do not initiate which was explained by faulty blood island in which cell migration was abrogated [41, 42]. Similarly, mutant heterozygous for VEGF die by E11 and showed impaired vasculogenesis and angiogenesis. These embryos showed severe abnormalities, such as underdeveloped brain and heart, decreased number of nucleated red blood cells in blood islands and aberrant vasculature in nervous system and placenta [43].

Neuropilins are co-receptors for VEGF receptors. Nrp1 is found in ECs of arteries, while neuropilin 2 (Nrp2) is found at the endothelium of lymphatic vessels and veins. Deletion of *Nrp1* in mice affects severely the central and peripheral nervous systems, as well as the yolk sac vasculature [44]. In contrast, depletion of *Nrp2* has no effects in the vasculature of arteries or veins, but it does affect angiogenesis of the lymphatic vasculature [45, 46]. In addition, mice harboring deletions in both neuropilins have shown obstruction in vasculogenesis in the yolk sac and in the formation of the primary vascular plexus [47].

4. Developmental angiogenesis

Angiogenesis is the formation of new blood vessels from existing vasculature. It occurs by mechanisms including sprouting angiogenesis and intussusceptive angiogenesis (**Figure 3**). Sprouting angiogenesis initiates with the selection of endothelial tip cells at the vessel wall. These cells react toward extracellular stimuli and secrete proteolytic enzymes to digest the surrounding ECM. Tip cells are connected to endothelial stalk cells to direct the vascular sprout [33, 48, 49]. Once the new tube is formed and a lumen is established, the vessel is stabilized by the recruitment of pericytes to capillaries or vascular smooth muscle cells (vSMC) to arteries and veins [6, 33], leading to re-establishment of mature blood vessels.

Intussusceptive angiogenesis, also known as splitting angiogenesis, results in the formation of intermediate intracapillary pillars. This mechanism is more efficient than sprouting angiogenesis since it does not require cell proliferation. Instead, it needs the reorganization of existing ECs. In this process, (i) ECs from opposite sides of the blood vessel make contacts, (ii) ECs from both ends reorganize and cause a splitting in the vessel wall, (iii) an interstitial pillar core is generated and (iv) myofibroblasts, pericytes and finally collagen invade the pillar and a basement membrane is formed [33, 49, 50].

a)   b)

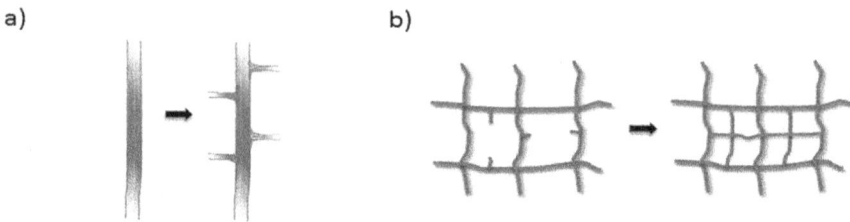

Figure 3. Mechanisms of angiogenesis. (**a**)Sprouting and (**b**)intussusceptive angiogenesis.

5. TGF-β in vasculogenesis and angiogenesis

5.1. Mutant phenotypes in mice lacking components of the TGF-B pathway

TGF-β mRNA was initially detected by PCR in preimplantation stages and in situ expression was present as early as E7.5, suggesting important roles in early development [51, 52]. In the embryo, proper TGF-β was detected in angioblast progenitors within the primitive heart mesoderm. Likewise, its expression was detected in extraembryonic tissues, including in the allantois mesoderm, and within blood islands of the yolk sac [53].

Deletion of the TGF-β1 gene in mice resulted in 50% lethality in utero, with the remaining 50% of mutant mice surviving up to three weeks postnatally. Histopathology analyses showed multifocal inflammatory cell infiltration and necrosis in several organs, especially the heart and stomach [53, 54]. It was subsequently shown that maternal contributions of *TGFB1* RNA and other genetic and epigenetic factors contributed to 50% postnatal survival [55].

The 50% of TGF-β mutants showed lethality and resorption by E10.5. Analysis of E8.5 embryos did not show significant morphological defects. However, analysis of E9.5 and E10.5 embryos resulted in a range of phenotypic defects within the yolk sac. While in some cases, vasculogenesis was delayed; in other cases, a dramatic reduction in size was observed and it was accompanied by weak and disorganized primary vessels, with some areas displaying complete vessel depletion. Analysis of the yolk sac vasculature indicated that the defects occurred during differentiation of ECs and hematopoietic cells. In contrast, the initial differentiation of mesodermal cells into ECs was not affected [52].

Genetic ablation of TβRII resulted in very similar phenotypes as in TGF-β1 mutants, with alterations in yolk sac vasculature and embryonic lethality by E10.5- E11.5 [56]. Mutants in endoglin also showed defects in vascular vessels within and outside the embryo. Embryo lethality was observed at E11.5, with mutants developing focal hemorrhage [57, 58]. Similarly, engineered mutations in mice that abrogate the expression of *ALK1, ALK5, SMAD1* or *SMAD5* resulted in defects in cardiovascular development [57, 59, 60].

5.2. Roles of TGF-β in angiogenesis

Early work to determine the roles for TGF-βs in ECs was contradictory. TGF-β signaling was initially found to inhibit cell migration and proliferation [61, 62], yet later studies indicated that it promotes cell proliferation [63–66]. The relative levels of expression of TGF-β seem to partially explain these discrepancies, with low doses promoting angiogenesis and higher levels resulting in growth inhibition of ECs and maturation of blood vessels [66, 67]. For instance, during blood vessel coverage by smooth muscle cells, TGF-β paracrine signaling from ECs to mesenchymal cells results in vascular smooth muscle cell and pericyte differentiation [6].

TGF-β also plays a role in the angiogenic process of hypoxic tissue. For instance, during infarction (stroke), neovascularization occurs primarily at the ischemic penumbra (periphery of the infarct), which correlates with high levels of both mRNA and active TGF-β protein [68]. Similarly, during organ transplant VEGF and TGF-β1, levels are increased in devascularized hypoxic tissue. TGF-β3 was also upregulated in hypoxic tissues, but to a lesser degree [69].

TGF-β regulates angiogenesis by different mechanisms; for example, it is involved in vessel proliferation and maturation by alternating two signaling cascades with opposite effects (ALK1 and ALK5). Likewise, TGF-β can promote its own expression, and it upregulates the expression of other angiogenic factors such as, platelet-derived growth factor (PDGF), interleukine-1, basic fibroblast growth factor (bFGF), tumor necrosis factor alpha and transforming growth factor alpha [70]. TGF-β can change the functions of other factors, such as VEGF, from prosurvival to pro-apoptotic [71]. Similarly, *in vitro* work has shown that in ECs TGF-β upregulates the expression of endothelin (*EDN1*), *PDGFA* and *PDGFB*, nitric oxide synthase

3 (*NOS3*), actin, alpha 2, smooth muscle, aorta (*ACTA2*), secreted protein acidic and cysteine rich (*SPARC*), *TSP-1*, fibronectin (*FN1*), collagens (*COL1A1, COL4A1,* and *COL5A1*), plasminogen activator (*PLAU*), serpin family E member 1 (*SERPINE1*) and integrins (*ITGB1, ITGB3, ITGAV, ITGA2* and *ITGA5*). It can also downregulate several genes, such as selectin-E (*SELE*), *KDR*, von Willebrand factor (*VWR*), thrombomodulin (*THBD*), monocyte chemo-attractant protein (*MCP1*), C-X-C motif chemokine ligand 1 (*CXCL1*), integrins (*ITGB1, ITGB3, ITGA5* and *ITGA6*), *TIMP1* and *PLAU* [70].

Levels of ALK1 and ALK5 determine TGF-β mitogenic or mitostatic responses in ECs. ALK5-Smad2/3 signaling stimulates transcription of ECM proteins such as fibronectin and plasminogen activator inhibitor type 1, which promote the resolution of angiogenesis by inducing vessel maturation. In contrast, signaling via the ALK1-Smad1/5/8 pathway generates anti-angiogenic responses [25, 51]. This requires a TGF-β accessory receptor, endoglin, which enhances ALK1 signaling and inhibits ALK5 cytostatic phenotype [72]. More recent work has shown that in the mouse eye retina the leucine-rich alpha-2-glycoprotein (Lrg1), which binds endoglin, promotes angiogenesis through Alk1-Smad1/5/8 in the presence of TGF-β [73].

5.2.1. TGF-β signaling in CNS development

In the mammalian CNS, neurons, astrocytes, pericytes and ECs closely interact to form a multicellular neurovascular unit [11]. During embryonic brain development, TGF-β is critical for sprouting angiogenesis of the CNS. In particular, TGF-β has been shown to work in conjunction with αv integrins to regulate paracrine signaling between neuroepithelial cells and ECs within neurovascular units. In mouse, embryos deletion of αv integrin showed vascular defects that were restricted mainly to the brain. This phenotype was recapitulated in β8 integrin mutant embryos. In contrast, deletion of β3 and β5 integrins did not cause brain vasculature abnormalities [74, 75]. Cell type-specific deletion of αv and β8 integrins in nervous system glial cells resulted in developmental intracerebral hemorrhage as well as postnatal motor dysfunction and seizures. Of note, the brain hemorrhage observed in embryos was absence in adult mice, suggesting that a compensatory mechanism that repairs hemorrhage occurs after birth [75, 76]. Interestingly, αv ablation in vascular ECs did not show a phenotype [75]. In later work, in which an outbred background was used to overcome the effects of β8−/− embryonic lethality, it was shown that adult mice lacking β8 integrin displayed neurovascular pathologies [77]. Most notably, adult β8 integrin mutants displayed a reduction in olfactory bulb size and abnormalities at the subventricular zone and rostral migratory stream. Neuroblasts generated in the subventricular zone utilize blood vessels as guides to migrate within the rostral migratory stream and differentiated to neurons within the olfactory bulbs. The size-reduced olfactory bulbs in adult β8−/− mice revealed essential roles for this integrin in promoting neuroblast migration along blood vessels. These defects correlated with a reduction in TGF-β signaling in neurospheres dissected from β8−/− mice [77].

The brain vascular defects observed in *Itgb8* null mutants are also shared by *Tgfb1* and *Tgfb3* loss of function mutants. In addition, mutating the integrin-binding RGD binding site in *Tgfb1* leads to early embryonic lethality [78]. Similarly, mice lacking both β6 and β8 integrins showed similar phenotypes as null mutants for *Tgfb1* and *Tgfb3* [78].

More recently, integrin β8 and Nrp1 have been shown to mediate neuroepithelial-endothelial cell interactions. β8 integrin in the neuroepithelium activates TGF-β signaling in ECs, while Nrp1 suppresses canonical TGF-β signaling, thus controlling normal sprouting angiogenesis [79]. Disruption of TGF-β signaling by targeting β8 integrin or Nrp1 results in excessive vessels sprouting and branching and formation of dysplastic glomeruloid-like vessels that are hemorrhagic [80].

The αvβ8-TGF-β connection in developmental angiogenesis in the brain also regulated neovascularization in the developing retina, where β8 integrin is expressed in astrocytes and Muller glial cells, a neuroepithelial cell type specifically found in the retina [81]. β8−/− retinas display abnormalities in the formation of the secondary vascular plexus, including impaired sprouting and formation of blood vessels with glomeruloid-like tufts. In addition, intraretinal hemorrhage was detected [81]. Furthermore, ablation of αv or β8 integrins but not of *Tgfbr2* in astrocytes resulted in defects in angiogenesis, and blocking TGF-β1 with neutralizing antibodies affected paracrine signaling to ECs [81]. This work was confirmed later in a study showing that *Tgfbr2* deletion in ECs of neonatal mice caused bleeding in the brain and vascular abnormalities, hemorrhage and deficiency in the formation of the deeper vascular network in the retina [82, 83]. Similarly, reduced Smad2 phosphorylation was observed in ECs from retina of *Tgfbr2* knockout mice [82].

6. TGF-β in pathological angiogenesis

Genetic mutations in TGF-β signaling components are associated with various human vascular pathologies. For example, mutations in the TβRIII/endoglin gene are linked to hereditary hemorrhagic telangiectasia (HHT) and Osler-Rendu-Weber syndrome. The disease is characterized, among others, by arteriovenous malformations (AVM) in the liver, brain and lung, telangiectases in skin and mucous membranes and recurrent epistaxis [84]. In trying to understand AVM, it was proposed that TGF-β paracrine signaling from ECs to vascular smooth muscle cells and/or pericytes was reduced. As a consequence, vascular smooth muscle cell differentiation was affected and this resulted in fragile, leaky blood vessels [85]. Alternatively, other suggested mechanisms underlying AVM endothelial cell apoptosis and depletion of smooth muscle cells [6]. In addition, it was discovered that brain AVM present decreased levels of integrin β8 which correlates with decreased TGF-β activation and signaling in ECs [86]. Mutations in human *ITGAV* and *ITGB8* genes also predispose some families to spontaneous brain hemorrhage [87].

In cancer, angiogenesis is not properly regulated as it occurs in developmental and physiological settings. Hypoxic conditions and proangiogenic factors released by tumor cells promote robust new blood vessel formation. The intratumoral vasculature is often disorganized and leaky with hypertension and acidosis. Similarly, tumor ECs display aneuploidy as well as centrosome and chromosomal amplifications [88]. The TGF-β pathway is affected by either mutations in the main signaling components, in particular SMADs, or by altered expression of repressive factors (e.g., FOXG1, PI3K-AKT and C-MYC) (**Figure 1**). Analysis of copy number alterations using data from The Center Genome Atlas (TCGA) and analyzed by cBioportal show that Smad2, 3 and 4 are mutated, deleted or amplified in several tumor types, but especially in pancreatic, colorectal and gastric cancers [89, 90].

During tumor growth and progression, TGF-β plays a dual role as both an angiogenic and angiostatic factor [6]. In early-stage tumors, higher TGF-β expression levels are correlative with a better prognosis. TGF-βs exert cell cycle arrest by downregulating c-Myc and Ids 1–3 in late G1 phase and by promoting the expression of cyclin-dependent protein kinase inhibitors [25]. As a proangiogenic factor, TGF-β pathway collaborates with VEGF, PDGF and bFGF in autocrine/paracrine signaling. In highly vascularized tumors, such as GBM and hepatocellular carcinoma (HCC), TGF-β levels are upregulated. In HCC cells, TGF-β induces the secretion of VEGF-A. Accordingly, inhibition of TGF-β by the TβRI/II synthetic kinase inhibitor LY2109761 showed decreased tumor size, vessel density and VEGF expression. This inhibitor also affected paracrine signaling between tumor cells and ECs. These effects on VEGF-A were dependent on SMAD2/3 expression levels [91]. Likewise, TGF-β inhibition in other cancer types such as colorectal cancer and GBM has also led to reduce intratumoral vascularization [59, 92–94]. Of note, the increase in angiogenesis caused by TGF-β in GBM was decreased by inhibition of the JNK pathway [95]. TGF-β family members also promote the secretion of MCP1 and TGF-α [96, 97], which impact inflammatory cells in the tumor microenvironment.

6.1. VEGF regulation by TGF-β

TGF-β promotes the expression of a major regulator of vasculogenesis and angiogenesis, VEGF. The VEGF family is comprised of a large group of secreted glycoproteins that interact with various cell surface receptors. VEGF-A is expressed as four different isoforms (121, 165, 189, 206 a.a.). Isoform 121 has low binding for heparan sulfate and diffuses away from its secreted location creating a chemogradient. Isoform 165 has higher affinity to heparan sulfate compared with 121, and it shows the highest mitogenic capacity among all isoforms. Finally, isoforms 189 and 206 have shown the highest binding capacity to bind heparan sulfates and are known to interact with other components of the ECM [33]. These ligands bind mainly three tyrosine kinase receptors (VEGFR) 1–3. VEGF-A has been a major therapeutic target in cancer due to its upregulation in many cancer types. Unfortunately, anti-angiogenic therapies that target VEGF-A, such as the neutralizing antibody Bevacizumab, have been unsuccessful in clinical studies where patients have shown resistance to anti-VEGF therapy. Similarly, in vitro studies performed in GBM cell lines indicated that irradiation enhances VEGF secretion [98–101].

FGF-2 induces VEGF expression in ECs via paracrine and autocrine signaling mechanisms [71]. TGF-β balances FGF-2 by suppressing the induction of plasminogen activator, a serine protease involved in the migration of cells, which is required in the formation of capillaries during angiogenesis [102]. In contrast, TGF-β induces ECs apoptosis as part of capillary remodeling and at the same time promotes ECs expression of VEGF [103]. VEGF-A is an ECs survival factor and protects ECs from apoptosis [104]. More recent work has shown that VEGF targets p38MAPK resulting in ECs survival. In contrast, in the presence of TGF-β, FGF-2 is activated, promoting VEGF upregulation, p38MAPK activation and apoptosis [71].

6.2. Upregulation of TGF-β in GBM

In GBM, an "angiogenic switch" marks the transition from low to more malignant tumors where ECs proliferate, resulting in a major increase in blood vessels. This excessive growth in vasculature was initially thought to be required for maintaining the aggressive growth rate of GBM. However, recent work suggests that these aberrant blood vessels are also required to maintain glioma stem cells (GSC), which are known to localize in close proximity to ECs in a perivascular niche. These cells secrete VEGF and express VEGFR2, and this complex is stabilized by NRP1. This axis is involved in the self-renewal, survival and tumorigenic capacity of GSCs [105]. Recent work has shown that TGF-β induces differentiation of GSCs into pericytes to support vessel formation and tumor growth [106].

TGF-β cooperates in glioma angiogenesis by enhancing the expression of FGF, VEGF, PDGF-β, and CD44. Increased expression of FGF promotes VEGF expression. High levels of TGF-β in gliomas correlate with poor prognosis, and it is known to work in conjunction with the PDGF-β to increase GSCs proliferation [107]. In vSMC, TGF-β expression increases the levels of PDGF-β, its receptor (βPDGFR) and of EGF receptor (EGFR). βPDGFR promotes VEGF expression and secretion in ECs and signals through PI3K [108].

Angiogenesis in GBM develops by two mechanisms: microvascular cell proliferation and sprouting. The origin of microvascular proliferation seems to arise from hypoxia, where cells migrate away from the hypoxic center as a result of an increase in the levels of migration-related genes. As a consequence, the center becomes necrotic and the cells surrounding it form a palisade, which secretes angiogenic factors such as VEGF. This promotes neighboring angiogenesis, known as glomeruloid-like microvascular proliferation, composed of both endothelial and smooth muscle cells. In contrast, the increase in angiogenic capillaries can be observed by staining with markers such as CD31 and Factor VIII-related antigen (**Figure** 4) [109].

TGF-β1-3 levels and endoglin-ALK1 signaling are elevated under hypoxic conditions. In addition, under hypoxia, *Snail* and *Slug* expression levels are increased. These genes are known to be involved in endothelial to mesenchymal transition and in sprouting angiogenesis and are regulated by TGF-β in ECs [110].

Integrins are important activators of the TGF-β pathway. They are important in regulating tumor angiogenesis by serving as receptors for ECM components, such as laminin, tenascin, fibronectin and collagens [111]. αvβ3 is a receptor for various secreted ECM proteins, such as von Willebrand factor, TSP-1, fibrinogen, proteolyzed collagen, fibronectin and vitronectin, and it is involved in angiogenesis and vascular remodeling. For instance, αvβ3 integrin associates with MMP-2 in blood vessels of melanoma tumors, and this binding facilitates collagen degradation in vitro [112]. In GBM, TGF-β enhances αvβ3 integrin adhesion and expression and promotes integrin-mediated motility [111].

αvβ8 is expressed in GBM cell lines and primary tumors samples. GBM cell lines overexpressing αvβ8 show an increase in proliferation but when injected into the brain generate tumors with a decrease in vascularity. Silencing αv or β8 integrin in transformed astrocytes or in human GBM cell lines leads to decreased in TGF-β signaling, resulting in increased tumor size, intratumoral hemorrhage and decreased tumor cell invasiveness [113, 114].

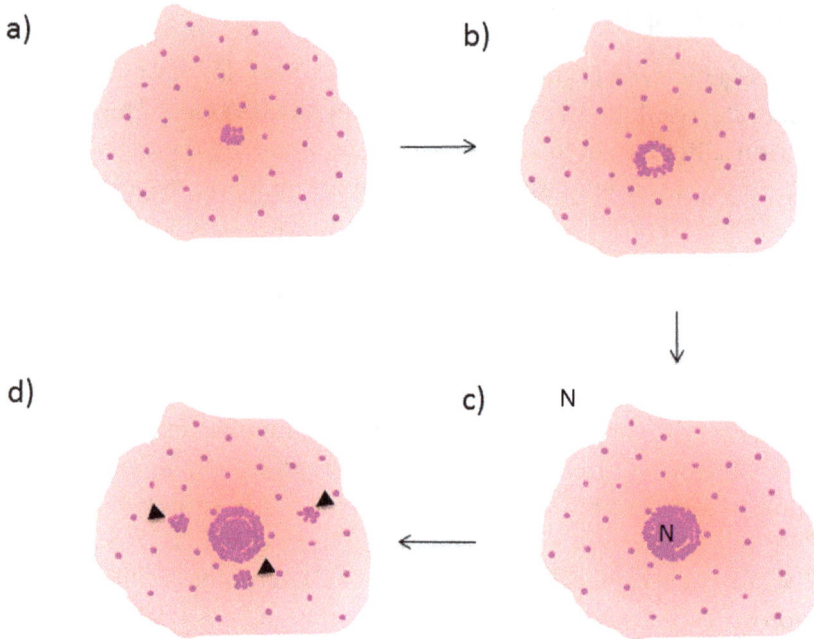

Figure 4. Microvascular proliferation. **(a)**Hypoxia center, **(b)**cell migration, **(c)**necrosis (N) and **(d)**glomeruloid microvascular proliferation (arrow heads).

In summary, TGF-β signaling is a crucial pathway in the angiogenesis of normal and tumor cells facilitating interactions between endothelial and epithelial cells. The vast majority of research has been focused on the activation of TGF-β, but more work is necessary to understand how the pathway is repressed. This could help to move forward current therapeutic attempts to target components of the TGF-β signaling pathway.

Author details

Paola A. Guerrero and Joseph H. McCarty*

*Address all correspondence to: jhmccarty@mdanderson.org

Department of Neurosurgery, University of Texas MD Anderson Cancer Center, Houston, TX, USA

References

[1] de Larco JE, Todaro GJ. Growth factors from murine sarcoma virus-transformed cells. Proceedings of the National Academy of Sciences of the United States of America. 1978;75(8):4001–5.

[2] Moses HL, Branum EL, Proper JA, Robinson RA. Transforming growth factor production by chemically transformed cells. Cancer Research. 1981;41(7):2842–8.

[3] Roberts AB, Anzano MA, Lamb LC, Smith JM, Sporn MB. New class of transforming growth factors potentiated by epidermal growth factor: isolation from non-neoplastic tissues. Proceedings of the National Academy of Sciences of the United States of America. 1981;78(9):5339–43.

[4] Moses HL, Roberts AB, Derynch R. The Discovery and Early Days of TGF-B: A Historical Perspective. Cold Spring Harbor Perspectives in Biology. 2016; 8(7): pii: a021865.

[5] Massague J. TGFbeta signalling in context. Nature Reviews Molecular Cell Biology. 2012;13(10):616–30.

[6] ten Dijke P, Arthur HM. Extracellular control of TGFbeta signalling in vascular development and disease. Nature Reviews Molecular Cell Biology. 2007;8(11):857–69.

[7] Shi M, Zhu J, Wang R, Chen X, Mi L, Walz T, et al. Latent TGF-beta structure and activation. Nature. 2011;474(7351):343–9.

[8] Robertson IB, Rifkin DB. Regulation of the bioavailability of TGF-beta and TGF-beta related proteins. Cold Spring Harbor Perspectives in Biology. 2016;8(6).pii: a021907

[9] Mu D, Cambier S, Fjellbirkeland L, Baron JL, Munger JS, Kawakatsu H, et al. The integrin alpha(v)beta8 mediates epithelial homeostasis through MT1-MMP-dependent activation of TGF-beta1. Journal of Cell Biology. 2002;157(3):493–507.

[10] Ludbrook SB, Barry ST, Delves CJ, Horgan CM. The integrin alphavbeta3 is a receptor for the latency-associated peptides of transforming growth factors beta1 and beta3. Biochemical Journal. 2003;369(Pt 2):311–8.

[11] McCarty JH. Integrin-mediated regulation of neurovascular development, physiology and disease. Cell Adhesion & Migration. 2009;3(2):211–5.

[12] Munger JS, Huang X, Kawakatsu H, Griffiths MJ, Dalton SL, Wu J, et al. The integrin alpha v beta 6 binds and activates latent TGF beta 1: a mechanism for regulating pulmonary inflammation and fibrosis. Cell. 1999;96(3):319–28.

[13] Annes JP, Chen Y, Munger JS, Rifkin DB. Integrin alphaVbeta6-mediated activation of latent TGF-beta requires the latent TGF-beta binding protein-1. Journal of Cell Biology. 2004;165(5):723–34.

[14] Fontana L, Chen Y, Prijatelj P, Sakai T, Fassler R, Sakai LY, et al. Fibronectin is required for integrin alphavbeta6-mediated activation of latent TGF-beta complexes containing LTBP-1. FASEB Journal: Official Publication of the Federation of American Societies for Experimental Biology. 2005;19(13):1798–808.

[15] Wang R, Zhu J, Dong X, Shi M, Lu C, Springer TA. GARP regulates the bioavailability and activation of TGFbeta. Molecular Biology of the Cell. 2012;23(6):1129–39.

[16] Edwards JP, Thornton AM, Shevach EM. Release of active TGF-beta1 from the latent TGF-beta1/GARP complex on T regulatory cells is mediated by integrin beta8. Journal of Immunology. 2014;193(6):2843–9.

[17] Lyons RM, Keski-Oja J, Moses HL. Proteolytic activation of latent transforming growth factor-beta from fibroblast-conditioned medium. Journal of Cell Biology. 1988;106(5):1659–65.

[18] Abe M, Oda N, Sato Y. Cell-associated activation of latent transforming growth factor-beta by calpain. Journal of Cellular Physiology. 1998;174(2):186–93.

[19] Maeda S, Dean DD, Gay I, Schwartz Z, Boyan BD. Activation of latent transforming growth factor beta1 by stromelysin 1 in extracts of growth plate chondrocyte-derived matrix vesicles. Journal of Bone and Mineral Research: The Official Journal of the American Society for Bone and Mineral Research. 2001;16(7):1281–90.

[20] Wipff PJ, Hinz B. Integrins and the activation of latent transforming growth factor beta1 — an intimate relationship. European Journal of Cell Biology. 2008;87(8–9):601–15.

[21] Seoane J, Le HV, Shen L, Anderson SA, Massague J. Integration of Smad and forkhead pathways in the control of neuroepithelial and glioblastoma cell proliferation. Cell. 2004;117(2):211–23.

[22] Anido J, Saez-Borderias A, Gonzalez-Junca A, Rodon L, Folch G, Carmona MA, et al. TGF-beta receptor inhibitors target the CD44(high)/Id1(high) glioma-initiating cell population in human glioblastoma. Cancer Cell. 2010;18(6):655–68.

[23] Frederick JP, Liberati NT, Waddell DS, Shi Y, Wang XF. Transforming growth beta-mediated transcriptional repression of c-myc is dependent on direct binding of Smad3 to a novel repressive Smad binding element. Molecular and Cellular Biology. 2004;24(6):2546–59.

[24] Seoane J, Le HV, Massague J. Myc suppression of the p21(Cip1) Cdk inhibitor influences the outcome of the p53 response to DNA damage. Nature. 2002;419(6908):729–34.

[25] Tian M, Neil JR, Schiemann WP. Transforming growth factor-beta and the hallmarks of cancer. Cellular Signalling. 2011;23(6):951–62.

[26] Yan X, Liu Z, Chen Y. Regulation of TGF-beta signaling by Smad7. Acta Biochimica et Biophysica Sinica. 2009;41(4):263–72.

[27] Massague J, Wotton D. Transcriptional control by the TGF-beta/Smad signaling system. EMBO Journal. 2000;19(8):1745–54.

[28] Xu J, Derynck R. Does Smad6 methylation control BMP signaling in cancer? Cell Cycle. 2014;13(8):1209–10.

[29] Xu J, Wang AH, Oses-Prieto J, Makhijani K, Katsuno Y, Pei M, et al. Arginine methylation initiates BMP-induced Smad signaling. Molecular Cell. 2013;51(1):5–19.

[30] Choy L, Skillington J, Derynck R. Roles of autocrine TGF-beta receptor and Smad signaling in adipocyte differentiation. Journal of Cell Biology. 2000;149(3):667–82.

[31] Caprioli A, Minko K, Drevon C, Eichmann A, Dieterlen-Lievre F, Jaffredo T. Hemangioblast commitment in the avian allantois: cellular and molecular aspects. Developmental Biology. 2001;238(1):64–78.

[32] Choi K, Kennedy M, Kazarov A, Papadimitriou JC, Keller G. A common precursor for hematopoietic and endothelial cells. Development. 1998;125(4):725–32.

[33] Patel-Hett S, D'Amore PA. Signal transduction in vasculogenesis and developmental angiogenesis. International Journal of Developmental Biology. 2011;55(4–5):353–63.

[34] Cox CM, Poole TJ. Angioblast differentiation is influenced by the local environment: FGF-2 induces angioblasts and patterns vessel formation in the quail embryo. Developmental Dynamics: An Official Publication of the American Association of Anatomists. 2000;218(2):371–82.

[35] Dyer MA, Farrington SM, Mohn D, Munday JR, Baron MH. Indian hedgehog activates hematopoiesis and vasculogenesis and can respecify prospective neurectodermal cell fate in the mouse embryo. Development. 2001;128(10):1717–30.

[36] Pepicelli CV, Lewis PM, McMahon AP. Sonic hedgehog regulates branching morphogenesis in the mammalian lung. Current Biology: CB. 1998;8(19):1083–6.

[37] Rowitch DH, B SJ, Lee SM, Flax JD, Snyder EY, McMahon AP. Sonic hedgehog regulates proliferation and inhibits differentiation of CNS precursor cells. Journal of Neuroscience: The Official Journal of the Society for Neuroscience. 1999;19(20):8954–65.

[38] Brown LA, Rodaway AR, Schilling TF, Jowett T, Ingham PW, Patient RK, et al. Insights into early vasculogenesis revealed by expression of the ETS-domain transcription factor Fli-1 in wild-type and mutant zebrafish embryos. Mechanisms of Development. 2000;90(2):237–52.

[39] Byrd N, Becker S, Maye P, Narasimhaiah R, St-Jacques B, Zhang X, et al. Hedgehog is required for murine yolk sac angiogenesis. Development. 2002;129(2):361–72.

[40] Fong GH, Rossant J, Gertsenstein M, Breitman ML. Role of the Flt-1 receptor tyrosine kinase in regulating the assembly of vascular endothelium. Nature. 1995;376(6535):66–70.

[41] Shalaby F, Rossant J, Yamaguchi TP, Gertsenstein M, Wu XF, Breitman ML, et al. Failure of blood-island formation and vasculogenesis in Flk-1-deficient mice. Nature. 1995;376(6535):62–6.

[42] Shalaby F, Ho J, Stanford WL, Fischer KD, Schuh AC, Schwartz L, et al. A requirement for Flk1 in primitive and definitive hematopoiesis and vasculogenesis. Cell. 1997;89(6):981–90.

[43] Ferrara N, Carver-Moore K, Chen H, Dowd M, Lu L, O'Shea KS, et al. Heterozygous embryonic lethality induced by targeted inactivation of the VEGF gene. Nature. 1996;380(6573):439–42.

[44] Kawasaki T, Kitsukawa T, Bekku Y, Matsuda Y, Sanbo M, Yagi T, et al. A requirement for neuropilin-1 in embryonic vessel formation. Development. 1999;126(21):4895–902.

[45] Chen H, Bagri A, Zupicich JA, Zou Y, Stoeckli E, Pleasure SJ, et al. Neuropilin-2 regulates the development of selective cranial and sensory nerves and hippocampal mossy fiber projections. Neuron. 2000;25(1):43–56.

[46] Giger RJ, Cloutier JF, Sahay A, Prinjha RK, Levengood DV, Moore SE, et al. Neuropilin-2 is required in vivo for selective axon guidance responses to secreted semaphorins. Neuron. 2000;25(1):29–41.

[47] Takashima S, Kitakaze M, Asakura M, Asanuma H, Sanada S, Tashiro F, et al. Targeting of both mouse neuropilin-1 and neuropilin-2 genes severely impairs developmental yolk sac and embryonic angiogenesis. Proceedings of the National Academy of Sciences of the United States of America. 2002;99(6):3657–62.

[48] Adams RH, Alitalo K. Molecular regulation of angiogenesis and lymphangiogenesis. Nature Reviews Molecular Cell Biology. 2007;8(6):464–78.

[49] Ribatti D, Nico B, Crivellato E. Morphological and molecular aspects of physiological vascular morphogenesis. Angiogenesis. 2009;12(2):101–11.

[50] Adair TH, Montani JP. Angiogenesis. Integrated Systems Physiology: from Molecule to Function to Disease. San Rafael (CA) 2010.

[51] Rossant J, Howard L. Signaling pathways in vascular development. Annual Review of Cell and Developmental Biology. 2002;18:541–73.

[52] Dickson MC, Martin JS, Cousins FM, Kulkarni AB, Karlsson S, Akhurst RJ. Defective haematopoiesis and vasculogenesis in transforming growth factor-beta 1 knockout mice. Development. 1995;121(6):1845–54.

[53] Akhurst RJ, Lehnert SA, Faissner A, Duffie E. TGF beta in murine morphogenetic processes: the early embryo and cardiogenesis. Development. 1990;108(4):645–56.

[54] Shull MM, Ormsby I, Kier AB, Pawlowski S, Diebold RJ, Yin M, et al. Targeted disruption of the mouse transforming growth factor-beta 1 gene results in multifocal inflammatory disease. Nature. 1992;359(6397):693–9.

[55] Letterio JJ, Geiser AG, Kulkarni AB, Roche NS, Sporn MB, Roberts AB. Maternal rescue of transforming growth factor-beta 1 null mice. Science. 1994;264(5167):1936–8.

[56] Oshima M, Oshima H, Taketo MM. TGF-beta receptor type II deficiency results in defects of yolk sac hematopoiesis and vasculogenesis. Developmental Biology. 1996;179(1):297–302.

[57] Arthur HM, Ure J, Smith AJ, Renforth G, Wilson DI, Torsney E, et al. Endoglin, an ancillary TGFbeta receptor, is required for extraembryonic angiogenesis and plays a key role in heart development. Developmental Biology. 2000;217(1):42–53.

[58] Li DY, Sorensen LK, Brooke BS, Urness LD, Davis EC, Taylor DG, et al. Defective angiogenesis in mice lacking endoglin. Science. 1999;284(5419):1534–7.

[59] Neuzillet C, Tijeras-Raballand A, Cohen R, Cros J, Faivre S, Raymond E, et al. Targeting the TGFbeta pathway for cancer therapy. Pharmacology & Therapeutics [Internet]. 2015;147:22–31 pp. Available from: http://www.ncbi.nlm.nih.gov/pubmed/25444759.

[60] Lechleider RJ, Ryan JL, Garrett L, Eng C, Deng C, Wynshaw-Boris A, et al. Targeted mutagenesis of Smad1 reveals an essential role in chorioallantoic fusion. Developmental Biology. 2001;240(1):157–67.

[61] Baird A, Durkin T. Inhibition of endothelial cell proliferation by type beta-transforming growth factor: interactions with acidic and basic fibroblast growth factors. Biochemical and Biophysical Research Communications. 1986;138(1):476–82.

[62] Frater-Schroder M, Muller G, Birchmeier W, Bohlen P. Transforming growth factor-beta inhibits endothelial cell proliferation. Biochemical and Biophysical Research Communications. 1986;137(1):295–302.

[63] Iruela-Arispe ML, Sage EH. Endothelial cells exhibiting angiogenesis in vitro proliferate in response to TGF-beta 1. Journal of Cellular Biochemistry. 1993;52(4):414–30.

[64] Sutton AB, Canfield AE, Schor SL, Grant ME, Schor AM. The response of endothelial cells to TGF beta-1 is dependent upon cell shape, proliferative state and the nature of the substratum. Journal of Cell Science. 1991;99 (Pt 4):777–87.

[65] RayChaudhury A, D'Amore PA. Endothelial cell regulation by transforming growth factor-beta. Journal of Cellular Biochemistry. 1991;47(3):224–9.

[66] Li C, Guo B, Bernabeu C, Kumar S. Angiogenesis in breast cancer: the role of transforming growth factor beta and CD105. Microscopy Research and Technique. 2001;52(4):437–49.

[67] Hofer E, Schweighofer B. Signal transduction induced in endothelial cells by growth factor receptors involved in angiogenesis. Thrombosis and Haemostasis. 2007;97(3):355–63.

[68] Krupinski J, Kumar P, Kumar S, Kaluza J. Increased expression of TGF-beta 1 in brain tissue after ischemic stroke in humans. Stroke; A Journal of Cerebral Circulation. 1996;27(5):852–7.

[69] Dissen GA, Lara HE, Fahrenbach WH, Costa ME, Ojeda SR. Immature rat ovaries become revascularized rapidly after autotransplantation and show a gonadotropin-dependent increase in angiogenic factor gene expression. Endocrinology. 1994;134(3):1146–54.

[70] Pepper MS. Transforming growth factor-beta: vasculogenesis, angiogenesis, and vessel wall integrity. Cytokine & Growth Factor Reviews. 1997;8(1):21–43.

[71] Ferrari G, Pintucci G, Seghezzi G, Hyman K, Galloway AC, Mignatti P. VEGF, a pro-survival factor, acts in concert with TGF-beta1 to induce endothelial cell apoptosis. Proceedings of the National Academy of Sciences of the United States of America. 2006;103(46):17260–5.

[72] Lebrin F, Goumans MJ, Jonker L, Carvalho RL, Valdimarsdottir G, Thorikay M, et al. Endoglin promotes endothelial cell proliferation and TGF-beta/ALK1 signal transduction. EMBO Journal. 2004;23(20):4018–28.

[73] Wang X, Abraham S, McKenzie JA, Jeffs N, Swire M, Tripathi VB, et al. LRG1 promotes angiogenesis by modulating endothelial TGF-beta signalling. Nature. 2013;499(7458):306–11.

[74] McCarty JH, Monahan-Earley RA, Brown LF, Keller M, Gerhardt H, Rubin K, et al. Defective associations between blood vessels and brain parenchyma lead to cerebral hemorrhage in mice lacking alpha v integrins. Molecular and Cellular Biology. 2002;22(21):7667–77.

[75] McCarty JH, Lacy-Hulbert A, Charest A, Bronson RT, Crowley D, Housman D, et al. Selective ablation of alphav integrins in the central nervous system leads to cerebral hemorrhage, seizures, axonal degeneration and premature death. Development. 2005;132(1):165–76.

[76] Proctor JM, Zang K, Wang D, Wang R, Reichardt LF. Vascular development of the brain requires beta8 integrin expression in the neuroepithelium. Journal of Neuroscience: The Official Journal of the Society for Neuroscience. 2005;25(43):9940–8.

[77] Mobley AK, Tchaicha JH, Shin J, Hossain MG, McCarty JH. Beta8 integrin regulates neurogenesis and neurovascular homeostasis in the adult brain. Journal of Cell Science. 2009;122(Pt 11):1842–51.

[78] Aluwihare P, Mu Z, Zhao Z, Yu D, Weinreb PH, Horan GS, et al. Mice that lack activity of alphavbeta6- and alphavbeta8-integrins reproduce the abnormalities of Tgfb1- and Tgfb3-null mice. Journal of Cell Science. 2009;122(Pt 2):227–32.

[79] Hirota S, Clements TP, Tang LK, Morales JE, Lee HS, Oh SP, et al. Neuropilin 1 balances beta8 integrin-activated TGFbeta signaling to control sprouting angiogenesis in the brain. Development. 2015;142(24):4363–73.

[80] Glinka Y, Stoilova S, Mohammed N, Prud'homme GJ. Neuropilin-1 exerts co-receptor function for TGF-beta-1 on the membrane of cancer cells and enhances responses to both latent and active TGF-beta. Carcinogenesis. 2011;32(4):613–21.

[81] Hirota S, Liu Q, Lee HS, Hossain MG, Lacy-Hulbert A, McCarty JH. The astrocyte-expressed integrin alphavbeta8 governs blood vessel sprouting in the developing retina. Development. 2011;138(23):5157–66.

[82] Allinson KR, Lee HS, Fruttiger M, McCarty JH, Arthur HM. Endothelial expression of TGFbeta type II receptor is required to maintain vascular integrity during postnatal development of the central nervous system. PLoS One. 2012;7(6):e39336.

[83] Nguyen HL, Lee YJ, Shin J, Lee E, Park SO, McCarty JH, et al. TGF-beta signaling in endothelial cells, but not neuroepithelial cells, is essential for cerebral vascular development. Laboratory Investigation; A Journal of Technical Methods and Pathology. 2011;91(11):1554–63.

[84] Marchuk DA, Srinivasan S, Squire TL, Zawistowski JS. Vascular morphogenesis: tales of two syndromes. Human Molecular Genetics. 2003;12(Spec No 1):R97–112.

[85] Carvalho RL, Jonker L, Goumans MJ, Larsson J, Bouwman P, Karlsson S, et al. Defective paracrine signalling by TGFbeta in yolk sac vasculature of endoglin mutant mice: a paradigm for hereditary haemorrhagic telangiectasia. Development. 2004;131(24):6237–47.

[86] Su H, Kim H, Pawlikowska L, Kitamura H, Shen F, Cambier S, et al. Reduced expression of integrin alphavbeta8 is associated with brain arteriovenous malformation pathogenesis. American Journal of Pathology. 2010;176(2):1018–27.

[87] Dardiotis E, Siokas V, Zafeiridis T, Paterakis K, Tsivgoulis G, Dardioti M, et al. Integrins AV and B8 gene polymorphisms and risk for intracerebral hemorrhage in Greek and Polish populations. Neuromolecular Medicine. 2016.

[88] Chung AS, Ferrara N. Targeting the tumor microenvironment with SRC kinase inhibition. Clinical Cancer Research: An Official Journal of the American Association for Cancer Research. 2010;16(3):775–7.

[89] Cerami E, Gao J, Dogrusoz U, Gross BE, Sumer SO, Aksoy BA, et al. The cBio cancer genomics portal: an open platform for exploring multidimensional cancer genomics data. Cancer Discovery. 2012;2(5):401–4.

[90] Gao J, Aksoy BA, Dogrusoz U, Dresdner G, Gross B, Sumer SO, et al. Integrative analysis of complex cancer genomics and clinical profiles using the cBioPortal. Science Signaling. 2013;6(269):pl1.

[91] Mazzocca A, Fransvea E, Lavezzari G, Antonaci S, Giannelli G. Inhibition of transforming growth factor beta receptor I kinase blocks hepatocellular carcinoma growth through neo-angiogenesis regulation. Hepatology. 2009;50(4):1140–51.

[92] Akbari A, Amanpour S, Muhammadnejad S, Ghahremani MH, Ghaffari SH, Dehpour AR, et al. Evaluation of antitumor activity of a TGF-beta receptor I inhibitor (SD-208) on human colon adenocarcinoma. Daru: Journal of Faculty of Pharmacy, Tehran University of Medical Sciences. 2014;22:47.

[93] Zhang M, Herion TW, Timke C, Han N, Hauser K, Weber KJ, et al. Trimodal glioblastoma treatment consisting of concurrent radiotherapy, temozolomide, and the novel TGF-beta receptor I kinase inhibitor LY2109761. Neoplasia. 2011;13(6):537–49.

[94] Zhang M, Kleber S, Rohrich M, Timke C, Han N, Tuettenberg J, et al. Blockade of TGF-beta signaling by the TGFbetaR-I kinase inhibitor LY2109761 enhances radiation response and prolongs survival in glioblastoma. Cancer Research. 2011;71(23):7155–67.

[95] Yang XJ, Chen GL, Yu SC, Xu C, Xin YH, Li TT, et al. TGF-beta1 enhances tumor-induced angiogenesis via JNK pathway and macrophage infiltration in an improved zebrafish embryo/xenograft glioma model. International Immunopharmacology. 2013;15(2):191–8.

[96] Deckers MM, van Bezooijen RL, van der Horst G, Hoogendam J, van Der Bent C, Papapoulos SE, et al. Bone morphogenetic proteins stimulate angiogenesis through osteoblast-derived vascular endothelial growth factor A. Endocrinology. 2002;143(4):1545–53.

[97]   Ma J, Wang Q, Fei T, Han JD, Chen YG. MCP-1 mediates TGF-beta-induced angiogenesis by stimulating vascular smooth muscle cell migration. Blood. 2007;109(3):987–94.

[98]   Hovinga KE, Stalpers LJ, van Bree C, Donker M, Verhoeff JJ, Rodermond HM, et al. Radiation-enhanced vascular endothelial growth factor (VEGF) secretion in glioblastoma multiforme cell lines—a clue to radioresistance? Journal of Neuro-oncology. 2005;74(2):99–103.

[99]   Lund EL, Hog A, Olsen MW, Hansen LT, Engelholm SA, Kristjansen PE. Differential regulation of VEGF, HIF1alpha and angiopoietin-1, -2 and -4 by hypoxia and ionizing radiation in human glioblastoma. International Journal of Cancer. 2004;108(6):833–8.

[100] Gupta VK, Jaskowiak NT, Beckett MA, Mauceri HJ, Grunstein J, Johnson RS, et al. Vascular endothelial growth factor enhances endothelial cell survival and tumor radioresistance. Cancer Journal. 2002;8(1):47–54.

[101] Harmey JH, Bouchier-Hayes D. Vascular endothelial growth factor (VEGF), a survival factor for tumour cells: implications for anti-angiogenic therapy. BioEssays: News and Reviews in Molecular, Cellular and Developmental Biology. 2002;24(3):280–3.

[102] Saksela O, Moscatelli D, Rifkin DB. The opposing effects of basic fibroblast growth factor and transforming growth factor beta on the regulation of plasminogen activator activity in capillary endothelial cells. Journal of Cell Biology. 1987;105(2):957–63.

[103] Pollman MJ, Naumovski L, Gibbons GH. Endothelial cell apoptosis in capillary network remodeling. Journal of Cellular Physiology. 1999;178(3):359–70.

[104] Bostrom K, Zebboudj AF, Yao Y, Lin TS, Torres A. Matrix GLA protein stimulates VEGF expression through increased transforming growth factor-beta1 activity in endothelial cells. Journal of Biological Chemistry. 2004;279(51):52904–13.

[105] Hamerlik P, Lathia JD, Rasmussen R, Wu Q, Bartkova J, Lee M, et al. Autocrine VEGF-VEGFR2-Neuropilin-1 signaling promotes glioma stem-like cell viability and tumor growth. Journal of Experimental Medicine. 2012;209(3):507–20.

[106] Cheng L, Huang Z, Zhou W, Wu Q, Donnola S, Liu JK, et al. Glioblastoma stem cells generate vascular pericytes to support vessel function and tumor growth. Cell. 2013;153(1):139–52.

[107] Bruna A, Darken RS, Rojo F, Ocana A, Penuelas S, Arias A, et al. High TGFbeta-Smad activity confers poor prognosis in glioma patients and promotes cell proliferation depending on the methylation of the PDGF-B gene. Cancer Cell. 2007;11(2):147–60.

[108] Roy LO, Poirier MB, Fortin D. Transforming growth factor-beta and its implication in the malignancy of gliomas. Targeted Oncology. 2015;10(1):1–14.

109]   Louis DN. Molecular pathology of malignant gliomas. Annual Review of Pathology. 2006;1:97–117.

[110] Doerr M, Morrison J, Bergeron L, Coomber BL, Viloria-Petit A. Differential effect of hypoxia on early endothelial-mesenchymal transition response to transforming growth beta isoforms 1 and 2. Microvascular Research. 2016;108:48–63.

[111] Platten M, Wick W, Wild-Bode C, Aulwurm S, Dichgans J, Weller M. Transforming growth factors beta(1) (TGF-beta(1)) and TGF-beta(2) promote glioma cell migration via Up-regulation of alpha(V)beta(3) integrin expression. Biochemical and Biophysical Research Communications. 2000;268(2):607–11.

[112] Brooks PC, Stromblad S, Sanders LC, von Schalscha TL, Aimes RT, Stetler-Stevenson WG, et al. Localization of matrix metalloproteinase MMP-2 to the surface of invasive cells by interaction with integrin alpha v beta 3. Cell. 1996;85(5):683–93.

[113] Tchaicha JH, Mobley AK, Hossain MG, Aldape KD, McCarty JH. A mosaic mouse model of astrocytoma identifies alphavbeta8 integrin as a negative regulator of tumor angiogenesis. Oncogene. 2010;29(31):4460–72.

[114] Tchaicha JH, Reyes SB, Shin J, Hossain MG, Lang FF, McCarty JH. Glioblastoma angiogenesis and tumor cell invasiveness are differentially regulated by beta8 integrin. Cancer Research. 2011;71(20):6371–81.

9

VEGF-Mediated Signal Transduction in Tumor Angiogenesis

Lucia Napione, Maria Alvaro and Federico Bussolino

Abstract

The vascular endothelial growth factor-A (VEGF) plays a crucial role in tumor angiogenesis. Through its primary receptor VEGFR-2, VEGF exerts the activity of a multitasking cytokine, which is able to stimulate endothelial cell survival, invasion and migration into surrounding tissues, proliferation, as well as vascular permeability and inflammation. The core components of VEGF signaling delineate well-defined intracellular routes. However, the whole scenario is complicated by the fact that cascades of signals converge and branch at many points in VEGF signaling, thus depicting a complex signal transduction network that is also finely regulated by different mechanisms. In this chapter, we present a careful collection of the best-characterized VEGF-induced signal transduction pathways, attempting to offer an overview of the complexity of VEGF signaling in the context of tumor angiogenesis.

Keywords: VEGF, signaling, angiogenesis, endothelial cells

1. Introduction

It has been over four decades that Judah Folkman hypothesized, demonstrated and emphasized the critical importance of angiogenesis in tumor growth [1]. His experimental studies showed that in the absence of vascularization a tumor would grow only to a finite size of few thousand cells, restricted by the inability of oxygen and nutrients to penetrate the tissue beyond the diffusion limits of approximately 1–2 mm. To overcome this passive diffusion-limited size, the tumor must perturb the physiological state of its environment inducing the so-called angiogenic switch that implicates the transition from quiescent to active endothelium leading to the vascularization of the growing cell mass. The angiogenic switch was initially hypothesized to be triggered by the production and release of a growth factor called TAF (tumor angiogenesis factor) by tumor cells [2]. Indeed, the explosive growth in tumor angiogenesis research identified and characterized a number of angiogenic inducers. Among them, vascular endothelial growth factor (VEGF) is recognized as the major tumor angiogenesis factor [3].

VEGF family consists of five secreted proteins (VEGF-A, VEGF-B, VEGF-C, VEGF-D and placental growth factor). In terms of endothelial biology and tumor angiogenesis, VEGF-A (hereafter referred as VEGF)—in particular VEGF-A$_{165}$—is considered to be the most physiologically relevant form. VEGF angiogenic potential is strictly dependent on its multifunctional activity. Indeed, the coordinated arrangement of endothelial cells to form and maintain new vascular tubes requires the induction of vascular permeability, endothelial cell migration, proliferation and survival. These biological responses take place in the endothelium via a complex network of intracellular signal transduction pathways, mainly mediated by VEGF-induced VEGF receptor 2 (VEGFR-2) activation [4].

In this chapter, after a short historical synopsis of Judah Folkman's hypotheses and main discoveries in the field of tumor angiogenesis, we will present a careful collection of the best characterized VEGF-induced signal transduction mechanisms, attempting to offer an overview of the complexity of VEGF signaling. The most intriguing aspect is that cascades of kinases, activity of other enzymes and recruitment of adapter proteins converge and branch at many points in VEGF signaling, emphasizing how linear pathways can integrate to form a complex signal transduction network. If multitasking and integrated signaling go some way toward an understanding of the functional versatility of VEGF, it becomes quite complicated to elucidate how specific information is processed through these pathways and how signaling events are regulated in order to trigger a specific cellular behavior.

2. Historical synopsis of Judah Folkman's hypotheses and main discoveries in the field of tumor angiogenesis

Judah Folkman's scientific achievements in angiogenesis research revolutionized biomedical research and clinical drug development. Until the early 1970s and for some years thereafter, the conventional wisdom was that tumor vasculature was an inflammatory reaction to dying tumor cells. In 1971, Folkman articulated several "visionary" hypotheses on tumor angiogenesis which are now widely accepted. His ideas were based not only on his own work, but also on some studies of a small number of investigators [5–7]. As well summarized in a Cancer Research Commentary recently written by Augustin [8], Folkman published his hypothesis article in 1971, (i) predicting that tumors would be restricted to microscopic size in the absence of angiogenesis, (ii) suggesting that tumors secrete diffusible angiogenic molecules, (iii) describing a model of tumor dormancy due to the blocked angiogenesis, (iv) proposing the term anti-angiogenesis for the prevention of new capillary sprouts from being recruited into a growing tumor, (v) envisaging the future discovery of angiogenesis inhibitors and (vi) proposing the idea that an antibody to a tumor angiogenic factor could be an anticancer drug.

Folkman and collaborators obtained the first evidence of the existence of the avascular and vascular phases of solid tumor growth in 1963, on the basis of experiments in isolated perfused organs [9]. A rabbit's thyroid gland was seeded with cancer cells from mice and perfused with a blood substitute. Tiny tumors formed, but they grew to the same size, then stopped and never became vascularized. When tumors were transplanted into live mice, they rapidly vascularized and grew vigorously. This lab work and some clinical observations (in particular those regarding retinoblastoma in children) help Folkman develop and sustain the hypothesis that tumor growth is angiogenesis dependent.

In the decade following the 1971 report, research in the tumor angiogenesis field attracted little scientific interest, but Folkman and his team preserved in their investigations, providing convincing evidences for dependence of tumor growth on neovascularization [10–14]. This was achieved in particular thanks to the development and use of bioassays devoted to angiogenesis research, such as the model of eye transplant and chick embryo chorioallantoic membrane. Of note, one of the major steps in allowing scientific appreciation of the role of tumor angiogenesis and demonstrating angiogenesis in vitro was developing methods for passage of endothelial cells. In 1979, Folkman's laboratory reported long-term passage of endothelial cells [15], and the following year, they demonstrated angiogenesis in vitro using endothelial cell cultures exposed to tumor conditioned media [16].

After the developments of the late 1970s, many other scientists entered the field of angiogenesis and Folkman's skeptics became his competitors [17]. In particular, the 1980s were an intense period of hunting for the hypothesized TAF [8]. In 1983, Dvorak and collaborators reported the isolation of a tumor-derived factor that they called "vascular permeability factor" (VPF) on the basis of its capability to induce blood vessel leakage [18]. However, at that time, VPF was not completely purified and therefore not fully identified. In 1989, Ferrara purified a novel angiogenic protein that he termed "vascular endothelial growth factor" (VEGF) on the basis of its observed growth-promoting activity toward only vascular endothelial cells [19]. Around the same time, Folkman's laboratory isolated an angiogenic protein that resulted to be identical to that purified by Ferrara [20]. By 1990, it was realized that VEGF and VPF were in fact the same protein. There is no doubt that it was the discovery of VEGF to set in motion a revolution in the field of angiogenic research.

From 1980 to 2005, Folkman's laboratory reported the discovery of eleven angiogenesis inhibitors, eight of them are endogenous angiogenesis inhibitors [21]. Effort persisted in this area and new anti-angiogenic molecules are continuously being developed. They essentially fall into two distinct types: (i) antibody directed toward angiogenic factors such as VEGF, for example, Avastin (Bevacizumab, Genentech) and (ii) small molecules inhibiting cellular signaling by targeting multiple receptor tyrosine kinases among them VEGFR-2, for example, Sutent (Sunitinib, Pfizer) and Nexavar (Sorafenib, Bayer and Onyx Pharmaceuticals) [17].

Targeting VEGF and VEGFR-2 offers benefit to patients with at least some types of cancer and provides proof of principle that attacking the vasculature is a valid approach to cancer therapy [22]. At present, however, despite important results, the overall clinical benefits of anti-VEGF/VEGFR-2 therapy are still relatively modest: not all cancer patients respond to anti-VEGF treatments, and when they do increased survival may only be measured in weeks or months [17]. This is realistically due to a number of different and not yet fully clarified reasons, which open discussion going beyond the topic of this chapter. Here, we will only mention, as reported by Van Epps in 2005, that one of Folkman's hopes for the future was that anti-angiogenesis therapy could be initiated—based on diagnostic biomarkers—even before the tumor reveals its location in the body, thus stopping cancer before it really gets started [23, 24].

3. VEGF-mediated signal transduction

In vivo angiogenic response to VEGF is mainly mediated via activation of VEGFR-2, expressed primarily in endothelial cells. VEGFR-2 activation initiates several intricate signaling paths, which eventually lead to different endothelial responses: cell survival, proliferation, migration, invasion into the surrounding tissue, vascular permeability and vascular inflammation [25]. These responses involve (i) a number of pivotal effectors such as phosphoinositide 3 kinase (PI3K), phospholipase Cγ (PLCγ), SRC, focal adhesion kinase (FAK) and Rho family of GTPases; (ii) several multifunctional docking proteins and adaptors; and (iii) VEGFR-2 partners such as Neuropilin 1 (NRP1), integrins and vascular endothelial (VE)-cadherin. It is apparent that these proteins orchestrate a complex signaling network leading to the integration of the different VEGF-induced endothelial responses that allows tumor angiogenesis to take place. **Figure 1** illustrates, in a simplified manner, VEGF-mediated signal transduction, showing signal core components along with the main well-defined intracellular routes leading to different endothelial responses.

3.1. VEGFR-2 activation

VEGFR-2 is a tyrosine kinase receptor (RTK). Binding of VEGF to VEGFR-2 promotes receptor dimerization, allowing trans/autophosphorylation of intracellular tyrosine residues. Among the 19 tyrosine residues present in the intracellular domain of VEGFR-2, there are five major phosphorylation sites: Y951, Y1054, Y1059, Y1175 and Y1214. The Y1054 and Y1059 are located in the kinase domain activation loop, and their phosphorylation is critical for receptor catalytic activity [26]. Y951 is located in the kinase insert domain, and its phosphorylation serves as a binding site for T cell-specific adaptor (TSAD) also known as VEGFR-2-associated protein (VRAP) [27, 28]. The Y1175 and Y1214 are located in the carboxy-terminal domain. Phosphorylation of Y1175 creates a binding site for PLCγ [29], p85 subunit of PI3K [30], the adaptor proteins SHB [31] and SCK [32]. This residue is well-recognized as a critical mediator of VEGFR-2 signaling. Phosphorylated Y1214 has been described to bind the adaptor protein NCK [33].

VEGFR-2 activation and downstream signaling are modulated by different mechanisms. The main of them involve (i) receptor interaction with NRP1, specific integrins and VE-cadherin

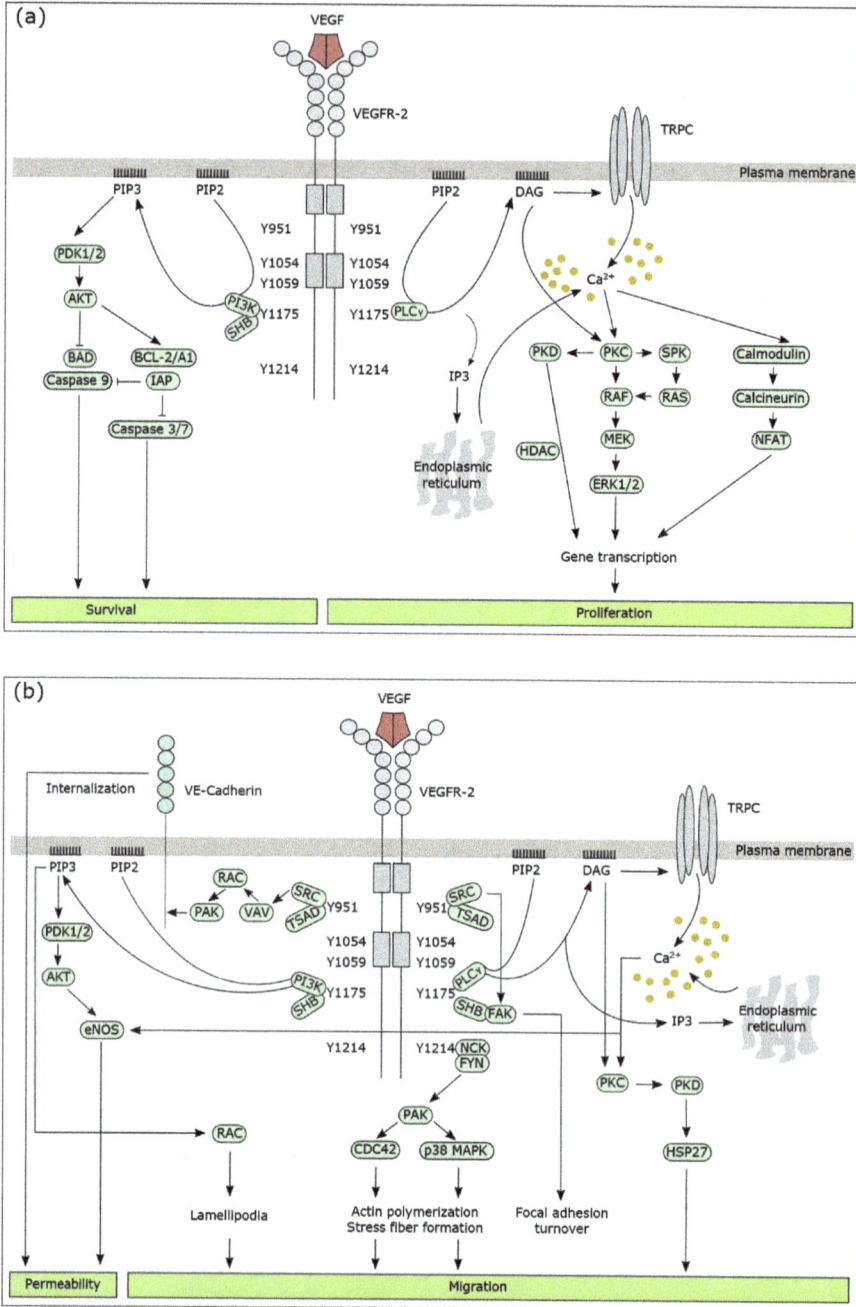

Figure 1. Signal transduction mediated by VEGF/VEGFR-2. Core signaling pathways involved in VEGF-induced (a) cell survival and proliferation and (b) vascular permeability and cell migration. See text for details.

(see Section 3.7) and (ii) the activity of the protein tyrosine phosphatases (PTPs) such as vascular endothelial PTP (VEPTP), SRC homology 2 domain PTP (SHP2) and PTP1B [34]. VEGFR-2 activation may also be influenced by the presence of heparin sulfate glycoproteins that modulate VEGF-VEGFR-2 binding and signaling amplitude [35, 36]. Indeed, a change in ligand-receptor affinity may highly influence RTK signaling. We recently reported that

VEGF-VEGFR2 affinity may vary from low to high based on the endothelial cell density state that we also reported to influence the number of total and surface VEGFR-2 [37]. In particular, by combining wet-lab experiments, theoretical insights and mathematical modeling, we found that ligand-receptor affinity is reduced in long-confluent compare to sparse endothelial cells, which recapitulate in vitro the condition of quiescent and angiogenic endothelium in vivo.

3.2. PLCγ signaling

Activated VEGFR-2 directly recruits PLCγ, which is in turn phosphorylated [38, 39]. Phosphorylated PLCγ hydrolyzes the membrane phospholipid phosphatidylinositol-4,5-bi-phosphate (PIP2), generating diacylglycerol (DAG) and inositol 1,4,5-trisphosphate (IP3). This latter mobilizes Ca^{2+} from the endoplasmic reticulum, thus leading to an increase in intracellular Ca^{2+}. IP3-mediated Ca^{2+} increase supports DAG-induced activation of PKC, from which it is triggered the RAF1-MEK-ERK1/2 mitogen-activated protein (MAP) kinase cascade, that is, the best characterized pathway propagated downstream to VEGF/VEGFR-2/PLCγ axis resulting, in particular, in endothelial cell proliferation trough the ERK1/2-dependent regulation of gene transcription.

Most RTKs are known to utilize the classical GRB2-SOS-RAS activation of the RAF1-MEK-ERK1/2 cascade. Conflicting results exist in the literature with respect to the interaction of VEGFR-2 with SHC or GRB2, which recruit the RAS activating nucleotide-exchange factor SOS to the receptor, and the significance of the classical RAS-mediated MAP kinase cascade downstream to VEGFR-2 is unclear [32, 40]. Indeed, it is well-accepted that, after VEGF stimulation, most of the MAP kinase activation is mediated via the PLCγ-activated PKC as first reported by Takahashi and coworkers [39, 41]. These authors described the pathway as RAS-independent; however, considering the same pathway, Shu and colleagues reported the involvement of sphingosine kinase (SPK), found to link PKC to RAS activation in a manner independent of RAS nucleotide-exchange factor [42].

VEGF-induced activation of PKC also results in activation of protein kinase D (PKD), found to influence ERK1/2 activation and cell proliferation [43]. In response to VEGF, gene repressive action of histone deacetylases (HDAC) 5 and 7 in endothelial cells is overcome by the PLCγ-PKC-PKD pathway-dependent HDAC 5 and 7 phosphorylation and nuclear export, resulting in the regulation of gene transcription, cell proliferation and migration [44, 45]. Moreover, VEGF-induced PKC-dependent activation of PKD has also been reported to induce HSP27 phosphorylation and mediate cell migration without involving the p38 MAP kinase (p38 MAPK)/MAP kinase-activated protein kinase 2 signaling cascade [46].

As mentioned above, PLCγ activation induced an increase in intracellular Ca^{2+}. Ca^{2+} signaling is crucial in VEGF/VEGFR-2 signal transduction, not only for PLCγ/PKC-mediated pathways but also for activation of other molecular players such as, in particular, the endothelial nitric oxide synthase (eNOS) and the nuclear factor of activated T-cell (NFAT) family of transcription factors. eNOS plays a crucial role in the control of vascular homeostasis and permeability; its activity is regulated by a complex combination of protein–protein interactions and signal transduction cascades involving Ca^{2+} mobilization and phosphorylation events

[47]. VEGF stimulates both Ca^{2+} and phosphorylation-dependent regulation of eNOS activity. VEGF stimulation in endothelial cells first leads to the Ca^{2+}-calmodulin disruption of the caveolin-eNOS complex and promotes the association between eNOS and the chaperon protein HSP90; eNOS-bound HSP90 can then recruit VEGF-activated AKT to the complex, which in turn can phosphorylate eNOS, resulting in potentiation of its activity [48]. NFAT proteins—extensively studied in the immune system—are functional in several cell types, including cancer cells, endothelial cells and infiltrating immune cells [49]. The multiple functions attributed to NFAT include cell growth, survival, invasion and angiogenesis. These transcription factors are activated through a Ca^{2+}- and calmodulin-activated calcineurin-dependent mechanism. In endothelial cells, VEGF stimulates receptor-mediated activation of PLCγ leading to an increase in intracellular Ca^{2+}, calcineurin activation and NFAT nuclear translocation that in turn leads to the transactivation of genes that are essential for angiogenesis [49, 50], such as COX-2 resulting in synthesis of PGE2, a mediator of endothelial cell migration and tube formation [51]. Moreover, in endothelial cells, VEGF-mediated NFAT activation induces a gene repertoire that includes an inherent inflammatory component, similar to that of interleukin 1 [52]. In addition, it has been recently reported that endothelial cells decode VEGF-mediated Ca^{2+} signaling patterns to produce distinct functional responses: cell proliferation and cell migration involving NFAT and myosin light chain kinase, respectively [53].

VEGFR-2/PLCγ signaling also involves TRPC channels, which are Ca^{2+}-permeable nonselective cation channels. Indeed, VEGF induces Ca^{2+} elevation through both Ca^{2+} release from intracellular stores and extracellular Ca^{2+} entry. In particular, VEGFR-2/PLCγ axis activates TRPC3 and TRPC6 in a DAG-dependent manner [54]. TRPC6 has been reported to be required for VEGF-mediated Ca^{2+} increase and the subsequent signaling that lead to processes associated with angiogenesis, such as cell migration, proliferation and tube formation [55, 56].

Overall, PLCγ appears as a regulator of a number of pathways, leading to cell proliferation and migration and contributing to vascular permeability. Thus, a better understanding of its downregulation may be of interest in further elucidating the regulation of VEGF-induced signaling, as well as in the development of new anti-angiogenic therapies. Indeed, very little is known about the regulation of PLCγ activity. Singh and colleagues have been reported that VEGF-induced PLCγ ubiquitination inhibits its tyrosine phosphorylation, thus providing a negative feedback to prevent sustained PLCγ stimulation [57]. In addition, we have previously reported the essential role of PTPs on VEGF-induced PLCγ activation, suggesting the existence of at least one—not yet characterized—PTP directly targeting PLCγ and counteracting receptor-mediated signal [37].

3.3. PI3K signaling

VEGF/VEGFR-2 axis activates PI3K in different ways, including direct or indirect (i.e., through adaptor and scaffold proteins) binding of PI3K to the receptor, and the involvement of SRC (see Sections 3.4 and 3.6). The activated PI3K converts the plasma membrane lipid PIP2 to phosphatidylinositol-3,4,5-trisphosphate (PIP3), and signaling proteins with pleckstrin homology (PH) domains accumulate at site of PI3K activation by directly binding to PIP3 [58]. Among these signaling proteins of particular interest are the serine-threonine kinases

AKT and phosphoinositide-dependent kinase 1 (PDK1). Phosphorylation of AKT by PDK1 and PDK2 allows the full activation of AKT, resulting in the phosphorylation of a number of proteins [59]. Other PH domain-containing proteins that are activated by PIP3 include GDP-GTP exchange factors for the small GTPase RAC [58, 60].

PI3K/AKT pathway is considered the main mechanism by which VEGF induces endothelial cell survival. AKT mediates both short- and long-term cell survival effects by inhibiting (through direct phosphorylation) pro-apoptotic proteins such as BAD, caspase 9 and forkhead transcription factors, and by upregulating anti-apoptotic proteins such as BCL-2 [61, 62]. In 1998, Gerber and coworkers were the first to report that VEGF regulates endothelial cell survival through the PI3K/AKT signal transduction pathway and that VEGF also induces expression of the anti-apoptotic proteins BCL-2 and A1 in endothelial cells [63, 64]. In the following year, Tran and colleagues reported a marked induction of the IAP family anti-apoptotic proteins survivin and XIAP—which inhibit caspase 3, 7 and 9—by VEGF in endothelial cells [65].

Although crucial for its function in cell survival, AKT is not simply a regulator of cell survival but a multifunctional protein playing a pivotal role in both cancer cells and endothelial cells. In addition to cell survival, AKT activation has been linked to tumor angiogenesis via several other biological processes, including vascular permeability, cell proliferation, synthesis and release of matrix metalloproteinases and induction of VEGF production by cancer cells [59]. Beyond the pro-survival effect and considering the VEGF/VEGFR-2 signal transduction in the endothelium, the main contribution exerted by AKT resides in the direct phosphorylation of eNOS, thus contributing to the control of endothelial permeability [48, 66].

3.4. SRC and FAK

The SRC family of protein tyrosine kinases (SFKs) plays key roles in regulating signal transduction by a diverse set of cell surface receptors in the context of a variety of cellular environments [67]. Endothelial SFKs includes SRC, YES and FYN. Many of the VEGF-mediated pathways involve SRC activity. Moreover, SRC is intimately involved in the modulation of the activity of FAK through direct phosphorylation (see below). VEGFR-2 activates SRC according to different mechanisms: (i) by direct binding to Y951 in the receptor [27], (ii) through the adaptor protein TSAD [68] or (iii) involving the scaffold protein GAB1 and GAB2 [69].

VEGF-induced SRC activity is involved in the activation of different signaling proteins, such as PI3K, FAK and eNOS. Holmqvist and colleagues reported that activated VEGFR-2 recruits SHB and SRC and that this latter phosphorylates SHB, which allows the subsequent activation of PI3K and phosphorylation of FAK at Y576 [31]. Duval and coworkers reported that VEGF induces phosphorylation of VEGFR-2-associated HSP90, which is dependent on receptor internalization and on SRC kinase activation; furthermore, they demonstrated that SRC directly phosphorylates HSP90 and that this event is essential for VEGF-stimulated eNOS association to HSP90 and thus NO release from endothelial cells [70]. In response to VEGF, Src may also activate members of the MAP kinase cascade such as RAF1 [71] and b-RAF [72]; this latter is activated in a manner dependent of SRC-mediated phosphorylation of the scaffold protein IQ motif-containing GTPase-activating protein 1 (IQGAP1).

In parallel with the effect exerted on intracellular signaling proteins, SRC plays a pivotal role in the disorganization of cadherin-dependent cell-cell contacts and in integrin-VEGFR-2 cross-activation. In response to VEGF, SRC phosphorylates VE-cadherin in adherens junctions, allowing endothelial cell migration and inducing vascular permeability [73–76]. Mahabeleshwar and coworkers reported that there is an intimate and coordinated relationship between VEGFR-2 and αvβ3 integrin involving SRC activity [77]. In particular, they demonstrated that (i) adhesion- and growth factor-induced β3 integrin tyrosine phosphorylation is directly mediated by SRC, (ii) SRC-dependent β3 integrin tyrosine phosphorylation is critical for interaction between VEGFR-2 and β3 integrin, and (iii) SRC mediates growth factor-induced β3 integrin activation, ligand binding and αvβ3 integrin-dependent cellular adhesion, directional migration of endothelial cells and initiation of angiogenic programming in endothelial cells.

As mentioned above, SRC is involved in the modulation of FAK activity through direct phosphorylation. The non-receptor tyrosine kinase FAK—well recognized as an important regulator of cell migration—is localized in focal adhesions, established as a consequence of integrin ligation to the extracellular matrix. Upon integrin-dependent cell adhesion, phosphorylation of FAK and its catalytic activity are stimulated. FAK possesses six tyrosyl residues (i. e., Y397, Y407, Y576, Y577, Y861 and Y925) that are differentially phosphorylated by diverse agonists and that are implicated in transmitting different signals and effects. Y397 is an autophosphorylation site that recruits SH2 domain-containing proteins, including members of SKFs, PLCγ and the p85 subunit of PI3K [78]. It appears that SRC is first recruited to Y397 and then involved in transphosphorylation of other tyrosyl residues within FAK, such as Y576 and Y577; this confers maximal activation of FAK and signaling in response to adhesion [79, 80]. In particular, upon VEGF stimulation, Y576 and Y861 are both phosphorylated in a SRC-dependent manner [31, 81], while Y407 is phosphorylated in a SRC-independent manner that involves the recruitment of HSP90 to the receptor, followed by the activation of RHOA and that of RHO activated kinase (ROCK) [81]. This results in phosphorylation of FAK on S732 that allows FAK-related kinase PYK2-mediated phosphorylation of FAK on Y407, promoting cell migration [82].

3.5. Rho family GTPases

The RHO family GTPases—shuttling between inactive GDP-bound and active GTP-bound forms—include RHO, RAC and CDC42, which are known to regulate primarily the reorganization of actin cytoskeletal systems such as actin stress fibers and focal adhesions, lamellipodia and filopodia, respectively [83]. A growing body of evidence indicates a crucial role for VEGF-induced RHO GTPases activity in endothelial cell during the processes involved in angiogenesis such as, in particular, cell migration and vascular permeability [84]. VEGF/VEGFR-2 axis stimulates the activities of RHO [81, 85], RAC [86, 87] and CDC42 [88]. As reported in Section 3.4, VEGF-induced RHO activity stimulates FAK activation promoting cell migration [81]. VEGF-induced RAC activation has been linked to both endothelial permeability and cell migration. Gavard and Gutkind reported that RAC takes part in a signaling pathway by which VEGF stimulation promotes the rapid endocytosis of VE-cadherin, thereby disrupting the endothelial barrier function [86]. In particular, they demonstrated that VEGFR-2 activates RAC through the SRC-dependent phosphorylation of the nucleotide-exchange factor VAV2 and that RAC activation, in turn, promotes the p21-activated kinase (PAK)-mediated phosphorylation of VE-cadherin resulting in the recruitment of beta-arrestin 2 to phosphorylated VE-cadherin, thereby promoting its internalization into clathrin-coated vesicles and the consequent disassembly of intercellular junctions. To complement this study, Garrett and coworkers reported that VEGF-induced SRC-dependent VAV2 phosphorylation and downstream activation of RAC1 are also responsible for endothelial cell migration and wound closure [87]. The involvement of CDC42 in VEGF signaling has been reported in particular by Lamalice and colleagues [33, 88]. They proposed a model according to which, upon VEGFR-2 activation phosphorylated Y1214 within the receptor recruits the adaptor protein NCK that becomes phosphorylated providing a recruitment site for FYN that is also phosphorylated and required for the phosphorylation of NCK and that of the p21-activated protein kinase PAK-2, an effector of CDC42; then, this early molecular complex containing VEGFR-2·NCK·FYN·PAK-2 triggers the sequential activation of CDC42 and p38 MAPK leading to actin polymerization, stress fiber formation and endothelial cell migration.

3.6. Key docking, adaptor and scaffold proteins

As it emerges from what above described, it is evident that, beyond a number of kinases and other enzymes, VEGFR-2 signaling involves several key docking, adaptor and scaffold proteins including SHB, TSAD, NCK, IQGAP1 and GAB1. In the following, we briefly summarize their main involvement downstream to VEGF/VEGFR-2 axis.

The adapter protein SHB contains at least four different domains responsible for protein-protein interactions (i.e., the proline-rich motifs in its N-terminus, the phospho-tyrosine binding (PTB) domain, potential tyrosine phosphorylation sites and the C-terminal SH2 domain) and has been shown to operate downstream of several RTKs exerting versatile effects on a number of signaling pathways [89]. SHB binds to phosphorylate Y1175 in VEGFR-2 and is phosphorylated by SRC; this allows the subsequent activation of PI3K and phosphorylation of FAK at Y576 in the kinase domain, regulating the migratory response in endothelial cells [31]. Along this pathway, it is possible that SHB is required for VEGF-mediated activation of FAK by allowing SRC to phosphorylate Y576. Indeed, it has been demonstrated that the PTB domain of SHB can bind directly to FAK and regulate its activity in response to FGFR-1 activation in endothelial cells [90].

TSAD is an adaptor protein containing a SH2 domain, tyrosines in protein binding motifs and a proline-rich domain allowing SH3-dependent interactions. TSAD interacts with and modulates the activity of some SFKs such as LCK and SRC [68, 91], and has been found to control actin polymerization events in both T cells and endothelial cells [27, 92]. TSAD binds to phosphorylate Y951 in VEGFR-2 via its SH2 domain and to SRC via its proline-rich domain. TSAD has been reported as an important docking mechanism for SRC to VEGFR-2, involved in the regulation of cell migration, endothelial cell junctions and vascular permeability, but not cell proliferation [27, 68].

NCK is an adapter protein consisting of one SH2 domain and three SH3 domains. A main function of NCK is to link receptor and receptor-associated tyrosine kinases with proteins that directly or indirectly regulate remodeling and reorganization of the actin cytoskeleton [93]. According to the model proposed by Lamalice and colleagues, upon phosphorylation on Y1214 in VEGFR-2, NCK is recruited to the receptor thus allowing the formation of a molecular complex containing VEGFR-2·NCK·FYN·PAK-2 that convey the sequential activation of CDC42 and p38 MAPK leading to actin polymerization, stress fiber formation and endothelial cell migration [33]. Moreover, it has been reported that NCK participates with PAK in the signaling pathway by which VEGF stimulates the assembly of focal adhesions [94].

The multidomain scaffold protein IQGAP1 binds to several structural and signaling proteins. For example, interactions of the IQGAP1 calponin homology domain (CHD) with F-actin and the GAP-related domain (GRD) with small GTPases regulate the cytoskeleton to promote actin binding or polymerization that regulates cell migration, stability of cell-cell contacts and cytokinesis; moreover, IQGAPs also scaffold molecules form signaling complexes, such as components of the MAP kinase cascade, thus promoting their activity [95]. Along VEGF signal transduction, IQGAP1 becomes phosphorylated by SRC and activates b-RAF, contributing to cell proliferation [72]. Moreover, IQGAP1 has been implicated in regulation of cell migration and cell-cell contacts [96, 97]. In particular, Yamaoka-Tojo and colleagues suggested that IQGAP1 may function as a scaffold to link VEGFR-2 to the adherens junctions through binding to VEGFR-2 and VE-cadherin/β-catenin complex, thereby dissociating α-catenin from the adherens junctional complex and contributing to VEGF-stimulated loss of cell-cell contacts in endothelial cell [97].

GAB1 is the prototype of a subfamily of large multiadapter proteins sharing an N-terminal PH domain, two proline-rich regions involved in constitutive binding to GRB2 and multiple tyrosine phosphorylation sites [98]. Downstream to VEGF/VEGFR-2 axis, GAB1—recruited through an amplification loop involving PIP3 and its PH domain—has been proposed to be a primary actor in coupling VEGFR-2 to PI3K/AKT [98]. In response to VEGF, it has been reported that GAB1 is phosphorylated and associates not only with PI3K, but also with GRB2, SHP2, SHC and PLCγ influencing the signaling downstream to VEGFR-2 and, in particular, cell migration and capillary formation [99].

3.7. Neuropilin 1, integrins and Vascular Endothelial Cadherin

VEGF signaling is complicated by the fact that VEGFR-2 interact with additional cellular proteins such as, in particular, NRP1, specific integrins and VE-cadherin [100]. This modulates the signal strength induced by VEGFR-2 on the basis of the extracellular cues arising from the soluble ligand, cell-substratum and cell-cell interactions.

NRP1 is a transmembrane receptor for VEGF and the neuronal guidance cue SEMA3A, with essential roles in both vascular and neuronal development, as well as in pathological angiogenesis [101, 102]. The precise mechanism of VEGF-VEGFR-2-NRP1 interaction and the functional consequences of this molecular complex are still being explored. The most widely accepted model of NRP1 function in angiogenesis postulates that it forms a VEGF-dependent complex with VEGFR-2 to enhance the activation of a wide variety of intracellular signal transduction pathways, including those that involve ERK1/2, AKT, SRC and p38 MAPK [103]. Moreover, it has been reported that NRP1 promotes VEGFR-2 trafficking through RAB11 vesicles thereby specifying signal output [104].

Integrins link intracellular signaling pathways induced by soluble factor to output elicited by cellular interactions with extracellular matrix. Specific integrins, particularly integrin β1 and β3, act as important partners for VEGFR-2. An intimate and coordinated relationship between VEGFR-2 and αvβ3 has been reported by Mahabeleshwar and coworkers (see Section 3.4) [77]. In particular, the relationship between VEGFR-2 and β3 integrin appears to be synergistic, because VEGFR-2 activation induces β3 integrin tyrosine phosphorylation, which, in turn, is crucial for maximum phosphorylation of VEGFR-2 [77]. Exposure of endothelial cells to matrix-bound VEGF promotes VEGFR-2-integrin β1 complex formation, redistribution to focal adhesion, prolonged activation of VEGFR-2 with differential phosphorylation of Y1214 and extended activation kinetics of p38 MAPK [105].

VE-cadherin is involved in the formation of adherens junctions in endothelial cells and plays a crucial role in VEGF signaling. In resting endothelial cells, VE-cadherin complexes with VEGFR-2 at cell-cell contacts and attenuates VEGFR-2 phosphorylation through the phosphatase DEP1 [106]. Upon VEGF stimulation, VEC is phosphorylated and in turn internalized, thereby disrupting the endothelial barrier function (see Sections 3.4 and 3.5).

3.8. VEGFR-2 internalization

It is well known that VEGFR-2 undergoes internalization and trafficking upon VEGF stimulation. Emerging evidences suggest that VEGFR-2 internalization and trafficking are tightly controlled processes that influence the sensitivity of endothelial cells to VEGF and the signaling propagated downstream to the receptor. Although the mechanisms regulating VEGFR-2 internalization and trafficking and their exerted effects on signaling are still not fully understood, it is apparent that a pivotal role is played by VEGFR-2 interaction with specific protein partners such as, in particular but not only, VE-cadherin and NRP1.

In endothelial cells, VEGFR-2 is located in different subcellular pools, including receptors diffusely distributed in the plasma membrane, engaged in cell-cell junctions through the interaction with VE-cadherin and associated with various intracellular compartments. Resting endothelial cells have two surface pools of VEGFR-2: a stable pool that is complexed with VE-cadherin, and a flux pool that is constantly cycling between the surface and the endocytic compartment in a VEGF independent manner [107, 108]. VE-cadherin prevents internalization of VEGFR-2 by physical interaction and recruitment of the DEP-1 phosphatase [106]. VEGF stimulation results in clathrin-dependent internalization of VEGFR-2. The clathrin-coated vesicles fuse with early endosomes and then proceed through a series of steps that can either direct their recycling back to the plasma membrane via the fast (RAB4) or slow (RAB11) recycling pathways or target them for degradation into lysosome via the RAB7 pathway [109]. Ballmer-Hofer and colleagues reported that when complexed with NRP1, internalized VEGFR-2 is recycled through RAB4 and RAB11 positive vesicles; while in the absence of NRP1, internalized VEGFR-2 bypassed RAB11 vesicles and rapidly accumulated in RAB7 vesicles indicative of receptor degradation [104]. They also showed that VEGFR-2 is dephosphorylated before entry into the RAB11 compartment and then targeted to the plasma membrane where it presumably initiates a new round of ligand binding and receptor activation thereby prolonging VEGF signaling to downstream targets [104]. Furthermore, there are also evidences that when activated VEGFR-2—not yet dephosphorylated—is trapped inside endosomes, it is still capable of stimulating some downstream signaling proteins such as those belonging to the MAP kinase cascade [110].

4. Synopsis of VEGF-induced endothelial responses and their role in tumor angiogenesis

VEGF/VEGFR-2 signal transduction leads to six major endothelial responses: cell survival, invasion and migration into the surrounding tissue, proliferation, vascular permeability and vascular inflammation. These endothelial responses are tightly integrated to allow tumor angiogenesis to progress successfully.

Vascular permeability—crucial for normal tissue homeostasis—is a prerequisite for VEGF-induced angiogenesis. Endothelial permeability is mediated by the so-called transcellular and paracellular pathways, that is, solutes and cells can pass through (transcellular) or between (paracellular) endothelial cells. Transcellular passage requires cell fenestration and/or a complex system of transport vesicles that includes organelles called vesiculo-vacuolar organelles, while the paracellular pathway depends on the coordinated opening and closure of endothelial cell-to-cell junctions, combined with cell retraction. VEGF is involved in both transcellular and paracellular permeability. VEGF/VEGFR-2 axis induces increased endothelial permeability mainly through SRC-mediated signaling of VE-cadherin internalization (see Sections 3.4 and 3.5) that disrupts the endothelial barrier function, and by activation of PLCγ that mediates an increase in intracellular Ca^{2+} resulting in Ca^{2+}-calmodulin-dependent regulation of eNOS (see Section 3.2). Activation of eNOS—also achieved by AKT-mediated phosphorylation—promotes an increase in vascular permeability by NO production that is followed by vasodilatation. VEGF-induced vascular permeability contributes to the dissemination of extracellular proteases and the deposition of a fibrin gel provisional stroma that changes the extracellular matrix of normal tissues from anti- to pro-angiogenic and stromagenic, favoring and supporting inward migration of endothelial cells and the growth of new endothelial sprouts [111]. In addition, the reduced vessel integrity may promote leukocyte extravasation and facilitate exit of metastasis from the primary tumors.

VEGF-induced vascular permeability goes in parallel with vascular inflammation. Although VEGF is not an inflammatory cytokine, VEGF-induced gene transcription—in particular through NFAT activation—includes a conspicuous inflammatory component (see Section 3.2). This could conceivably promote attraction of inflammatory cells that may contribute to the angiogenic response. Indeed, it is well established that tumor angiogenesis is linked to inflammation. On the one hand, tumor cells can be killed by the immune system; on the other hand, tumor can use leukocytes to supports its expansion.

Endothelial cell invasion into the surrounding tissue is made possible by means of the release of MMPs, which degrade the basal membrane and the extracellular matrix and allow the migration of endothelial cells to form capillary sprouts. Endothelial cells express different MMPs, and it has been reported that their expression is induced by VEGF and regulated by Ets transcription factors [112, 113]. Signaling pathways, such as MAP kinase cascade, PI3K/AKT axis, and Ca^{2+}-specific signals, converge on the Ets transcription factors, controlling their activity.

VEGF-induced endothelial cell migration and proliferation are tightly regulated and coordinated spatio-temporal behaviors, which—in parallel with sustained cell survival—enable angiogenic sprouting and capillary lumen formation, necessary to create the new vessels devoted to support tumor growth and metastasis spread. VEGF-induced endothelial survival and proliferation are stimulated primarily via PI3K/AKT and PLCγ/ERK pathways, respectively, involving—as above described—several signaling intermediates. VEGF-induced endothelial cell migration appears to be regulated by a larger number of pathways, including the involvement of PLCγ, PI3K, RHO GTPases, SRC and FAK activities.

5. Conclusions

In this chapter, we attempted in particular to describe the best characterized signal transduction events downstream to VEGF/VEGFR-2 axis involved in tumor angiogenesis. Multiple VEGF-induced signaling pathways take part in the promotion of different biological responses in endothelial cells. Although it is possible to recognize distinct patterns along VEGF-induced signaling, they are intricate, characterized by the involvement of a number of enzymes and adaptor/scaffold proteins—whose activity converges and branches at many point—and by the presence of VEGFR-2 molecular partners influencing endothelial cell sensitivity to VEGF and receptor signal output. This depicts a complex signal network induced by VEGF, where the apparent redundancy in operating signaling pathways is likely to reflect a need for a fine-tuning and a differential control of the biological effects in response to VEGF [25]. Although past decade has seen an important advancement in our understanding of VEGF signaling, there is still a lack of insight in many aspects of VEGF/VEGFR-2 signal transduction, in particular for what concerns its fine regulation. A further elucidation of the multifaced VEGF signaling network in the context of endothelial biology is crucial for developing new potential anti-angiogenic therapies. In parallel with current therapies that directly target VEGF and VEGFR-2, agents able to influence key molecular player—proximal, median or distal to VEGFR-2—could be of clinical interest.

Acknowledgement

Publication costs have been supported by "Associazione Italiana per la Ricerca sul Cancro" (AIRC), project code 12182.

Author details

Lucia Napione[1,2,*], Maria Alvaro[1,2] and Federico Bussolino[1,2]

*Address all correspondence to: lucia.napione@ircc.it

1 Laboratory of Vascular Oncology, Candiolo Cancer Institute – IRCCS, Candiolo, Italy

2 Department of Oncology, University of Torino, Candiolo, Italy

References

[1] Folkman J. Tumor angiogenesis: therapeutic implications. N Engl J Med. 1971; 285(21):1182–6.

[2] Folkman J. Proceedings: tumor angiogenesis factor. Cancer Res. 1974;34(8):2109–13.

[3] Ferrara N, Gerber HP, LeCouter J. The biology of VEGF and its receptors. Nat Med. 2003;9(6):669–76.

[4] Koch S, Claesson-Welsh L. Signal transduction by vascular endothelial growth factor receptors. Cold Spring Harb Perspect Med. 2012;2(7):a006502.

[5] Algire G, Chalkley H. Vascular reactions of normal and malignant tissues in vivo. I. Vascular reactions of mice to wounds and to normal and neoplastic implants. J Natl Cancer Inst. 1945. p. 73–85.

[6] Greenblatt M, Shubi P. Tumor angiogenesis: transfilter diffusion studies in the hamster by the transparent chamber technique. J Natl Cancer Inst. 1968;41(1):111–24.

[7] Warren BA, Shubik P. The growth of the blood supply to melanoma transplants in the hamster cheek pouch. Lab Invest. 1966;15(2):464–78.

[8] Augustin HG. Commentary on Folkman: "How is blood vessel growth regulated in normal and neoplastic tissue?". Cancer Res. 2016;76(10):2854–6.

[9] Ribatti D. Judah Folkman, a pioneer in the study of angiogenesis. Angiogenesis. 2008; 11(1):3–10.

[10] Gimbrone MA, Leapman SB, Cotran RS, Folkman J. Tumor dormancy in vivo by prevention of neovascularization. J Exp Med. 1972;136(2):261–76.

[11] Gimbrone MA, Leapman SB, Cotran RS, Folkman J. Tumor angiogenesis: iris neovascularization at a distance from experimental intraocular tumors. J Natl Cancer Inst. 1973;50(1):219–28.

[12] Gimbrone MA, Cotran RS, Leapman SB, Folkman J. Tumor growth and neovascularization: an experimental model using the rabbit cornea. J Natl Cancer Inst. 1974;52(2):413–27.

[13] Knighton D, Ausprunk D, Tapper D, Folkman J. Avascular and vascular phases of tumour growth in the chick embryo. Br J Cancer. 1977;35(3):347–56.

[14] Brem S, Brem H, Folkman J, Finkelstein D, Patz A. Prolonged tumor dormancy by prevention of neovascularization in the vitreous. Cancer Res. 1976;36(8):2807–12.

[15] Folkman J, Haudenschild CC, Zetter BR. Long-term culture of capillary endothelial cells. Proc Natl Acad Sci U S A. 1979;76(10):5217–21.

[16] Folkman J, Haudenschild C. Angiogenesis in vitro. Nature. 1980;288(5791):551–6.

[17] Stephenson J, Goddard J, Al-Taan O, Dennison A, Morgan B. Tumor Angiogenesis: a growth area—from John Hunter to Judah Folkman and beyond. J Cancer Res: Hindawi Publishing Corporation; 2013. pp. 1–6.

[18] Senger DR, Galli SJ, Dvorak AM, Perruzzi CA, Harvey VS, Dvorak HF. Tumor cells secrete a vascular permeability factor that promotes accumulation of ascites fluid. Science. 1983;219(4587):983–5.

[19] Leung DW, Cachianes G, Kuang WJ, Goeddel DV, Ferrara N. Vascular endothelial growth factor is a secreted angiogenic mitogen. Science. 1989;246(4935):1306–9.

[20] Rosenthal RA, Megyesi JF, Henzel WJ, Ferrara N, Folkman J. Conditioned medium from mouse sarcoma 180 cells contains vascular endothelial growth factor. Growth Factors. 1990;4(1):53–9.

[21] Folkman J. Endogenous angiogenesis inhibitors. APMIS. 2004;112(7–8):496–507.

[22] Sitohy B, Nagy JA, Dvorak HF. Anti-VEGF/VEGFR therapy for cancer: reassessing the target. Cancer Res. 2012;72(8):1909–14.

[23] Van Epps H. What tumors need: a brief history of angiogenesis. J Exp Med. 2005. p. 1024.

[24] Folkman J. Angiogenesis: an organizing principle for drug discovery? Nat Rev Drug Discov. 2007;6(4):273–86.

[25] Claesson-Welsh L, Welsh M. VEGFA and tumour angiogenesis. J Intern Med. 2013;273(2): 114–27.

[26] Kendall RL, Rutledge RZ, Mao X, Tebben AJ, Hungate RW, Thomas KA. Vascular endothelial growth factor receptor KDR tyrosine kinase activity is increased by autophosphorylation of two activation loop tyrosine residues. J Biol Chem. 1999;274(10):6453–60.

[27] Matsumoto T, Bohman S, Dixelius J, Berge T, Dimberg A, Magnusson P, et al. VEGF receptor-2 Y951 signaling and a role for the adapter molecule TSAd in tumor angiogenesis. EMBO J. 2005;24(13):2342–53.

[28] Wu LW, Mayo LD, Dunbar JD, Kessler KM, Ozes ON, Warren RS, et al. VRAP is an adaptor protein that binds KDR, a receptor for vascular endothelial cell growth factor. J Biol Chem. 2000;275(9):6059–62.

[29] Takahashi T, Yamaguchi S, Chida K, Shibuya M. A single autophosphorylation site on KDR/Flk-1 is essential for VEGF-A-dependent activation of PLC-gamma and DNA synthesis in vascular endothelial cells. EMBO J. 2001;20(11):2768–78.

[30] Dayanir V, Meyer RD, Lashkari K, Rahimi N. Identification of tyrosine residues in vascular endothelial growth factor receptor-2/FLK-1 involved in activation of phosphatidylinositol 3-kinase and cell proliferation. J Biol Chem. 2001;276(21):17686–92.

[31] Holmqvist K, Cross MJ, Rolny C, Hägerkvist R, Rahimi N, Matsumoto T, et al. The adaptor protein shb binds to tyrosine 1175 in vascular endothelial growth factor (VEGF) receptor-2 and regulates VEGF-dependent cellular migration. J Biol Chem. 2004;279(21):22267–75.

[32] Warner AJ, Lopez-Dee J, Knight EL, Feramisco JR, Prigent SA. The Shc-related adaptor protein, Sck, forms a complex with the vascular-endothelial-growth-factor receptor KDR in transfected cells. Biochem J. 2000;347(Pt 2):501–9.

[33] Lamalice L, Houle F, Huot J. Phosphorylation of Tyr1214 within VEGFR-2 triggers the recruitment of Nck and activation of Fyn leading to SAPK2/p38 activation and endothelial cell migration in response to VEGF. J Biol Chem. 2006;281(45):34009–20.

[34] Kappert K, Peters KG, Böhmer FD, Ostman A. Tyrosine phosphatases in vessel wall signaling. Cardiovasc Res. 2005;65(3):587–98.

[35] Gitay-Goren H, Soker S, Vlodavsky I, Neufeld G. The binding of vascular endothelial growth factor to its receptors is dependent on cell surface-associated heparin-like molecules. J Biol Chem. 1992;267(9):6093–8.

[36] Jakobsson L, Kreuger J, Holmborn K, Lundin L, Eriksson I, Kjellén L, et al. Heparan sulfate in trans potentiates VEGFR-mediated angiogenesis. Dev Cell. 2006;10(5):625–34.

[37] Napione L, Pavan S, Veglio A, Picco A, Boffetta G, Celani A, et al. Unraveling the influence of endothelial cell density on VEGF-A signaling. Blood. 2012;119(23):5599–607.

[38] Olsson AK, Dimberg A, Kreuger J, Claesson-Welsh L. VEGF receptor signalling—in control of vascular function. Nat Rev Mol Cell Biol. 2006;7(5):359–71.

[39] Takahashi T, Shibuya M. The 230 kDa mature form of KDR/Flk-1 (VEGF receptor-2) activates the PLC-gamma pathway and partially induces mitotic signals in NIH3T3 fibroblasts. Oncogene. 1997;14(17):2079–89.

[40] Kroll J, Waltenberger J. The vascular endothelial growth factor receptor KDR activates multiple signal transduction pathways in porcine aortic endothelial cells. J Biol Chem. 1997;272(51):32521–7.

[41] Takahashi T, Ueno H, Shibuya M. VEGF activates protein kinase C-dependent, but Ras-independent Raf-MEK-MAP kinase pathway for DNA synthesis in primary endothelial cells. Oncogene. 1999;18(13):2221–30.

[42] Shu X, Wu W, Mosteller RD, Broek D. Sphingosine kinase mediates vascular endothelial growth factor-induced activation of ras and mitogen-activated protein kinases. Mol Cell Biol. 2002;22(22):7758–68.

[43] Wong C, Jin ZG. Protein kinase C-dependent protein kinase D activation modulates ERK signal pathway and endothelial cell proliferation by vascular endothelial growth factor. J Biol Chem. 2005;280(39):33262–9.

[44] Ha CH, Wang W, Jhun BS, Wong C, Hausser A, Pfizenmaier K, et al. Protein kinase D-dependent phosphorylation and nuclear export of histone deacetylase 5 mediates vascular endothelial growth factor-induced gene expression and angiogenesis. J Biol Chem. 2008;283(21):14590–9.

[45] Wang S, Li X, Parra M, Verdin E, Bassel-Duby R, Olson EN. Control of endothelial cell proliferation and migration by VEGF signaling to histone deacetylase 7. Proc Natl Acad Sci U S A. 2008;105(22):7738–43.

[46] Evans IM, Britton G, Zachary IC. Vascular endothelial growth factor induces heat shock protein (HSP) 27 serine 82 phosphorylation and endothelial tubulogenesis via protein kinase D and independent of p38 kinase. Cell Signal. 2008;20(7):1375–84.

[47] Shaul PW. Regulation of endothelial nitric oxide synthase: location, location, location. Annu Rev Physiol. 2002;64:749–74.

[48] Brouet A, Sonveaux P, Dessy C, Balligand JL, Feron O. Hsp90 ensures the transition from the early Ca^{2+}-dependent to the late phosphorylation-dependent activation of the endothelial nitric-oxide synthase in vascular endothelial growth factor-exposed endothelial cells. J Biol Chem. 2001;276(35):32663–9.

[49] Mancini M, Toker A. NFAT proteins: emerging roles in cancer progression. Nat Rev Cancer. 2009;9(11):810–20.

[50] Suehiro J, Kanki Y, Makihara C, Schadler K, Miura M, Manabe Y, et al. Genome-wide approaches reveal functional vascular endothelial growth factor (VEGF)-inducible nuclear factor of activated T cells (NFAT) c1 binding to angiogenesis-related genes in the endothelium. J Biol Chem. 2014;289(42):29044–59.

[51] Hernández GL, Volpert OV, Iñiguez MA, Lorenzo E, Martínez-Martínez S, Grau R, et al. Selective inhibition of vascular endothelial growth factor-mediated angiogenesis by cyclosporin A: roles of the nuclear factor of activated T cells and cyclooxygenase 2. J Exp Med. 2001;193(5):607–20.

[52] Schweighofer B, Testori J, Sturtzel C, Sattler S, Mayer H, Wagner O, et al. The VEGF-induced transcriptional response comprises gene clusters at the crossroad of angiogenesis and inflammation. Thromb Haemost. 2009;102(3):544–54.

[53] Noren DP, Chou WH, Lee SH, Qutub AA, Warmflash A, Wagner DS, et al. Endothelial cells decode VEGF-mediated Ca^{2+} signaling patterns to produce distinct functional responses. Sci Signal. 2016;9(416):ra20.

[54] Cheng HW, James AF, Foster RR, Hancox JC, Bates DO. VEGF activates receptor-operated cation channels in human microvascular endothelial cells. Arterioscler Thromb Vasc Biol. 2006;26(8):1768–76.

[55] Ge R, Tai Y, Sun Y, Zhou K, Yang S, Cheng T, et al. Critical role of TRPC6 channels in VEGF-mediated angiogenesis. Cancer Lett. 2009;283(1):43–51.

[56] Hamdollah Zadeh MA, Glass CA, Magnussen A, Hancox JC, Bates DO. VEGF-mediated elevated intracellular calcium and angiogenesis in human microvascular endothelial cells in vitro are inhibited by dominant negative TRPC6. Microcirculation. 2008;15(7):605–14.

[57] Singh AJ, Meyer RD, Navruzbekov G, Shelke R, Duan L, Band H, et al. A critical role for the E3-ligase activity of c-Cbl in VEGFR-2-mediated PLCgamma1 activation and angiogenesis. Proc Natl Acad Sci U S A. 2007;104(13):5413–8.

[58] Cantley LC. The phosphoinositide 3-kinase pathway. Science. 2002;296(5573):1655–7.

[59] Jiang BH, Liu LZ. PI3K/PTEN signaling in angiogenesis and tumorigenesis. Adv Cancer Res. 2009;102:19–65.

[60] Missy K, Van Poucke V, Raynal P, Viala C, Mauco G, Plantavid M, et al. Lipid products of phosphoinositide 3-kinase interact with Rac1 GTPase and stimulate GDP dissociation. J Biol Chem. 1998;273(46):30279–86.

[61] Vivanco I, Sawyers CL. The phosphatidylinositol 3-kinase AKT pathway in human cancer. Nat Rev Cancer. 2002;2(7):489–501.

[62] Pugazhenthi S, Nesterova A, Sable C, Heidenreich KA, Boxer LM, Heasley LE, et al. Akt/protein kinase B up-regulates Bcl-2 expression through cAMP-response element-binding protein. J Biol Chem. 2000;275(15):10761–6.

[63] Gerber HP, McMurtrey A, Kowalski J, Yan M, Keyt BA, Dixit V, et al. Vascular endothelial growth factor regulates endothelial cell survival through the phosphatidylinositol 3′-kinase/Akt signal transduction pathway. Requirement for Flk-1/KDR activation. J Biol Chem. 1998;273(46):30336–43.

[64] Gerber HP, Dixit V, Ferrara N. Vascular endothelial growth factor induces expression of the antiapoptotic proteins Bcl-2 and A1 in vascular endothelial cells. J Biol Chem. 1998;273(21):13313–6.

[65] Tran J, Rak J, Sheehan C, Saibil SD, LaCasse E, Korneluk RG, et al. Marked induction of the IAP family antiapoptotic proteins survivin and XIAP by VEGF in vascular endothelial cells. Biochem Biophys Res Commun. 1999;264(3):781–8.

[66] Dimmeler S, Fleming I, Fisslthaler B, Hermann C, Busse R, Zeiher AM. Activation of nitric oxide synthase in endothelial cells by Akt-dependent phosphorylation. Nature. 1999;399(6736):601–5.

[67] Parsons SJ, Parsons JT. Src family kinases, key regulators of signal transduction. Oncogene. 2004;23(48):7906–9.

[68] Sun Z, Li X, Massena S, Kutschera S, Padhan N, Gualandi L, et al. VEGFR2 induces c-Src signaling and vascular permeability in vivo via the adaptor protein TSAd. J Exp Med. 2012;209(7):1363–77.

[69] Caron C, Spring K, Laramée M, Chabot C, Cloutier M, Gu H, et al. Non-redundant roles of the Gab1 and Gab2 scaffolding adapters in VEGF-mediated signalling, migration, and survival of endothelial cells. Cell Signal. 2009;21(6):943–53.

[70] Duval M, Le Boeuf F, Huot J, Gratton JP. Src-mediated phosphorylation of Hsp90 in response to vascular endothelial growth factor (VEGF) is required for VEGF receptor-2 signaling to endothelial NO synthase. Mol Biol Cell. 2007;18(11):4659–68.

[71] Alavi A, Hood JD, Frausto R, Stupack DG, Cheresh DA. Role of Raf in vascular protection from distinct apoptotic stimuli. Science. 2003;301(5629):94–6.

[72] Meyer RD, Sacks DB, Rahimi N. IQGAP1-dependent signaling pathway regulates endothelial cell proliferation and angiogenesis. PLoS One. 2008;3(12):e3848.

[73] Eliceiri BP, Paul R, Schwartzberg PL, Hood JD, Leng J, Cheresh DA. Selective requirement for Src kinases during VEGF-induced angiogenesis and vascular permeability. Mol Cell. 1999;4(6):915–24.

[74] Weis S, Shintani S, Weber A, Kirchmair R, Wood M, Cravens A, et al. Src blockade stabilizes a Flk/cadherin complex, reducing edema and tissue injury following myocardial infarction. J Clin Invest. 2004;113(6):885–94.

[75] Wallez Y, Cand F, Cruzalegui F, Wernstedt C, Souchelnytskyi S, Vilgrain I, et al. Src kinase phosphorylates vascular endothelial-cadherin in response to vascular endothelial growth factor: identification of tyrosine 685 as the unique target site. Oncogene. 2007;26(7):1067–77.

[76] Dejana E, Tournier-Lasserve E, Weinstein BM. The control of vascular integrity by endothelial cell junctions: molecular basis and pathological implications. Dev Cell. 2009;16(2):209–21.

[77] Mahabeleshwar GH, Feng W, Reddy K, Plow EF, Byzova TV. Mechanisms of integrin-vascular endothelial growth factor receptor cross-activation in angiogenesis. Circ Res. 2007;101(6):570–80.

[78] Mitra SK, Hanson DA, Schlaepfer DD. Focal adhesion kinase: in command and control of cell motility. Nat Rev Mol Cell Biol. 2005;6(1):56–68.

[79] Calalb MB, Polte TR, Hanks SK. Tyrosine phosphorylation of focal adhesion kinase at sites in the catalytic domain regulates kinase activity: a role for Src family kinases. Mol Cell Biol. 1995;15(2):954–63.

[80] Owen JD, Ruest PJ, Fry DW, Hanks SK. Induced focal adhesion kinase (FAK) expression in FAK-null cells enhances cell spreading and migration requiring both auto- and activation loop phosphorylation sites and inhibits adhesion-dependent tyrosine phosphorylation of Pyk2. Mol Cell Biol. 1999;19(7):4806–18.

[81] Le Boeuf F, Houle F, Huot J. Regulation of vascular endothelial growth factor receptor 2-mediated phosphorylation of focal adhesion kinase by heat shock protein 90 and Src kinase activities. J Biol Chem. 2004;279(37):39175–85.

[82] Le Boeuf F, Houle F, Sussman M, Huot J. Phosphorylation of focal adhesion kinase (FAK) on Ser732 is induced by rho-dependent kinase and is essential for proline-rich tyrosine kinase-2-mediated phosphorylation of FAK on Tyr407 in response to vascular endothelial growth factor. Mol Biol Cell. 2006;17(8):3508–20.

[83] Takai Y, Sasaki T, Matozaki T. Small GTP-binding proteins. Physiol Rev. 2001;81(1): 153–208.

[84] van der Meel R, Symons MH, Kudernatsch R, Kok RJ, Schiffelers RM, Storm G, et al. The VEGF/Rho GTPase signalling pathway: a promising target for anti-angiogenic/anti-invasion therapy. Drug Discov Today. 2011;16(5–6):219–28.

[85] Sulpice E, Ding S, Muscatelli-Groux B, Bergé M, Han ZC, Plouet J, et al. Cross-talk between the VEGF-A and HGF signalling pathways in endothelial cells. Biol Cell. 2009;101(9):525–39.

[86] Gavard J, Gutkind JS. VEGF controls endothelial-cell permeability by promoting the beta-arrestin-dependent endocytosis of VE-cadherin. Nat Cell Biol. 2006;8(11): 1223–34.

[87] Garrett TA, Van Buul JD, Burridge K. VEGF-induced Rac1 activation in endothelial cells is regulated by the guanine nucleotide exchange factor Vav2. Exp Cell Res. 2007;313(15):3285–97.

[88] Lamalice L, Houle F, Jourdan G, Huot J. Phosphorylation of tyrosine 1214 on VEGFR2 is required for VEGF-induced activation of Cdc42 upstream of SAPK2/p38. Oncogene. 2004;23(2):434–45.

[89] Annerén C, Lindholm CK, Kriz V, Welsh M. The FRK/RAK-SHB signaling cascade: a versatile signal-transduction pathway that regulates cell survival, differentiation and proliferation. Curr Mol Med. 2003;3(4):313–24.

[90] Holmqvist K, Cross M, Riley D, Welsh M. The Shb adaptor protein causes Src-dependent cell spreading and activation of focal adhesion kinase in murine brain endothelial cells. Cell Signal. 2003;15(2):171–9.

[91] Granum S, Andersen TC, Sørlie M, Jørgensen M, Koll L, Berge T, et al. Modulation of Lck function through multisite docking to T cell-specific adapter protein. J Biol Chem. 2008;283(32):21909–19.

[92] Berge T, Sundvold-Gjerstad V, Granum S, Andersen TC, Holthe GB, Claesson-Welsh L, et al. T cell specific adapter protein (TSAd) interacts with Tec kinase ITK to promote CXCL12 induced migration of human and murine T cells. PLoS One. 2010;5(3):e9761.

[93] Lettau M, Pieper J, Gerneth A, Lengl-Janssen B, Voss M, Linkermann A, et al. The adapter protein Nck: role of individual SH3 and SH2 binding modules for protein interactions in T lymphocytes. Protein Sci. 2010;19(4):658–69.

[94] Stoletov KV, Ratcliffe KE, Spring SC, Terman BI. NCK and PAK participate in the signaling pathway by which vascular endothelial growth factor stimulates the assembly of focal adhesions. J Biol Chem. 2001;276(25):22748–55.

[95] Hedman AC, Smith JM, Sacks DB. The biology of IQGAP proteins: beyond the cytoskeleton. EMBO Rep. 2015;16(4):427–46.

[96] Yamaoka-Tojo M, Ushio-Fukai M, Hilenski L, Dikalov SI, Chen YE, Tojo T, et al. IQGAP1, a novel vascular endothelial growth factor receptor binding protein, is involved in reactive oxygen species-dependent endothelial migration and proliferation. Circ Res. 2004;95(3):276–83.

[97] Yamaoka-Tojo M, Tojo T, Kim HW, Hilenski L, Patrushev NA, Zhang L, et al. IQGAP1 mediates VE-cadherin-based cell-cell contacts and VEGF signaling at adherence junctions linked to angiogenesis. Arterioscler Thromb Vasc Biol. 2006;26(9):1991–7.

[98] Dance M, Montagner A, Yart A, Masri B, Audigier Y, Perret B, et al. The adaptor protein Gab1 couples the stimulation of vascular endothelial growth factor receptor-2 to the activation of phosphoinositide 3-kinase. J Biol Chem. 2006;281(32):23285–95.

[99] Laramée M, Chabot C, Cloutier M, Stenne R, Holgado-Madruga M, Wong AJ, et al. The scaffolding adapter Gab1 mediates vascular endothelial growth factor signaling and is required for endothelial cell migration and capillary formation. J Biol Chem. 2007;282(11):7758–69.

[100] Cébe-Suarez S, Zehnder-Fjällman A, Ballmer-Hofer K. The role of VEGF receptors in angiogenesis; complex partnerships. Cell Mol Life Sci. 2006;63(5):601–15.

[101] Raimondi C, Ruhrberg C. Neuropilin signalling in vessels, neurons and tumours. Semin Cell Dev Biol. 2013;24(3):172–8.

[102] Fantin A, Herzog B, Mahmoud M, Yamaji M, Plein A, Denti L, et al. Neuropilin 1 (NRP1) hypomorphism combined with defective VEGF-A binding reveals novel roles for NRP1 in developmental and pathological angiogenesis. Development. 2014;141(3):556–62.

[103] Plein A, Fantin A, Ruhrberg C. Neuropilin regulation of angiogenesis, arteriogenesis, and vascular permeability. Microcirculation. 2014;21(4):315–23.

[104] Ballmer-Hofer K, Andersson AE, Ratcliffe LE, Berger P. Neuropilin-1 promotes VEGFR-2 trafficking through Rab11 vesicles thereby specifying signal output. Blood. 2011;118(3):816–26.

[105] Chen TT, Luque A, Lee S, Anderson SM, Segura T, Iruela-Arispe ML. Anchorage of VEGF to the extracellular matrix conveys differential signaling responses to endothelial cells. J Cell Biol. 2010;188(4):595–609.

[106] Grazia Lampugnani M, Zanetti A, Corada M, Takahashi T, Balconi G, Breviario F, et al. Contact inhibition of VEGF-induced proliferation requires vascular endothelial cadherin, beta-catenin, and the phosphatase DEP-1/CD148. J Cell Biol. 2003;161(4):793–804.

[107] Gampel A, Moss L, Jones MC, Brunton V, Norman JC, Mellor H. VEGF regulates the mobilization of VEGFR2/KDR from an intracellular endothelial storage compartment. Blood. 2006;108(8):2624–31.

[108] Scott A, Mellor H. VEGF receptor trafficking in angiogenesis. Biochem Soc Trans. 2009;37(Pt 6):1184–8.

[109] Simons M, Gordon E, Claesson-Welsh L. Mechanisms and regulation of endothelial VEGF receptor signalling. Nat Rev Mol Cell Biol. 2016;17(10):611–25.

[110] Lampugnani MG, Orsenigo F, Gagliani MC, Tacchetti C, Dejana E. Vascular endothelial cadherin controls VEGFR-2 internalization and signaling from intracellular compartments. J Cell Biol. 2006;174(4):593–604.

[111] Nagy JA, Dvorak AM, Dvorak HF. Vascular hyperpermeability, angiogenesis, and stroma generation. Cold Spring Harb Perspect Med. 2012;2(2):a006544.

[112] Oda N, Abe M, Sato Y. ETS-1 converts endothelial cells to the angiogenic phenotype by inducing the expression of matrix metalloproteinases and integrin beta3. J Cell Physiol. 1999;178(2):121–32.

[113] Heo SH, Choi YJ, Ryoo HM, Cho JY. Expression profiling of ETS and MMP factors in VEGF-activated endothelial cells: role of MMP-10 in VEGF-induced angiogenesis. J Cell Physiol. 2010;224(3):734–42.

10

Angiogenesis-Related Factors in Early Pregnancy Loss

Marina M. Ziganshina, Lyubov V. Krechetova,

Lyudmila V. Vanko, Zulfiya S. Khodzhaeva,

Ekaterina L. Yarotskaya and Gennady T. Sukhikh

Abstract

The habitual loss of early pregnancy is one of the major problems of obstetrics now-adays, provided that the cause of more than 50% of all early pregnancy losses is unknown. Adequate angiogenesis is one of the main indicators of proper formation of placental system, making the basis of fetal life support. The objective description of angiogenesis in physiological development of pregnancy and in pathological conditions is complicated by the difficulties in obtaining and characterizing placental tissue in early pregnancy. Thus, angiogenesis-related factors are promising indicators to characterize angiogenesis in pregnancy. This chapter draws attention to alteration in angiogenesis-related factors in peripheral blood of patients with habitual early pregnancy losses. Investigation of factors (vascular endothelial growth factor (VEGF), sFlt-1, sKDR, metalloproteinase (MMP)-2, MMP-9, tissue inhibitor (TIMP)-1, TIMP-2 and placental growth factor (PLGF)), which specifically and nonspecifically regulate angiogenesis in pregnancy, was performed in the most significant terms for placentogenesis: 6 weeks, 7–8 weeks and 11–14 weeks of pregnancy. It was found that in a missed abortion there was a significant imbalance of angiogenesis-related factors compared with normal pregnancy. These results reflect a disturbance of angiogenesis in a missed abortion and point to the importance of the studied factors in the pathogenesis of early pregnancy losses.

Keywords: Angiogenesis, angiogenic factors, pregnancy, angiogenesis inhibitors, matrix metalloproteinases, pro- and antiangiogenic factors ratio, VEGF/VEGF-R1, VEGF/VEGF-R2, MMP-9/TIMP-1

1. Introduction

Adequate formation of uteroplacental and fetal placental blood flow is the determining factor of physiological pregnancy and fetal development. Successful uterine-placental vascular morphogenesis and embryonic morphogenesis of fetal blood system are the basis of these processes. There are two stages of vascular morphogenesis: vasculogenesis—primary formation and development of blood vessels *de novo* from committed mesodermal cells—and angiogenesis—formation of new blood vessels from existing vascular structures, which reflect the formation of vascular system of a fetus and placenta during pregnancy [1–4].

"Early pregnancy" period includes several time intervals when the most significant for angiogenesis events occur, determining further course and outcome of pregnancy. During gestation up to 6 weeks, the primary fetal circulatory system and placental bed with the development of villi are formed, and extensive vascularization of placental villous tree occurs. The 6–8th weeks of pregnancy are marked by the start of transition to the placental circulation, as well as by the most expressed invasion of extravillous trophoblast into maternal spiral arteries (first wave of trophoblast invasion). The period of 11–13 weeks is considered to be borderline and is characterized by the completion of embryogenesis, the starting period of fetal development, fading of the first wave of trophoblast invasion and further increase in the volume of uteroplacental blood flow [4–8].

During trophoblast invasion into endometrium, interactions with components of the extracellular matrix, which is mediated by cell adhesion molecules, occur. Proteinases participate in the degradation of extracellular matrix and cell migration deep into the myometrium through the uterine spiral arteries. Cytotrophoblast cells change their phenotype from epithelial to endothelial, producing a large number of soluble factors contributing to the development of the vasculature [9, 10].

Growth factors play the key role in vessels formation. They serve as cell mitogens, as attractants in the formation of vascular architectonics, and most important, as morphogens. The main regulators of angiogenesis are members of the family of vascular endothelial growth factor (VEGF). In addition to direct activators of angiogenesis, there is a large group of factors, whose effect on angiogenesis is nonspecific. It includes matrix metalloproteinases (MMPs) and their tissue inhibitors (TIMPs) [11–14].

Decidual NK-cells in early pregnancy, at the stage preceding the invasion of trophoblast into the maternal arteries, produce VEGF, placental growth factor (PLGF) and matrix metalloproteinases (MMPs), in particular MMP-2 and MMP-9 [15–17]. These MMPs are collagenases of IV type which specifically hydrolyze the collagen of basement membranes and thereby facilitate cell invasion through the basement membranes and stimulate angiogenesis [18–21]. Decidual NK-cells are the main source of MMP-2 and TIMP-2 from the group of tissue inhibitors of matrix metalloproteinases (TIMPs) [22–24].

Trophoblast also produces factors regulating processes of vessels formation. Particularly, MMP-9, TIMP-1, TIMP-2 and TIMP-3 are produced by the cells of extravillous trophoblast. Villous cytotrophoblast cells and invasive endovascular trophoblast produce MMP-2 which is considered a key regulator of cell invasion in early gestation (up to 8 weeks), according to some authors [17, 19].

Production of anti-angiogenic factors is an integral part of the normal angiogenesis. As a result of the molecular dialog during vascularization, production of inhibitors serves as a hamper for excessive trophoblast invasion, as well as an obstacle for the further development of the vascular bed and for vascularization of pathologically changed tissue sites. Angiogenic factors are specifically expressed in endothelium and in the placenta during pregnancy. These include receptors VEGF-R1 (Flt-1), VEGF-R2 (Flk-1, KDR) and VEGF-R3 (Flt-4). Soluble forms of these receptors are able to bind growth factors in circulation, slowing or blocking angiogenesis [25].

Humoral factors involved in vascular formation processes are more accessible for research in maternal circulation, and change of their content in mother's blood reflects changes in the content of these factors in the fetal blood circulation and tissues. In this regard, a complex study of angiogenesis-related factors and their ratios is crucial for understanding and predicting vascular morphogenesis disorders during pregnancy.

2. Characteristics of the groups and study design

The prospective study included 66 patients with early stage pregnancy.

The control group consisted of 20 patients with normal pregnancy. All the patients had one or two previous pregnancies uneventfully completed at term.

The main subgroup A consisted of 16 patients with the history of miscarriage and current threatening miscarriage. All patients from the main subgroup A gave live births at term. The main subgroup B included 30 patients whose pregnancy ended as «missed abortion».

In patients of the control group and of the main subgroup A, the study of angiogenesis-related factors in peripheral blood samples was performed within 6 weeks, at 7–8 weeks and at 11–14 weeks of pregnancy. In the main subgroup B, the investigation was conducted at the time of diagnosis of «missed abortion» (8 patients were examined before 6 weeks, 14 patients—at 7-8 weeks and 8 patients—at 11-14 weeks).

The criteria for inclusion into the main groups were as follows: history of two and more early pregnancy losses, no childbirth in current marriage, singleton natural pregnancy.

Exclusion criteria were endometriosis, POS, uterine fibroids, induced pregnancy and/or extragenital conditions (diabetes mellitus, psoriasis and systemic autoimmune diseases, and malignancies), FV L and FII G20210A gene mutations, and activation of bacterial viral infections. Groups were matched for the patient's age.

Diagnosis of recurrent miscarriage was established according to the International Classification of Diseases 10th Edition (ICD-10-CM). Pregnancy was diagnosed based on the ultrasonography study and HCG.

The samples of peripheral blood for investigation of angiogenesis-related factors were obtained from the cubital vein not later than 5 days after ultrasonic detection of cessation of pregnancy development in the patients of the main subgroup B in case of intact chorion (absence of retroplacental and/or retro amniotic hematomas, vaginal tract bleedings). Prior to investigation, the serum was stored at the temperature of «-80°C».

3. Methods

Determination of serum levels of VEGF, VEGF-R1 (sFlt-1), VEGF-R2 (sKDR), MMP-2, MMP-9, TIMP-1, TIMP-2 and PLGF was performed by enzyme-linked immunosorbent assay (ELISA) using standard test systems: Bender MedSystems GmbH (Austria) and R&D Systems (USA). The optical density was measured using the plate reader BioTek (USA) at the wavelength of 450 nm. Construction of the calibration curve and calculation of the concentrations of VEGF, sFlt-1, sKDR, MMP-2, MMP-9, TIMP-1, TIMP-2 and PLGF were performed by linear regression equation in logarithmic coordinates.

The statistical processing was carried out using statistical analysis package for Microsoft Office Excel 2007 and software package Statistica for Windows 7.0, Statsoft Inc. (USA). Control of the normality of obtained parameters in studied groups was performed with Shapiro-Wilk W test. The significance of differences of mean values of the measured parameters was evaluated using unpaired t-test with different dispersions. Differences were considered significant at a significance level $p < 0.05$.

4. Results

Results of the study of angiogenesis-related factors are presented in **Tables 1** and **2**.

4.1. Time course of angiogenesis-related factors in patients with normal pregnancy

It was found that VEGF had the maximum concentration in blood at terms up to 6 weeks of gestation: Contents of this factor was significantly higher (more than 10 times) compared with further points of study. Concentration of PLGF at terms up to 6 weeks and at 7–8 weeks remained unchanged but increased more than two times by 11–14 weeks; this is consistent with the published data [24]. This trend in changing of VEGF and PLGF during early pregnancy probably provides pro-angiogenic effect because under the decrease in VEGF, PLGF is able to synergistically enhance angiogenesis promoted by VEGF [26].

Level of sVEGF-R1 was minimal at the starting point of the study but significantly increased reaching maximum values at 11-14 weeks. In contrast, the concentration of sVEGF-R2 was decreased only at 7-8 weeks of pregnancy. It is known that VEGF interacts with receptors VEGF-R1 and VEGF-R2, while VEGF-R1 is the only receptor for PLGF [27]. These factors compete for binding with VEGF-R1. Under increased secretion of VEGF and PLGF, this leads to exhaustion of VEGF-R1 and predominance of VEGF-R2 in circulation. PLGF is also supposed to be able to replace VEGF in the VEGF/VEGF-R1 complex, activating the

Factor (u.m.)	Groups	Factor's values in terms of study		
		Up to 6 weeks	7–8 weeks	11–14 weeks
VEGF (pg/ml)	Control	100.5 ± 24.5	$5.5 \pm 1.3^{\#}$	$8.9 \pm 3.2^{\#}$
	Main subgroup A	202.7 ± 82.3	$5.9 \pm 0.9^{\#}$	$4.2 \pm 1.2^{\#}$
	Main subgroup B	49.6 ± 28.6	4.7 ± 1.9	3.2 ± 0.4
VEGF-R1 (ng/ml)	Control	0.4 ± 0.1	$1.1 \pm 0.2^{\#}$	$1.7 \pm 0.4^{\#}$
	Main subgroup A	$0.9 \pm 0.1^{*}$	$1.4 \pm 0.1^{*\#}$	$1.7 \pm 0.1^{\#} \bullet$
	Main subgroup B	$0.4 \pm 0.1^{**}$	$5.8 \pm 2.6^{*\#}$	$0.5 \pm 0.2^{*,**} \bullet$
VEGF-R2 (ng/ml)	Control	9.4 ± 1.9	$4.9 \pm 0.6^{\#}$	$9.3 \pm 1.5 \bullet$
	Main subgroup A	8.4 ± 1.9	$10.6 \pm 0.4^{*}$	10.5 ± 0.6
	Main subgroup B	12.5 ± 2.0	$11.6 \pm 1.5^{*}$	12.5 ± 2.0
PLGF (pg/ml)	Control	12.2 ± 1.4	13.2 ± 2.5	$28.9 \pm 4.1^{\#} \bullet$
	Main subgroup A	$7.5 \pm 0.6^{*}$	$9.9 \pm 0.8^{\#}$	$22.5 \pm 2.5^{\#} \bullet$
	Main subgroup B	$8.5 \pm 0.7^{*}$	9.5 ± 2.0	$8.8 \pm 2.4^{*,**}$

*Comparison with the control group;
**comparison with the main subgroup A;
#the differences within one group in comparison with the data obtained before 6 weeks.
•the differences within one group in comparison with data obtained at 7-8 weeks (# < 0.05).

Table 1. Blood levels of pro- and antiangiogenic factors of the first trimester of pregnancy.

Factor (u.m.)	Groups	Factor's values in terms of study		
		up to 6 weeks	7–8 weeks	11–14 weeks
MMP-2 (ng/ml)	Control	330.6 ± 31.1	331.8 ± 13.2	364.2 ± 30.9
	Main subgroup A	$415.3 \pm 21.9^{*}$	$411.1 \pm 30.0^{*}$	392.6 ± 34.8
	Main subgroup B	$526.8 \pm 16.0^{*,**}$	$378.7 \pm 33.7^{\#}$	$271.8 \pm 21.9^{*,\,**\#} \bullet$
MMP-9 (ng/ml)	Control	556.5 ± 71.4	$379.6 \pm 50.1^{\#}$	558.8 ± 92.8
	Main subgroup A	537.2 ± 78.6	500.1 ± 51.1	578.9 ± 109.0
	Main subgroup B	296.1 ± 132.6	403.6 ± 79.3	$278.0 \pm 67.7^{*,**}$
TIMP-1 (ng/ml)	Control	435.6 ± 31.0	$357.5 \pm 26.1^{\#}$	388.5 ± 23.9
	Main subgroup A	440.3 ± 62.1	$458.8 \pm 34.1^{*}$	$344.0 \pm 42.3 \bullet$
	Main subgroup B	$321.4 \pm 27.9^{*}$	403.9 ± 48.9	342.0 ± 27.4
TIMP-2 (ng/ml)	Control	22.6 ± 2.1	19.4 ± 1.5	21.0 ± 1.5
	Main subgroup A	23.3 ± 2.4	21.2 ± 2.6	$29.4 \pm 4.1^{*}$
	Main subgroup B	$30.4 \pm 1.4^{*,**}$	$25.3 \pm 3.0^{*}$	$18.1 \pm 1.3^{**\#} \bullet$

*Comparison with the control group;
**comparison with the main subgroup A;
#the differences within one group in comparison with the data obtained before 6 weeks.
•the differences within one group in comparison with data obtained at 7-8 weeks ($p < 0.05$).

Table 2. Blood levels of matrix metalloproteinases and their tissue inhibitors in the first trimester of pregnancy.

expression of VEGF-R2 [28]. According to the published data, VEGF-R2 is a key receptor in angiogenesis [29] although its affinity to VEGF is quite lower than VEGF-R1 [30].

It is known that normally pro-angiogenic molecules are less than their inhibitors; nevertheless, intensive vascularization of placenta and of fetal developing organs occurs in pregnancy. This situation can be described as "pro-angiogenic state." However, it is quite difficult to quantify it, as the described models of angiogenic factors-receptor interactions do not give guide on the factor/inhibitor ratio, allowing to specify the pro-angiogenic state or block of angiogenesis [26, 31]. Therefore, trends observed in normal pregnancy may serve as references for challenging cases.

Blood levels of MMP-2 and TIMP-2 vary insignificantly in the studied terms of normal pregnancy. Significant decrease in MMP-9 and TIMP-1 concentration was found at 7–8 weeks compared with the terms before 6 weeks of pregnancy.

Normally, MMPs blood level is insignificant. Soluble forms of MMPs are present in blood as inactive proenzymes and transfer into active forms after propeptide cleavage under the impact of activation factors including inhibitors. Constant concentrations in the system "protease-antiprotease" (MMP-2/TIMP-2) may indicate extracellular matrix remodeling and vascular morphogenesis which intensively go at these terms; degradation of interstitial collagens and basement membrane collagens under the participation of these factors is obvious.

4.2. Time course of angiogenesis-related factors in patients of the main subgroup A

Blood levels of PLGF and sVEGF-R1 in patients of main subgroup A significantly increased with gestational age. In contrast, concentration of VEGF was maximum at the starting point of the study but significantly decreased (more than 30 times) by 7-8 weeks and then remained at the same level till 11–14 weeks of gestation.

Lack of significant differences in dynamics of MMP-2, MMP-9, TIMP-2 and sVEGF-R2 was observed during entire pregnancy. Concentration of TIMP-1 significantly decreased by 11–14 weeks.

Thus, in the main subgroup A, we found significant fluctuations of certain soluble factors. For several factors (VEGF, PLGF, MMP-2, TIMP-2), trends of this levels alterations at the same study points coincided with those observed during normal pregnancy; there was no statistically significant differences between the groups and the most studied terms. At the same time, for sVEGF-R1, sVEGF-R2, MMP-9 and TIMP-1, the trends were significantly different from the control group. However, these differences do not seem sufficient to cause dramatic consequences in pregnancy. Probably for successful outcome of pregnancy, a balanced production of VEGF and PLGF, key angiogenic factors for pregnancy [14, 24, 32], is necessary, as well as the balance between MMP-2 and TIMP-2, because MMP-2 is the key regulator of trophoblast invasion [17, 19] especially in early pregnancy.

4.3. Angiogenesis-related factors in the main subgroup B

4.3.1. Blood levels of angiogenesis-related factors in patients with missed abortion before 6 weeks of gestation

Missed abortion before 6 weeks was characterized by significant differences of the levels of angiogenesis-related factors: sVEGF-R1, PLGF, MMP-2, TIMP-1 and TIMP-2. Thus, with missed abortion, the level of PLGF was lower than in the control group; however, there was no significant difference with the main subgroup A. Blood level of sVEGF-R1 did not differ from the values of the control group. However, comparison with the main subgroup A showed that in complicated pregnancy which further accomplished with childbirth, level of sVEGF-R1 was higher than in missed abortion. These results may indicate the existence of subtle mechanisms of regulation in the system "ligand/receptor," where the most important aspect is not a certain level of material content of the molecule, but the impacts of the factors on each other.

The concentrations of MMP-2 in the main subgroups A and B were significantly higher than in the control group. The maximum level of MMP-2 in blood was detected in missed abortion. TIMP-1 and TIMP-2 levels in the control group and main subgroup A differed insignificantly; in the main subgroup B, the level of TIMP-1 was significantly lower and the level of TIMP-2 was significantly higher at these terms.

Thus, more distinct differences specific for missed abortion were found in the group of factors "protease-antiprotease." The content of the factors in the system MMP-2–TIMP-2 at this term is, probably, critical for pregnancy. It is known that MMP-2 and TIMP-2 are most important at early terms of gestation during trophoblast invasion into maternal tissues [19]. Constant expression of MMP-2 and TIMP-2 was detected in apical layer of the syncytiotrophoblast and decidual NK-cells [19]. The published data suggest a possibility of syncytium activation by MMP-2, and the participation of this molecule in the processing of paracrine factors synthesized by these cells [19, 21]. There is a probability of change in the balance of production of biologically active molecules determining the development of pregnancy, due to the excessive production of MMP-2 or TIMP-2.

Pregnancy-initiated angiogenesis is closely associated with tissue remodeling and vascularization. Changes occurring in the endometrium decidualization include as follows: infiltration of tissues by immune cells (uNK-cells and macrophages), extracellular matrix remodeling with cell invasion through the matrix and membrane, and lysis of muscle-elastic tissue elements. In this period, the most important processes are formation of the placental bed and vascularization of the villi [6, 8, 10]. It is known that embryos which stopped to develop at 3–5 weeks had vascular villi, large hydropic dystrophy of the villous stroma and no embryonic blood vessels [33–35]. The disbalance of angiogenic factors, causing autocrine and paracrine effects to each other and to the cells, leads to microenvironment that is not compatible with the development of pregnancy. Excessive protease activity under these conditions may also reflect degenerative processes in the uterus before abortion.

4.3.2. Blood levels of angiogenesis-related factors in patients with missed abortion at 7–8 weeks

Pathological changes specific for missed abortion at 7–8 weeks were reflected by the significant increase in VEGF-R1, VEGF-R2 and TIMP-2 levels compared with the control group.

The interval of 7–8 weeks of gestation is marked by the first wave of trophoblast invasion into the mother's arteries and the start of uteroplacental blood flow. Extravillous trophoblast has a high invasive potential and expresses VEGF, PLGF and VEGF-R1 [36]. The receptor VEGF-R2 is expressed by the cells of fetoplacental complex [36, 37]. It should be noted that the level of VEGF-R1 is five times higher and VEGF-R2 more than two times differ from these factor levels in the control group. According to the published data, soluble forms of VEGF-R1 and VEGF-R2 are able to block angiogenesis and adversely affect the migration and proliferation of endothelial cells [27, 38, 39]. However, comparison with the main subgroup A did not show any significant differences in the studied period. Therefore, excessive levels of soluble forms of VEGF-R1 and VEGF-R2 in maternal circulation are not the main cause of this pathology at this term. It is known that adequate angiogenesis of villous tree and chorionic villi are critical stage and condition for further development of the placenta and fetus [1–4]. Inadequate start of restriction of uterine arteries at these terms initiates a chain of troubles in the system mother-placenta-fetus.

The key process of pregnancy is cytotrophoblast invasion into uterine arteries. At the same time, there is arteriolar lumen expansion under the impact of metalloproteinases. Excess of tissue inhibitors at 7–8 weeks, probably, leads to incomplete trophoblast invasion and insufficient lumen expansion which under the increased secretion of VEGF-R1 and VEGF-R2 can result in vasospasm and enhanced vascular permeability-specific manifestations of increased contents of these factors [36, 40] which adversely affect the embryo development.

4.3.3. Blood levels of angiogenesis-related factors in patients with missed abortion at 11–14 weeks of pregnancy

Missed abortion detected at of 11–14 weeks was characterized by a significant decrease in sVEGF-R1, PLGF, MMP-2 and MMP-9 compared with the control group and main subgroup A. Level of TIMP-2 was significantly lower than in the main subgroup A, but close to the control group.

The end of the first trimester of pregnancy is marked by the start of the fetal period of intrauterine human development, fading of the first wave of trophoblast invasion and preparation for a second wave at 16-18 weeks of pregnancy. Significant decrease in soluble forms of VEGF-R1 and PLGF in the main subgroup B could evidence the role of these factors in the pathologic processes leading to pregnancy loss. PLGF is the main regulatory factor in the first trimester of physiological pregnancy [2, 24] that acts as paracrine regulator of decidual angiogenesis and autocrine regulator of trophoblast function [24]. The synergy of effects of PLGF and VEGF on angiogenesis manifests with the morphogenesis of more mature and stable vasculature [24, 27]. Its effect is more significant in angiogenesis than in vasculogenesis [2]. Besides inhibition of angiogenesis, soluble form of the receptor VEGF-R1 also provides "support," and thus, the effect depends on the factor blood level. Probably in this situation, levels of sVEGF-R1 and PLGF are insufficient for adequate angiogenesis.

4.4. Ratio of angiogenesis-related factors

Dynamic balance in the system ligand/receptor provides a state of the system which empowers the implementation of its function, if this system tends towards the harmonic balance. The equilibrium point in such systems is always moving, because ligand/receptor pairs, being complex systems, are influenced by a variety of factors. In terms of the dynamic balance theory, ligand's positions in this study were occupied by the factors which specifically and nonspecifically affect angiogenesis, while the receptor's positions were occupied by its inhibitors. Studied ligands and receptors have multiple substrate specificity, but because their activity is affected by other factors that are present in the bloodstream and were not included in this study, investigation of ligand/receptor pairs in terms of classical concepts is difficult. Moreover, current models describing interactions of VEGF family members with the receptors [26] as well as of the matrix metalloproteinase family members with the inhibitors [31] do not provide quantitative binding characteristics of the system receptor/ligand for these molecules. The situation is complicated by the different levels of expression of these factors by various cell types. Therefore, the use of any index or ratio characterizing the dynamic situation in the selected time interval as a pro-angiogenic or nonproangiogenic state does not seem possible. To describe such situations, "surrogate" indexes characterizing the ligand/receptor ratio may be most appropriate to define any process, particularly angiogenesis. Such ratios are used to calculate the risk of development of pregnancy complications, such as preeclampsia [41–44].

Changes of the ligand/receptor pair ratio (VEGF/VEGF-R1, VEGF/VEGF-R2, PLGF/VEGF-R1, MMP-9/TIMP-1, MMP-2/TIMP-2) in the studied groups are presented in **Figure 1**.

4.4.1. VEGF/VEGF-R1 and VEGF/VEGF-R2 ratios

VEGF/VEGF-R1 ratio (**Figure 1A**) in the control group before 6 weeks was significantly higher than in the main subgroups A and B (0.562; 0.178 and 0.0312, respectively). In the control group, we observed significant differences between the terms before 6 weeks of gestation and other terms. Interestingly, the pattern of the VEGF/VEGF-R1 ratio change in the main subgroup A had tendencies similar to the control group. In the main subgroup B, the values of ligand/receptor pairs were significantly low, except for the last study term (0.0086) compared with the control group (0.006) and the main subgroup A (0.0024).

VEGF/VEGF-R2 ratio changed in a similar way (**Figure 1B**). Before 6 weeks of pregnancy, the significant changes were noted only in the main subgroup B (0.0023), compared with the control group (0.020) and the main subgroup A (0.011).

Tendencies of changes of VEGF/VEGF-R2 were similar in the control and the main subgroup A, demonstrating at the same time significant differences at 7-8 weeks. The main subgroup B was characterized by minimal values of the ratio which significantly differed in terms before 6 and 7–8 weeks compared with the other groups, but do not change within group in all terms of pregnancy.

It is known that realization of different mechanisms of angiogenesis depends on the type of receptor interacting with VEGF. Activation of VEGF-R2 leads to stimulation of angiogenesis

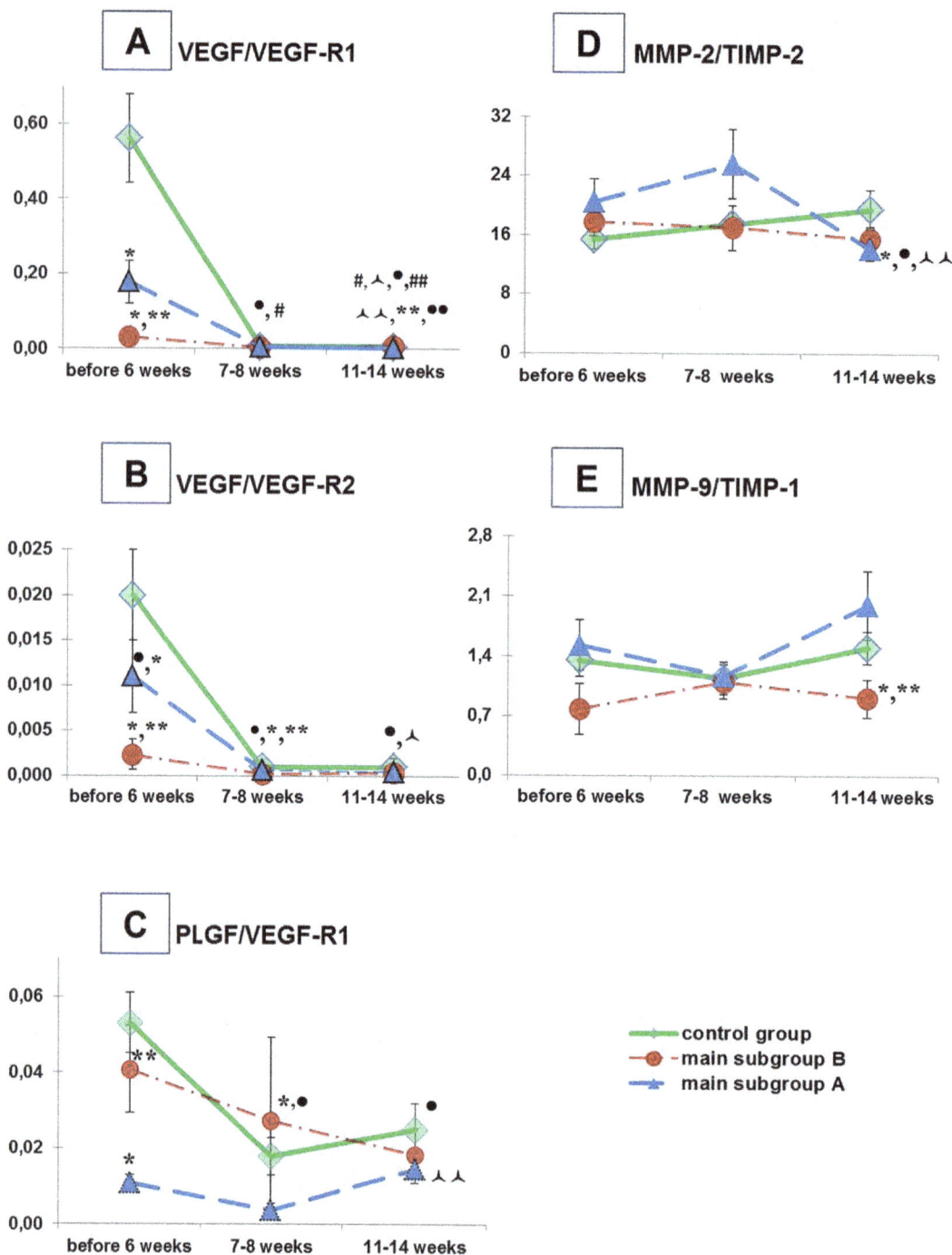

Figure 1. Factor/receptor (A, B, C) and factor/inhibitor (D, E) ratio in the blood of women at early terms of pregnancy. *Significant difference from the control group; **significant difference from the main subgroup A; 'significant differences inside the control group in comparison with terms before 6 weeks; ''significant difference inside the control group in comparison with terms 7-8 weeks; #significant difference inside the main subgroup A in comparison with terms before 6 weeks; ##significant difference inside the main subgroup A in comparison with terms 7-8 weeks; ⅄ significant difference inside the main subgroup B in comparison with terms before 6 weeks; ⅄ ⅄ significant difference inside the main subgroup B in comparison with terms 7-8 weeks ($p < 0.05$).

by triggering proliferation, migration, differentiation and inhibition of apoptosis of endothelial cells. Activated VEGF-R1 receptor stimulates intercellular interactions, branching of vascular network and regulates the trophoblast invasion into the spiral arteries [27]. Use of blocking antibodies for VEGF-R2 causes reduction in decidual angiogenesis and pregnancy loss in mice, while use of antibodies of similar effect for VEGF-R1 does not cause such effects [37]. In other studies, the lack of VEGF-R1 in experimental animals led to overdevelopment of disorganized vessels and clusters of endothelial cells, and the absence of VEGF-R2—to reduction in development of vasculature [2]. It has been demonstrated that interaction of VEGF/VEGF-R2 regulates the development of fetoplacental complex [27] and acts as a paracrine system in the processes of formation of primitive embryo vascular network [24, 29]. On the contrary, the formation of an active complex VEGF/VEGF-R1 mostly affects the processes of differentiation and migration of trophoblast and also regulates invasion [27].

4.4.2. PLGF/VEGF-R1 ratio

PLGF factor affects endothelium through specific binding with the receptor VEGF-R1 (**Figure 1C**). According to the published data, PLGF more impacts the processes of angiogenesis, than vasculogenesis; however, PLGF and VEGF-R1 also affect the mobilization of mesenchymal progenitors of endothelial cells, which are involved in vasculogenesis [2]. PLGF enhances angiogenesis acting synergistically with VEGF, and it is also able to replace VEGF in the complex with VEGF/VEGF-R1 releasing it for VEGF-R2 activation. It is also known that PLGF is a paracrine regulator of decidual angiogenesis and autocrine regulator of trophoblast's functions in differentiation and invasion [24] and also the main regulating factor in normal pregnancy in the first trimester [2, 24].

The ratio of PLGF/VEGF-R1 for each group of pregnant women had its own tendencies. There were significant differences between the main subgroup A and control group before 6 and at 7–8 weeks. However, there was notable misbalance of factors in ligand/receptor pair PLGF/VEGF-R1 manifesting with significant deviations from the average value of the factors ratio at 7-8 weeks of pregnancy in the main subgroup B. Moreover, low ratio values were noted in the ligand/receptor pair of the main subgroup A at all studied points. The reduced value of this ratio in the main subgroup A may be due to the changes in the dynamic system PLGF/VEGF-R1 (both toward the increase in sVEGF-R1 and toward the decrease in PLGF). Obtained ratio values for the given ligand/receptor pair for all groups at early terms of pregnancy may evidence the acceptable fluctuations of the values of the factors in this pair, which are nonsignificant for the development of pregnancy.

4.4.3. MMP-9/TIMP-1 and MMP-2/TIMP-2 ratio

Analysis of the obtained results showed no significant differences of ratios of free forms of MMPs and tissue inhibitors TIMPs (MMPs/TIMPs) between the groups at the most studied terms of pregnancy (**Figure 1D, E**). Significant differences were shown for the MMP-9/TIMP-1 ratio at 11-14 weeks for the main subgroup B (0.91) and the control group (1.48). The significant decrease in this ratio in the main subgroup B may evidence degradation processes and autolysis in missed abortion. The character of changes of the ligand/receptor ratio within studied groups confirms some stable dynamic equilibrium of the factors concentrations. Probably, nonspecific effects of the factors in the studied ligand/receptor pairs on angiogenesis processes are of somewhat conservative nature comprising prevention of excessive protease activity, and sufficient for an adequate angiogenesis at the studied terms of pregnancy. However, use of these ratios is not informative to characterize the pathologic processes at studied terms in patients of these groups, excluding the ratio MMP-9/TIMP-1 at 11-14 weeks of pregnancy. The observed reduction in MMP-9/TIMP-1 at 11-14 weeks may serve as an alert of the development of critical events.

5. Conclusions

This study revealed the features of humoral systems regulating angiogenesis during physiological pregnancy and in patients with successful and unsuccessful perinatal outcomes. We found that deviations in the peripheral blood contents of angiogenesis-related factors: VEGF-R1, VEGF-R2, MMP-9 and TIMP-1 in patients with the history of missed abortion do not reflect critical for angiogenesis events in the first trimester of pregnancy. However, a significant disbalance of soluble factors, regulating angiogenesis, detected in patients with missed abortion shows that matrix metalloproteinases and their tissue inhibitors play the leading role in pregnancy losses before 6 and 7–8 weeks. Analysis of ligand/receptor ratios complements the obtained results, as we have found a significant decrease in the VEGF/VEGF-R1 and VEGF/VEGF-R2 ratios before 6 weeks of pregnancy despite the fact that there were no significant differences between individual molecules forming these pairs. The nature of VEGF/VEGF-R1 and VEGF/VEGF-R2 ratios alterations within the groups at the studied terms suggests the presence of a single mechanism that regulates interactions between VEGF and its receptors VEGF-R1 and VEGF-R2. In patients with pregnancy losses at 11-14 weeks, we found low concentrations of PLGF and sVEGF-R1 and also of MMP-2 and MMP-9, and reduction in MMP-2/TIMP-2 ratio, which are probably insufficient for an adequate angiogenesis at this term. Since an adequate angiogenesis is the determining factor for the development of pregnancy, early identification of criteria alerting about a trouble in fetoplacental system will also have diagnostic and prognostic value. Detection of the markers is especially important in cases of habitual pregnancy loss of unknown origin, because the disturbance of angiogenesis may be one of the causes of missed abortion. Taking into account difficulties with obtaining placental tissue at the studied terms of pregnancy, the angiogenesis-related factors may serve as unbiased indicators of placental angiogenesis. The obtained results allow to presume various mechanisms of pregnancy pathology at early terms and to demonstrate the possibility of using the analysis of ligand/receptor pairs to characterize the angiogenesis processes in early pregnancy.

Acknowledgements

The authors express their deep appreciation and gratitude to employee of Department of Perinatal Pathology, Kulikova G.V and the Department of Library and Information Resources and Telemedicine, A.L. Komarovsky, V.I. Kulakov Research Center for Obstetrics, Gynecology and Perinatology of the Russian Ministry of Health, for his help in preparing this manuscript.

Author details

Marina M. Ziganshina*, Lyubov V. Krechetova, Lyudmila V. Vanko, Zulfiya S. Khodzhaeva, Ekaterina L. Yarotskaya and Gennady T. Sukhikh

*Address all correspondence to: mmz@mail.ru

Federal State Budget Institution "The Research Center for Obstetrics, Gynecology and Perinatology" of the Ministry of Healthcare of the Russian Federation, Moscow, Russia

References

[1] Demir R, Seval Y, Huppertz B. Vasculogenesis and angiogenesis in the early human placenta. Acta Histochem. 2007;109(4):257–65. doi:10.1016/j.acthis.2007.02.008

[2] Burton GI, Charnock-Jones DS, Jauniaux E. Regulation of vascular growth and function in the human placenta. Reproduction. 2009;138(6):895–902. doi:10.1530/REP-09-0092

[3] Zygmunt M, Herr F, Münstedt K, Lang U, Liang OD. Angiogenesis and vasculogenesis in pregnancy. Eur J Obstet Gynecol Reprod Biol. 2003;110(Suppl 1):S10–8. doi:10.1016/S0301-2115(03)00168-4

[4] Milovanov AP, Kirichenko AK. Molecular mechanisms of regulation of cytotrophoblastic invasion in uteroplacental region. Arkh Patol. 2001;63(5):3–8.

[5] Mihu CM, Susman S, Rus Ciucă D, Mihu D, Costin N. Aspects of placental morphogenesis and angiogenesis. Rom J Morphol Embryol. 2009;50(4):549–57. http://www.rjme.ro/RJME/resources/files/500409549557.pdf

[6] Kingdom J, Huppertz B, Seaward G, Kaufmann P. Development of the placental villous tree and its consequences for fetal growth. Eur J Obstet Gynecol Reprod Biol. 2000;92(1):35–43. doi:10.1016/S0301-2115(00)00423-1

[7] James JL, Carter AM, Chamley LW. Human placentation from nidation to 5 weeks of gestation. Part I: What do we know about formative placental development following implantation? Placenta. 2012;33(5):327–34. doi:10.1016/j.placenta.2012.01.020.

[8] Benirschke K, Burton GJ, Bergen RN. Pathology of the human placenta. 6th ed., Springer, NewYork, 2012.

[9] Kaufmann P, Black S, Huppertz B. Endovascular trophoblast invasion: implications for the pathogenesis of intrauterine growth retardation and preeclampsia. Biol Reprod. 2003;69(1):1–7. doi:10.1095/biolreprod.102.014977

[10] Pollheimer J, Knöfler M. The role of the invasive, placental trophoblast in human pregnancy. Wien Med Wochenschr. 2012;162(9–10):187–90. doi:10.1007/s10354-012-0071-6

[11] Raza SL, Cornelius LA. Matrix metalloproteinases: pro- and anti-angiogenic activities. J Investig Dermatol Symp Proc. 2000;5(1):47–54. doi:10.1046/j.1087-0024.2000.00004.x

[12] Rundhaug JE. Matrix metalloproteinases and angiogenesis. J Cell Mol Med. 2005;9(2):267–85. doi:10.1111/j.1582-4934.2005.tb00355.x

[13] Vrachnis N, Kalampokas E, Sifakis S, Vitoratos N, Kalampokas T, Botsis D, Iliodromiti Z. Placental growth factor (PlGF): a key to optimizing fetal growth. J Matern Fetal Neonatal Med. 2013;26(10):995–1002. doi:10.3109/14767058.2013.766694

[14] Andraweera PH, Dekker GA, Roberts CT. The vascular endothelial growth factor family in adverse pregnancy outcomes. Hum Reprod Update. 2012;18(4):436–57. doi:10.1093/humupd/dms011

[15] Lash GE, Schiessi B, Kirkley M, Innes BA, Cooper A, Searle RF et al. Expression of angiogenic growth factors by uterine natural killer cells during early pregnancy. J Leukoc Biol. 2006;80:572–580. doi:10.1189/jlb.0406250

[16] Quenby S, Nik H, Innes B, Lash G, Turner M, Drury J, Bulmer J. Uterine natural killer cells and angiogenesis in recurrent reproductive failure. Hum Reprod. 2009;24:45–54. doi:10.1093/humrep/den348

[17] Naruse K, Lash GE, Innes B, Otun HA, Searle RF, Robson SC, Bulmer JN. Localization of matrix metalloproteinase (MMP)-2, MMP-9 and tissue inhibitors for MMPs (TIMPs) in uterine natural killer cells in early human pregnancy. Hum Reprod. 2008;1:1–9. doi:10.1093/humrep/den408

[18] Anacker J, Feix S, Kapp M, et al. Expression pattern of matrix metalloprotenases (MMPs) in human deciduas during pregnancy. J Reprod Immunol. 2010;86:79–111.

[19] Bai SX, Wang YL, Qin L, Xiao ZJ, Herva R, Piao YS. Dynamic expression of matrix metalloproteinases (MMP-2,-9 and -14) and the tissue inhibitors of MMPs (TIMP-1,-2 and -3) at the implantation site during tubal pregnancy. Reproduction. 2005;129:103–113. doi:10.1530/rep.1.00283

[20] Cockle J, Gopichandran N, Walker J, Levene MI, Orsi NM. Matrix metalloproteinases and their tissue inhibitors in preterm perinatal complications. Reprod Sci. 2007;14:629–645. doi:10.1177/1933719107304563

[21] Smith SD, Dunk CE, Aplin J, Harris LK, Jones RL. Evidence for immune cell involvement in decidual spiral arteriole remodeling in early human pregnancy. Am J Pathol. 2009;174:1959–1971. doi:10.2353/ajpath.2009.080995

[22] Forbes K, Westwood M. Maternal growth factor regulation of human placental development and fetal growth. J Endocrinol. 2010;207:1–16. doi:10.1677/JOE-10-0174

[23] Florio P, Gabbanini M, Borges LE, Bonaccorsi L, Pinzauti S, Reis FM et al. Activins and related proteins in the establishment of pregnancy. Reprod Sci. 2010;17:320–330. doi:10.1177/1933719109353205

[24] Plaisier M, Dennert I, Rost E, Koolwijk P, van Hinsbergh VW, Helmerhorst FM. Decidual vascularization and the expression of angiogenic growth factors and proteases in first trimester spontaneous abortions. Hum Reprod. 2009;24:185–197. doi:10.1093/humrep/den296

[25] Sugimoto H, Hamano Y, Charytan D, Cosgrove D, Kieran M, Sudhakar A, Kalluri R. Neutralization of circulating vascular endothelial growth factor (VEGF) by anti-VEGF antibodies and soluble VEGF receptor 1 (sFlt-1) induced proteinuria. J Biol Chem. 2003;278:12605–12608. doi:10.1074/jbc.C300012200

[26] Gabhann FM, Popel AS. Model of competitive binding of vascular endothelial growth factor and placental growth factor to VEGF receptors on endothelial cells. Am J Physiol Heart Circ Physiol. 2004;286:H153–H164. doi:10.1152/ajpheart.00254.2003

[27] Wulff C, Weigand M, Kreienberg R, Fraser HM. Angiogenesis during primate placentation in health and disease. Reproduction. 2003;126:569–577. doi:10.1530/rep.0.1260569

[28] Dewerchin M, Carmeliet P. PlGF: a multitasking cytokine with disease-restricted activity. Cold Spring Harb Perspect Med. 2012;2(8). pii: a011056. doi:10.1101/cshperspect.a011056

[29] Plaisier M, Streefland E, Koolwijk P, van Hinsbergh VW, Helmerhorst FM, Erwich JJ. Angiogenic growth factors and their receptors in first-trimester human decidua of pregnancies further complicated by preeclampsia or fetal growth restriction. Reprod Sci. 2008;15:720–726. doi:10.1177/1933719108317300

[30] Molskness TA, Stouffer RL, Burry KA, Gorrill MJ, Lee DM, Patton PE. Circulating levels of free and total vascular endothelial growth factor (VEGF)-A, soluble VEGF recepror-1 and -2, and angiogenin during ovarian stimulation in non-human primates and women. Hum Reprod. 2004;19:822–830. doi:10.1093/humrep/deh132

[31] Olson MW, Gervasi DC, Mobashery S, Fridman R. Kinetic analysis of the binding of human matrix metalloproteinase-2 and -9 to tissue inhibitor of metalloproteinase (TIMP-1) and (TIMP-2). J Biol Chem. 1997;272:29975–29983. doi:10.1074/jbc.272.47.29975

[32] Kalkunte SS, Mselle NF, Norris WE, Wira CR, Sentman CL, Sharma S. Vascular endothelial growth factor C facilitates immune tolerance and endovascular activity of human uterine NK cells at the maternal-fetal interface. J Immunol. 2009;182:4085–4092. doi:10.4049/jimmunol.0803769

[33] Cherstvoi ED, Kirillova IA, Kravtsova GI, Laziuk GI. The prospective directions of research in teratology. Arkh Patol. 1990;52(4):3–9.

[34] Laziuk GI. Human Teratology. A Guide for Physicians. (in Russian) 1991. 480p.

[35] Carmeliet P, Ferreira V, Breier G, Pollefeyt S, Kieckens L, Gertsenstein M, et al. Abnormal blood vessel development and lethality in embryos lacking a single VEGF allele. Nature. 1996;380(6573):435–9. doi:10.1038/380435a0

[36] Wang A, Rana S, Karumanchi SA. Preeclampsia: the role of angiogenic factors in its pathogenesis. Physiology. 2009;24:147–158. doi:10.1152/physiol.00043.2008

[37] Douglas NC, Tang H, Gomez R, Pytowski B, Hicklin DJ, Sauer CM et al. Vascular endothelial growth factor receptor 2 (VEGF-2) functions to promote uterine decidual angiogenesis during early pregnancy in the mouse. Endocrinology. 2009;150:3845–3854. doi:10.1210/en.2008-1207

[38] Lorquet S, Berndt S, Blacher S, Pequeux C. Implication of VEGF receptor soluble forms, sVEGFR-1 and sVEGFR-2, in pathological angiogenesis. Abstracts of the 23rd Annual Meeting of the ESHRE1-4; July 2007; Lyon, France, pp.1174–1175.

[39] Wathen KA, Tuutti E, Stenman UH, Alfthan H, Halmesmäki E, Finne P, Ylikorkala O, Vuorela P. Maternal serum-soluble vascular endothelial growth factor receptor-1 in early pregnancy ending in preeclampsia or intrauterine growth retardation. J Clin Endocrinol Metab. 2006;91:180–184. doi:10.1210/jc.2005-1076

[40] Bates DO. Vascular endothelial growth factors and vascular permeability. Cardiovasc Res. 2010;87:262–271. doi:10.1093/cvr/cvq105

[41] Erez O, Romero R, Espinoza J, Fu W, Todem D, Kusanovic JP, et al. The change in concentrations of angiogenic and anti-angiogenic factors in maternal plasma between the first and second trimesters in risk assessment for the subsequent development of preeclampsia and small-for-gestation age. J Matern Fetal Neonatal Med. 2008;21:279–287. doi:10.1080/14767050802034545

[42] Verlohren S, Galindo A, Schlembach D, Zeisler H, Herraiz I, Moertl MG, et al. An automated method for determination of the sFlt-1/PLGF ratio in the assessment of preeclampsia. Am J Obstet Gynecol. 2010;202:161. e1-161.e11. doi:10.1016/j.ajog.2009.09.016

[43] Schoofs K, Grittner U, Engels T, Pape J, Denk B, Henrich W, Verlohren S. The importance of repeated measurements of the sFlt-1/PlGF ratio for the prediction of preeclampsia and intrauterine growth restriction. J Perinat Med. 2014;42(1):61–8. doi:10.1515/jpm-2013-0074

[44] Herraiz I, Simón E, Gómez-Arriaga PI, Martínez-Moratalla JM, García-Burguillo A, Jiménez EA, Galindo A. Angiogenesis-related biomarkers (sFlt-1/PLGF) in the prediction and diagnosis of placental dysfunction: an approach for clinical integration. Int J Mol Sci. 2015;16(8):19009–26. doi:10.3390/ijms160819009

11

Recent Advances in Angiogenesis Assessment Methods and their Clinical Applications

Imran Shahid, Waleed H. AlMalki,

Mohammed W. AlRabia, Muhammad Ahmed,

Mohammad T. Imam, Muhammed K. Saifullah and

Muhammad H. Hafeez

Abstract

Angiogenesis, a natural phenomenon of developing new blood vessels, is an integral part of normal developmental processes as well as numerous pathological states in humans. The angiogenic assays are reliable predictors of certain pathologies in particular tumor growth, metastasis, inflammation, wound healing, tissue regeneration, ischemia, cardiovascular, and ocular diseases. The angiogenic inducer and inhibitor studies rely on both in vivo and in vitro angiogenesis methods, and various animal models are also standardized to assess qualitative and quantitative angiogenesis. Analogously, the discovery and development of anti-angiogenic agents are also based on the choice of suitable angiogenic assays and potential drug targeted sites within the angiogenic process. Similarly, the selection of cell types and compatible experimental conditions resembling the angiogenic disease being studied are also potential challenging tasks in recent angiogenesis studies. The imaging analysis systems for data acquisition from in vivo, in vitro, and in ova angiogenesis assay to preclinic, and clinical research also requires novel but easy-to-use tools and well-established protocols. The proposition of this pragmatic book chapter overviews the recent advances in angiogenesis assessment methods and discusses their applications in numerous disease pathogenesis.

Keywords: angiogenesis techniques, *in vitro* angiogenesis, angiogenic mouse models, quantitative angiogenesis, transgenic animal models, angiogenesis in clinical practice, angiogenic inhibitors

1. Introduction

The growth of new microvessels from the parent ones is an integral part of new tissue growth in growing organisms. It plays an essential part in human health while playing key roles in wound healing and tissue development [1]. Similarly, the phenomenon is regularly triggered in certain pathological conditions including rheumatoid arthritis, endometriosis, diabetic retinopathy, macular degeneration, tumor growth, and inflammatory conditions in response to certain antigens and toxins [2]. However, almost every normal tissues lack this phenomenon in adulthood, except cyclical events in the female reproductive organs [3]. Physiological angiogenesis in tissues contains a natural balance between endogenous pro- and anti-angiogenic factors [3]. When this balance gets disturbed and shifts more toward the pro-angiogenic side in certain pathological states (inflammation, ischemia, hypoxia, and cancer), microvascular endothelial cells (ECs) initiate a cascade of angiogenic reactions which may be retracted or progressive and turn microvessels to an angiogenic phenotype [4]. A considerable diversity exists among microvascular endothelial cells in different tissues and organs, and species heterogeneity cannot be ignored in this scenario [4].

Where angiogenesis is useful for tissue growth and development, excessive vessel growth is really problematic and a hallmark to propagate many diseases while contributing to turning tumor cells into cancer, tumor metastasis, psoriasis, arthritis, diabetic retinopathy, and predominantly metabolic disease such as obesity, atherosclerosis, and certain infectious diseases [5]. Conversely, insufficient angiogenesis or neovascularization may cause ischemic tissue states in heart, brain, and peripheral muscles which may lead to high blood pressure, preeclampsia, neurodegeneration, and osteoporosis [5]. In such pathological states, pro-angiogenic therapies which promote compensatory angiogenesis show promise to treat such pathologies [6]. In parallel to that, angiogenic inhibitors found highly effective in clinical trials as successful strategic treatment approaches with or without conventional chemotherapy for the treatment of solid tumors and metastasis [7]. The potential beneficiary of such novel treatment strategies are patients with aberrant ocular angiogenesis and cancer patients, where defective sight and cancer progression are entirely angiogenesis-dependent [7]. Such treatment paradigms are also heralding a new era of the treatment for other commonly occurring angiogenesis-related diseases.

The formation of new vessels involves many different cell types, and an intricate interplay of various endogenous vascular growth factors, receptors, extracellular matrix (ECM) proteins and the humoral factors [8]. To design and develop potentially effective pro- and anti-angiogenic treatments and to understand molecular mechanisms involved in angiogenesis and neovascularization, numerous in vivo and in vitro assays and animal models of angiogenesis have been developed [9]. Similarly, preclinical angiogenesis assays have also used for drug screening, molecular structure activities, and dosage effects of certain approved anti-angiogenic compounds although such assays are not equivalent and relevant to human disease regarding efficacy [10]. The prime objective of this book chapter is to overview current major and newly introduced angiogenic assays with regard to major advantages and limitations from biological, technical, ethical, and economic perspectives. The major assays which we discuss here include corneal micropocket assay, CAM (chick chorioallantoic membrane) assay, rodent mesentery, Matrigel plug assays, whole-animal assays (zebrafish), and animal models of angiogenesis in the context of cardiovascular, ocular, and adipose tissue diseases. A precise note on genetically engineered animal models for vascular endogenous genes and their spatial, temporal, and conditional expression is also included [9]. It is beyond the scope of this chapter to cover every angiogenesis assays in details, so we briefly overview quantitative techniques and/or methods to assess/evaluate neovascularization in tissues. We also briefly discuss molecular mechanisms and cell signaling pathways involved in angiogenesis and potential anti-angiogenic therapies, their clinical impact, limitations, and future prospects.

2. Prerequisite for good angiogenesis assays

Before to choose an ideal assay for angiogenesis studies, the investigators and researchers must know the assay kinetics in terms of operating procedures, handling the environment, ethical justification, and assay economy [8]. In vivo angiogenic studies are more informative than in vitro due to complex cellular and molecular activities of angiogenic reactions while providing biology of the assay and showing experimental design are relevant [9]. Similarly, in trauma-based assays (either physical or chemical), where cell damage triggers inflammatory reactions which mimic the release of several pro-angiogenic cytokines, the sensitivity and specificity of the assay are reduced [10]. For such assays, specific precautions must be taken to avoid any inflammatory reaction or to minimize the traumatic tissue state. In parallel to that, the test substance/compound should be designed as being angiogenic in a noninflammatory state. A near to physiological dose of the test compound should be administered for inducing an angiogenic response while to modulate angiogenic assay conditions and dosage response, a dose range of the clinical use must be chosen [10].

Vehicles carrying the test compound in many assays may also affect the pharmacokinetics of the tested drug and alter the dose-response curves among different experimental animals within one group. For such circumstances, the best solution is to compare test animals/samples with vehicle-exposed counterparts [9]. However, for data interpretation, one must be fully acquainted with the fact that how the vehicle-administered tested animals differ from the untreated controls [10]. Spatial and temporal distributions of the tested compounds are also necessary and vital because failure to do so may produce or hinder to generate reliable and rigorous dose-response curves [10]. As in different pathological states newly formed, vessels are delicate in quality and poorly functional, the selection of angiogenic assessment methods (either qualitative or quantitative) also matters to evaluate the morphology and physiology of the neovascularization in diseased tissues [9]. For in vivo angiogenesis assays, histological microscopy provides the detailed information precisely. Mammalian systems adopted for in vivo angiogenesis assays and mouse models for certain cardiovascular, ocular, and cerebral diseases are comparatively more close to relating human pathophysiology than the embryonic CAM assay, embryonic zebrafish (*Xenopus laevis*), and invertebrate (*Hirudo medicinalis*) angiogenic assays [9, 10].

3. Key components of an ideal angiogenesis assay

It would be interesting to describe that despite the much progress in the field of angiogenesis research, there is no single angiogenic model available which may fully elucidate the entire process and molecular mechanisms of the angiogenic and neovascularization process. Some exogenous and endogenous factors hinder the efforts to develop such an ideal system. Due to cell diversity among different tissues where angiogenesis takes place and intricate interplay among different cell signaling pathways of angiogenic reactions, it is an uphill task to develop and validate a unique assay that is optimal for all situations. However, different modalities and ingenious ways with the passage of time in a particular assay facilitate and provide optimisms for better measurements of angiogenesis than the past. In this context, Vallee et al. [11] conclude that "The design and verification of [new] specific, reliable, repeatable, and precise methodology to measure angiogenesis are considered an imperative of high priority in the field of angiogenesis research." Similarly, Auerbach et al. [10] state "Perhaps the most consistent limitation in all these studies and approaches has been the availability of simple, reliable, reproducible, quantitative assays of the angiogenic response." Moreover, it is challenging although not impossible in several angiogenic assays that the quantification of newly formed vessels regarding numbers and lengths. Similarly, the spatial and temporal distribution of tested compound is also necessary to get strong dose-response curves. Performing an assay in a blinded manner may helpful in this prospect and also to alleviate the influence of any preconceived notions. Analogously, the technical skills to perform any angiogenesis assay are of utmost importance to ensure maximum success.

Despite all these qualms as described above, an ideal angiogenesis assay for quantification of newly formed vessels must feature the following characteristics; first [12], "the release rate [R] and the spatial and temporal concentration distribution [C] of tested compounds should be known to evaluate dose-response curves; second, if tumor cells are used as a source of angiogenic factors, oncogene expression and production of growth factors (either stimulants or inhibitors) must be genetically well defined before the assay proceeding; third, the assay must be designed in a way ensure to provide quantitative measuring parameters of the newly formed vessels (e.g., vascular length [L], surface area [A], volume [V], number of vessels in the network [N], fractal dimensions of the network [Df], and extent of basement membrane [BM]); fourth, the assay should be designed in a way to weigh quantitative measure of morphological characteristics of new vessels (e.g., endothelial cell migration [MR], proliferation rate [PR], canalization rate [CR], blood flow rate [F], and vascular permeability [P]); fifth, a clear demarcation must exist between new and parent vessels; sixth, tissue trauma must be minimized to prevent the formation of new vessels; seventh, in vitro assessment should be verified by in vivo procedures; eighth, angiogenesis assay for long term and with noninvasive monitoring should be preferred; last, the selected assay should be economical, ethically justifiable, robust, and reliable." [12].

4. Process of angiogenesis

Endothelial cell activation, proliferation, and directed migration to form new microvasculature (capillaries) from the parent ones should be a complex process involving many molecular and cell signaling pathway events [2]. Some key regulators to switch on or off gene expression are also participating and influence by positive and negative feedbacks of cellular processes. The normal physiological angiogenesis initiates by sprouting of capillaries under the effect of vascular endothelial growth factors (VEGFs) from parent vessels [13]. It continuous during embryonic development and transiently during female reproductive cycle but almost stops in adult tissues except for some wound healing states [13]. Pathologic angiogenesis remains persistent with the continuous proliferation of ECs in different tissue pathologies and particularly in cancer [3]. Many tumor cells are capable of attracting adjacent blood vasculature from nearby tissues [2]. It was evident by the fact that for solid tumors to grow a certain size, neovascularization is necessary otherwise such tumors rarely metastasize as found in thin melanomas which reside on the avascular basement membrane [2, 13]. Also, for tumor growth, the nutrient supply, oxygen, and waste removal are also essential. The new vasculature fulfills this task while providing immune cells, macrophages, and humoral factors to the vicinity of the tumor cells [2].

The parent vessel wall comprises endothelial cell lining, basement membrane, and pericytic cells. Pro-angiogenic growth factors (VEGF, TGF-α, TNF-α) from tumor cells bind to the receptors of ECs and initiate a cascade of cell signaling pathways and angiogenic reactions [2]. Activation and resolution of ECs are two key steps of the angiogenic cascade reactions. When ECs activate and stimulate to grow, the cells secrete proteases, heparanase, and other digestive enzymes that degrade the extracellular matrix (ECM) [13]. ECM degradation allows the secretion of many pro-angiogenic factors from the endothelial cell matrix, and the junctions between ECs become leaky; new microvessel sprouts grow in the direct toward the stimulus [2] (**Figure 1**). For further ECs to grow, proliferate, and migrate, hematopoietic-endothelial progenitor cells (HEPC) also play an essential role [13]. In resolution phase, the new microvasculature tends to mature with the help of pericytic cell adhesion, reconstitution of basement membrane, and

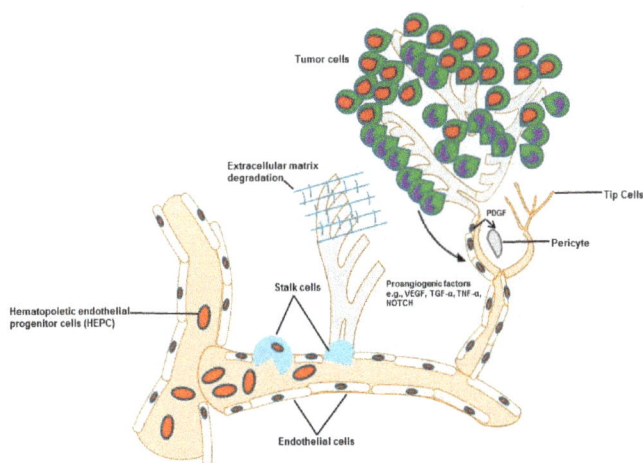

Figure 1. Process of angiogenesis from parent vessels: Angiogenesis sprouting initiates when vascular endothelial growth factors (e.g., VEGF-A) bind to VEGFR-2 receptors located on endothelial cells (ECs). ECs release matrix metalloproteinase (MMP) which degrades extracellular matrix (ECM) from which endothelial tip cells migrate. Vascular endothelial growth factors also regulate Notch cell signaling to inhibit proliferation of endothelial stalk cells. Platelet-derived growth factor (PDGF) released from ECs recruits smooth muscle cells (e.g., pericyte) to stabilize the neovasculature. TGF-α = transforming growth factor, TNF-α = tumor necrosis factor.

formation of cell junctions [14]. Interestingly, the resolution phase in tumor surrounding capillary network remains incomplete which results in irregular and tortuous microvasculature with partial ECs, increased cell permeability, and fragmentary basement membrane [15]. Tumor vasculature is disorganized with poor microcirculation, and vessel diameter changes without any differentiation into arterioles, capillaries, and venules [13]. Similarly, tumor vasculature is sprouting type, so assays which quantify sprouting angiogenesis are very useful to study the kinetics of tumor angiogenesis [15].

In the following section, we present the major and currently used preclinical angiogenesis assays in approximate chronological order of their first publication like chick chorioallantoic membrane (CAM), Matrigel plug, and corneal micropocket assays, while the others described in brief. [10]. CAM, Matrigel plug, and zebrafish assays are very useful for new angiogenic inhibitors screening. For a particular research focus, we provide advantages and disadvantages between different assays in a tabular form feasible for the readers (**Table 1**).

Assay name	Advantages	Disadvantages
In vivo angiogenesis assays		
Corneal micropocket assay	(a) Easy-to-identify newly formed vessels	(a) Atypical assay due to avascular tissue nature
	(b) Easy to perform in animals (e.g., mice, rat, and rabbit)	(b) Induction of nonspecific inflammation to test substance
	(c) Qualitatively permits noninvasive and long-term monitoring	(c) Inaccessible to endogenous blood-borne angiogenic factors
	(d) Immunologically, cross reaction is minimized	(d) Ethical problems as using a major sensory organ for angiogenic assay
	(e) New vessel formation by sprouting	(e) Oxygen exposure may affect angiogenesis
		(f) Not a suitable site for tumor growth
		(g) Tested compounds are few
Chick chorioallantoic membrane assay	(a) Simple to perform and low in cost	(a) Inflammation-mediated angiogenic reactions
	(b) Suitable to study pro- and anti-angiogenic compounds	(b) Very sensitive to change in O_2 tension
	(c) Tumor angiogenesis may assess	(c) Not suitable for metabolically activated compounds
		(d) Embryonic nonmammalian procedure
		(e) Newly formed vessels are difficult to identify
Rodent mesentery assays	(a) Natively sparsely vascularized	(a) Less significant for quantitative angiogenesis in mice than rats
	(b) Lacks physiological angiogenesis	(b) Real-time observation is limited

Assay name	Advantages	Disadvantages
	(c) Angiogenesis induction with little or no trauma	(c) Technically require skills and time consuming
	(d) Suitable for quantitative measurement of microvessel variables (e.g., spatial extension, density, vessel number and length)	
	(e) Suitable to study tumor angiogenesis	
	(f) Sprouting type of angiogenesis	
Sponge/matrix implant assay	(a) Simple and inexpensive to proceed	(a) Nonspecific inflammatory host responses
	(b) Replicate in hypoxic tumor microenvironment so convenient for tumor angiogenesis studies	(b) Implant/sponge composition may vary
	(c) Reproducible and continuous assessment of angiogenesis	(c) s.c is not a reliable route for tumor growth
		(d) Variable drug retention within implant
Disk angiogenesis assay	(a) Inexpensive and easy to perform	(a) Continuous or kinetic observation is limited
	(b) Quantitative assessment of angiogenesis	(b) Encapsulated by granulation tissue
	(c) Wound healing may access	
	(d) Multiple disks can be used at one time	
Matrigel plug assay	(a) Rapid screening of pro- and anti-angiogenic compounds	(a) Matrigel chemical composition is not defined
	(b) An experimental model for tissue regeneration	(b) Three-dimensional plugs are difficult to generate
	(c) Simple to proceed and rapid screening in chambers	(c) Avascular test tissue
Whole-animal models for angiogenic assays		
Xenopus laevis (Zebrafish)	(a) Embryonic and organogenic angiogenesis is assessed	(a) Expensive in breeding condition
	(b) Useful animal model for functional genomic analysis	(b) Non-mammalian and embryonic in nature
	(c) Simple to proceed and relatively fast	
	(d) Easy animal maintenance and significant number of tested animals per statistical analysis	
	(e) Single-drug dosing and small quantities of drugs are required	

Assay name	Advantages	Disadvantages
Mouse models of angiogenesis		
Adipose angiogenesis models		
1. ob/ob mice	(a) Deficient in leptin	(a) Expensive in terms of handling and treatment
	(b) Suitable to study angiogenesis in adipose tissue expansion	(b) Time consuming to assess angiogenesis
	(c) Helpful to test compounds related to metabolic disorders and obesity	
2. Db/db mice	(a) Excellent for role of angiogenesis in insulin resistance and obesity-related diabetes	(a) Difficult to handle and time consuming
Cardiovascular angiogenesis mouse models		
1. Hindlimb ischemic model	(a) Suitable to study arteries growth in tissue hypoxia	(a) Hind limb surgery is complicated
	(b) Can be performed in mice or rat	(b) Skilled and experienced person is required
	(c) Suitable to use for therapeutic agents which augment perfusion to ischemic limb	(c) Degree of tissue hypoxia may vary within experimental animals group
		(d) Residual blood flow may slightly differ in limb after surgery
2. Heart ischemic model	(a) Suitable for pathological and drug evaluation studies	(a) Inflammatory response–mediated angiogenesis
	(b) Efficient neovascularization	
Wound healing assays	(a) Suitable for vascular maturation/remodelling studies	(a) Inflammatory responsemediated angiogenesis
	(b) Surgery is very simple	(b) limited to skin regeneration
	(c) Pro- or anti-angiogenic compounds can be tested for vessel morphology or regenerative angiogenesis	(c) Regeneration through new tissue formation instead repairing and replacing damaged tissue
	(d) Very easy and robust assay	
Transgenic animal models		
1. Transgenic choroidal neovascularization model	(a) Controlling transgene conditional expression and evaluation of spatial and temporal vascular gene expression	(a) Ethically questionable
2. Transgenic zebrafish model	(b) Knock-down vascular endogenous gene expression	(b) Time consuming
		(c) Differential gene expression may observed within same animal

Table 1. The advantages and disadvantages of major *in vivo, in vitro* and animal models angiogenesis assays.

5. In vivo angiogenesis models

5.1. The corneal micropocket assay

The firm foundation of systematic angiogenesis research was initiated by Folkman and associates who introduced first time the corneal micropocket assay and chick chorioallantoic membrane (CAM assay) in 1974 [16, 17]. The corneal micropocket assay allows the growth of newly formed blood vessels in vivo, and the techniques were first time applied in rabbits and after that in mice and rat [16]. In this assay, a micropocket is made in the stroma where a pellet containing the growth factors is placed inside the micropocket on the corneal surface of the eye. The growth factors induce a reproducible angiogenic response, and by implanting multiple pellets of different growth factors into parallel micropockets, the various stimuli of angiogenic response may be assessed. The angiogenic response in this assay is entirely due to direct stimulation of blood vessels instead to indirect induction of inflammation reaction. The assay shows minimal inflammatory cellular activity. However, the tested compounds are slowly released from the polymer of the micropocket, and such formulations may cause irritation and ultimately lead to inflammatory reactions which may alter angiogenesis quantification. The micropocket itself is inaccessible to certain blood borne growth factors and blood progenitor cells which may influence angiogenesis. The new vasculature mainly forms through the sprouting from the adjacent limbal area. Being avascular in nature, the corneal assay is useful in visibility and accessibility of new vessel formation and topical application of test drugs and biomicroscopic grading of new vasculature. However, it makes the assay atypical because normal tissues are vascular with few exceptions [16].

5.2. Chick chorioallantoic membrane (CAM) assay

The assay was introduced by Folkman and associates, but embryologists used this method to evaluate embryonic tissue grafts for their developmental potential [17]. The assay is useful to study tumor angiogenesis as well as pro- and anti-angiogenesis compound screening [18]. Fertilized hen's egg incubated at 37°C for 3 days is prepared for grafting by removing enough egg albumin to reduce shell membrane adhesion. Carriers containing the tested compound are placed directly onto the CAM by making a rectangular opening in the eggshell. Slow-release polymer pellets, air-dried disks, and gelatin sponges can be used as tested compound carriers; however, Elvax 40 and Hydron which are used to form sponges and membranes remain inert when applied to the CAM [19]. The quantification of angiogenesis can be made 3–4 days after grafting [18–20]. The in ovo CAM assay is relatively simple to perform as described above. However, a complementary in vitro method has also been described during which the chicken embryos grow in Petri dishes after 3 days of incubation. The assay is technically in vitro, but strictly speaking, it presents a whole-animal assay. After three to six days' extra incubation, the CAM develops, and grafts can be assessed for subsequent development. In vitro CAM allows the quantification of blood vessels over a wider area than in ovo CAM assay. Similarly, a large number of samples can be evaluated at one time, and response occurs within a short period of time (i.e., 2–3 days). Furthermore, the test compound can be placed on the underside of the coverslips. Generally, in ovo CAM assay is performed more than in vitro CAM. The calculated time for CAM angiogenesis response is very critical as between day five and twelve, the experimentally induced acceleration or suppression of embryonic organogenic angiogenesis can be determined. From day 12 onward, endogenous organogenic angiogenesis under the influence of undefined growth factor may initiate, and identification of newly formed vessels under the effect of tested compound becomes vague [18].

5.3. Rodent mesentery assay

The rodent mesentery assay was introduced by K. Norrby and associates in 1986 and refined later on [21, 22]. The peculiarity of the assay is to use the small gut mesentery of small rodents which is considered ideal for the physiological measurement of angiogenesis. It can be exteriorized from the abdominal cavity, and it's "window" like thin membranous parts make it an ideal angiogenic test tissue by using intravital microscopy. Other potential advantage is that the intestinal mesentery of mouse, rat, guinea pig, rabbit, cat, and dog is almost identical. The test tissue is a 5–10 μm thin membrane which is covered by a single layer of mesothelial cells covered on both sides bordering onto a delicate basal membrane. The thin membrane sandwiches a tissue space that contains mast cells, histiocytes, fibroblasts, and some lymphocytes. It is the thinnest tissue found in the body of Sprague-Dawley (SD) rats. Avascular part of the test tissue contains predominantly 52% fibroblasts and 48% of the mesothelial cells in adult male SD rats. The connective tissue elements of varying size including collagen, elastin, and elastic fiber are also a part of mesentery test tissue [21].

A microscopic analysis clearly shows the cellular and vascular components of the mesenteric windows [22]. The microvessel number per mm circumference is increased in the 15-week-old male rat as compared to 5.5-week-old which demonstrates a slow progression of physiological angiogenesis to the peripheral part of the windows. The same phenomenon is noticed in female SD rats with an age increase; however, the increase in microvessel length, density, and vascularization is not seen in untreated male SD rats at the age of 7 weeks. The distal part of the mesentery (i.e., standard test tissue) of these rats shows no significant angiogenesis for 2–3 weeks which is the usual duration of angiogenesis assay. The test compound usually in the form of an intraperitoneal injection (i.p.) reaches all targeted microvessel of the test tissue because the mesothelial cell lining is highly permeable to a wide range of the molecular weight of the test compounds. The test tissue is unaffected by inflammation mediated angiogenesis as it is untouched mechanically, and no surgery is involved. The assay was tested for the first time for mast cell-induced angiogenesis and later on inflammatory cytokines, and humoral growth factors were also tested almost near to physiologic level doses [22].

The quantitative assessment of angiogenesis is performed by immunohistochemically using a specific primary monoclonal antibody against the rat endothelium. The assay allows clear cut identification of even the smallest newly formed vessels in the test tissue. Thus, the quantitative vessel parameters (as discussed on page 4) can be measured easily which are very vital to determine molecular activity, the effect of low molecular weight heparinized preparations, and dose-response curves. Computer imaging and microscopic morphometry may be used to further validate the immunohistochemistry findings in a blinded fashion [22].

5.4. The sponge implant assays

The assay was introduced by Andrade and associates by which tested compound is directly injected into a sponge which is implanted subcutaneously in the rat [23]. The assay is used for continuous assessment of the angiogenesis as sterile polyester sponge implants become vascularized, and the measurement of blood flow in sponge by using Xe^{133} clearance technique produces reproducible and objective angiogenesis. The exudate fluid for biochemical analysis may be extracted after local injection of angiogenic stimulator or inhibitors. The assay is useful to study tumor angiogenesis as the sponge implant may replicate the hypoxic tumor microenvironment although the composition of sponge implant may vary [9]. The potential disadvantage of the assay is a nonspecific inflammatory response to sponge implant which may infiltrate the sponge substance as the subcutaneous implant becomes encapsulate due to granulation tissue. A variable composition of sponge sometimes makes inter-experimental comparison difficult, and use of Xe^{133} becomes complicated [23].

5.5. Disk angiogenesis system (DAS)

The assay was introduced to study wound healing and solid tumor angiogenesis as well as the angiogenic response of soluble substances in mice [24]. A synthetic foam disk composed of polyvinyl alcohol foam and covered on both flat sides by filters is inserted into mice abdomen or thorax which is well tolerated. The disk is easy to assemble, and the tested compound or tumor cells suspension is placed at the center of the disk. The slow release of the tested drug or tumor cell suspension is managed by the use of agarose or ethylene-vinyl acetate copolymer. The disk is removed within a period of 7–21 days, during which microvascular growth occurs centripetally into the disc. Paraffin-prepared sections of the disk are used to microscopically view the vascular growth as well as fibroblasts and connective tissue components. The quantitative vessel parameters can be determined by point counting on histological sections, intravascular volume, and so on. The disadvantage of the assay is inflammation-mediated angiogenesis as the disk is always surrounded by fibroblasts whenever vascular growth occurs. Similarly, the kinetic observation of newly formed vessels is difficult because one disk provides information for only one point in time [9].

5.6. The Matrigel plug assay

The Matrigel plug assay was introduced by Passaniti and coworkers in 1992 [25]. The Matrigel was extracted from Engelberth-Holm-Swarm (EHS) tumor, which is rich in ECM proteins. It is a solubilized basement membrane preparation which liquefies at 4°C but reconstitutes into a gel at 37°C when injected subcutaneously into mice where it is slowly surrounded by granulation tissue. The gel induces highly vascularized response under the influence of angiogenic growth factors in particular bFGF [25]. The assay is noninvasive and easy to administer but time-consuming to handle.

The Matrigel composition is not fully defined. However, the major components include epidermal, transforming, platelet, nerve, and insulin-like growth factors (e.g., PDGF, TGF, and bFGF) laminin, collagen, heparin sulfate proteoglycans, and entactin [26]. For this reason, care should be taken while using Matrigel assay for the cellular activity studies. It was observed that when Matrigel with reduced growth factors is implanted, few cells invade the plug or gel. However, with known angiogenic growth factors (e.g., bFGF), mixed with Matrigel and injected subcutaneously, endothelial cells migrate into the gel and constitute vessel-like structures. A fine network of endothelial cell tubes enlarged by micro- and macro-vessel endothelial cells slowly progress to capillary networks in vivo [26].

For the quantitative assessment of angiogenesis, Matrigel and surrounded granulation tissue are removed after 1–3 weeks, and immunohistochemistry and histological sections are measured [27]. However, determining the profiles of capillary-like vessels is difficult. Similarly, the hemoglobin (Hb) test does not differentiate the blood flow in newly formed blood vessels and large parent vessels. Fluorochrome-labeled high molecular weight dextran and quantitative vascular specific indicators are alternative methods to assess neovascularization [27].

The assay is suitable for tissue regeneration experiment model where neovascularization is coupled with organogenesis, fibrosis, and monocytes/macrophages play a pivotal structural role. A possible drawback of the assay is that Matrigel plug contains only capillary network rather than no tissue without any pro- and anti-angiogenic factors to influence angiogenic reactions [28].

A variation of the Matrigel plug assay is the combination of Matrigel and sponge techniques. Five-hundred microliters of Matrigel is injected subcutaneously into mice and solidify for 20–30 min [27]. After that, the mice are anesthetized, skin overlying Matrigel is shaved, and a small nick is made. A similar nick is made to Matrigel plug, and a sterile polyvinyl sponge with the test compound is introduced into the center of the Matrigel plug with the help of tweezers. The same procedure may use for angiogenic growth factors or test tissue to be implanted in the Matrigel plug. By this modification, neovascularization is directional, and assay sensitivity is increased to measure direct angiogenesis as compared to standard Matrigel plug assay. However, the sponge/Matrigel combined assay is time-consuming, and the total number of assayed animals become limited [27].

5.7. Whole-animal angiogenesis model

Zebrafish was introduced in 1999 as a whole small angiogenesis model for the screening of pro-angiogenic compounds which directly influence the newly formed vessels [29]. The choice of the whole animal as a tested tissue was based on the remarkable similarity of zebrafish organs to those of a human at the physiological, anatomical, and molecular levels [30]. Moreover, the short generation time (approx. 3 months) and easy to house in small space and relatively large numbers also facilitate to evaluate many tested animals in one assay [31]. The external development of zebrafish embryos and optical transparency during embryonic stage assists continuous microscopic evaluations of different developmental processes from gastrulation to organogenesis [30]. Furthermore, external mode of fertilization also permits easy access to experiment design and assessment. Small tested compounds dissolve to water diffuse directly to fish embryo and induce distinct and dose-dependent angiogenic effects. Both pro- and anti-angiogenic compounds exhibit similar effects in zebrafish as exerted in mammals [31].

6. Animal models of angiogenesis

In biomedical research, mouse models are of utmost importance for a wide variety of medical tests including gene expression, gene knockout, and medical genetic analysis [32]. For this purpose, SCID, transgenic, and genetically engineered mouse models are of particular interests which allow sophisticated investigations for genetically induced pathological states and molecular pathogenesis of certain genetic disorders. Furthermore, such mouse models are useful to study genes essential for angiogenesis and vascular biology [32]. In parallel to that mice with conditional, global knockouts, over-expressing angiogenic factors are also considerable in this prospect [33]. As remarkable similarity exists between human and murine vasculatures, such tools are valuable to search possible molecular interactions among distinct angiogenic factors in the onset and progression of various human diseases [32, 33]. In the following section, we shed light on some practically used mouse models in the context of pathological angiogenesis which directly plays a part in human diseases.

6.1. Mouse model of angiogenesis in adipose tissue

Genetically engineered mouse model for adipose tissue angiogenesis is highly reproducible and produces robust results because the mice are inbred and share a highly similar genetic background. This approach is irrelevant to humans because high caloric intake and little physical exercise are the predisposing factors for developing obesity instead a little genetics involved. Thus, mice fed on high-fat diet present an ideal animal model to study non-genetically related obesity [34].

6.1.1. Ob/ob mice

The mouse carrying the obese mutation (ob) was first described in 1950, and later on, it was shown that the mutation located in the gene coding for a hormone leptin, which regulates appetite and food intake [35]. The hormone binds to leptin receptor (Ob-R) in the hypothalamus and subsequent cell signaling regulates food uptake, energy expenditure as well as fat and glucose metabolism. Ob/ob mice are deficient in leptin exhibit uncontrolled and continuous food intake which results in a gain of body weight. Consequently, mutated mice weight is three times higher, and body fat content elevates up to fivefold as compared to wild-type species. The mutated mice also show decreased physical activity and energy expenditure, infertility, and immune deficiencies. The mutation is recessive, so the heterozygotes do not display such phenotype [35]. Ob/ob mice can be used as an outstanding model to explore the role of angiogenesis in adipose tissue expansion, and with specific angiogenic inhibitors, obesity may be prevented in such mice [36]. As the leptin kinetics in mice to regulate food intake and obesity are homologous to human, such angiogenic model can be used to search novel therapeutic targets to treat obesity and metabolic disorders [37].

6.1.2. Db/db mice

The mouse strain C57BL/KsJ was first described with an autosomal recessive mutation diabetes (db) in 1966 [38]. Homozygous mice with such mutation are deficient for the leptin receptor and exhibit a phenotype that resembles human diabetes mellitus. The mice with such mutations are also characterized as an obese phenotype. Furthermore, such mice exhibit infertility and hyperglycemia while heterozygotes are typically lived as wild type. Db/db mice can be used to study molecular mechanisms involved in obesity-related diabetes and insulin insensitivity, and the role of angiogenesis and neovascularization can be elucidated in this regard [38].

6.2. Hindlimb ischemic model of angiogenesis

Most of the angiogenic models described above are very useful to study pathological angio-genesis and search for novel anti-angiogenic treatment in the form of angiogenic inhibitors. However, certain pathological states (e.g., myocardial infarction, stroke, and wound heal-ing/regeneration) in human body require accelerated blood vessel growth to reinstate the proper function of such vital organs [39]. In myocardial infarction, an occluded coronary artery obstructs blood flow to a part of the cardiac muscle tissue which leads to severe tissue hypoxia (ischemia). The cardiac muscle requires a regular supply of oxygen and glucose lev-els for normal function. To overcome tissue hypoxia, the growth of highly functional arteries is eagerly awaited in such situations. Hind limb ischemia in rat or mice presents an excellent model to study and manipulate newly formed vessels in particular arteries in response to tis-sue hypoxia [39].

In this assay, the arteries supply blood to one back limb of the mice is ligated to stop the blood circulation in the entire limb [40]. The occlusion of arteries leads to tissue ischemia and the initiation of arteriogenesis from collateral arteries. Pro-angiogenic factors and even anti-angiogenic compounds under investigation can be administered to the limb musculature to modulate the arteriogenic response. Doppler angiography is used to evaluate the blood circulation in the hind limb, and the procedure can be repeated in the same animal to know that how the blood flow improves over time. To study newly formed microvessels, the tissue can be excised and stained, and morphology of the blood vessels is elucidated [40].

The assay is the first in class to present therapeutic angiogenesis and widely used in funda-mental discoveries to demonstrate that how to generate highly functional and stable arteries therapeutically [39]. On the other side, the potential disadvantage of the assay is very compli-cated hind limb surgery and requires highly skilled professionals and experienced surgeons. Similarly, the proportion of blood flow in a hind limb may vary after surgery, and it may affect the degrees of tissue hypoxia which ultimately influence on the therapeutic activity of pro- and anti-angiogenic compounds under investigation [39].

6.3. Wound healing assays

The wound healing assay allows to study and evaluate both angiogenesis and vascular matu-ration/remodeling in injured or damaged tissues [41]. The assay is usually performed on the skin of mice because other accessible tissues (e.g., tail and ears) do not regenerate well. Two circular holes (approx. 5mm in diameter) are punched through the dorsal skin of anesthetized wild-type C57B16 mice. One hole would serve as control while drugs under investigation can be administered on the other. No bandages or sponge is required as no major blood vessels exist in this region of the skin and wound formation allows very little bleeding in the sur-rounding area. Wound sealing starts within two weeks, and complete wound healing occurs within a month [41].

Photography and measuring of wound area with calipers provide information about wound size, scar formation, and re-epithelization of the wound [41]. The drugs under investigation (either pro- or anti-angiogenic compounds) in this model may be administered either sys-temically by oral administration, injection, or topically. The drug effects can be determined by excision of the skin tissue, fixed, and stained with specific dyes. The tested compounds may influence regenerative angiogenesis, vessel morphology, and function. The assay is easy to setup, and surgery is very simple. The wound size remains uniform and homogenous for all animals used in one experiment [41].

The potential disadvantage of the assay is that angiogenesis is inflammation-dependent involving blood clotting phenomenon and other complex biological processes and occurs only in the skin [41]. Similarly, skin tissue regeneration is entirely different as compared to other highly vascular tissues such as the heart and nervous system and does not provide an adequate understanding of the role of angiogenesis in tissue regeneration. Furthermore, tis-sue regeneration is mainly due to reconstitute new tissue rather than repairing or replacing, which is hard to replace in ischemic insults which produce large patches of dead tissue [41].

6.4. Genetically engineered animal model for angiogenesis

Gene expression analysis and gene function studies are contributing widely to almost every research in life sciences, biomedical research, biotechnology, molecular pathology, and human health [42]. In vivo applied and functional genomic studies are particularly consid-ered by overexpressing a candidate gene or suppressing the gene expression for the purpose of gene knockout [43]. Such approaches are achieved and applicable by genome manipulation of wild-type animals [43]. Similarly, the generation of transgenic animals by injecting desired DNA constructs to fertilized eggs also presents some standard technology in gene expres-sion studies [44]. Transgenic animal models and DNA constructs (e.g., gene expression plas-mids and vectors) with desired gene expression are widely used to study gene function and molecular pathogenesis of diseases, and it create models to demonstrate the complex, intri-cate interplay between gene overexpression or suppression for the molecular epidemiology of human diseases [44]. In the following section, we briefly overview such novel approaches to be involved in the context of vascular angiogenesis.

The control of target gene expression in vascular cells of transgenic animals by cell or tis-sue expression plasmid with specific promoters is very helpful to study developmental and pathological gene function in the vasculature [42]. It was found that the promoters derived from the sequences of VEGFR-1, ICAM-2, vWF, or endoglin efficiently work in mouse endo-thelial cells both in vivo and in vitro with specific intensity and specificity [42]. Similarly, lacZ selective transgene expression was seen in ECs cells under the control of promoters derived from Tie 2 (angiopoietin receptor), ICAM-2, or VE-Cadherin [42]. However, the expression of a transgene in smooth muscle cells (SMCs) is difficult to achieve because most SMC mark-ers are expressed differentially, and SMC growth and cell differentiation are an exclusive process [42]. In contrast, transgenic mice may obtain using selective promoters expressing smooth muscle myosin heavy chain (SM-MHC), smooth muscle α-actin, and SM22α [42]. Such models provide valuable information about the function of a specific gene in a particular tissue, and controlling the expression of such genes may use as a therapeutic approach to certain disease and also for angiogenesis and cancer [42]. However, the transgene expression depends on promoter's characteristics to be used while constructing cell or tissue expression plasmids with the gene of interests including; promoters is constitutively active, capable to express and replicate gene of interest or to express in embryonic or in the adulthood stage [45]. Failure to do so may limit studies in molecular pathogenesis, leads to nonviable transgenic animals or compensatory responses. More powerful tools are being developed based on conditional transgene expression systems [45].

The inhibition of endogenous gene expression is also a potential method to suppress the gene function involved in the molecular pathogenesis of many genetic disorders and infectious diseases [46]. Many studies show that sequence-specific mRNA degradation by double-strand RNA strongly inhibits the function of that gene involved in pathogenesis or propagation of a particular disease [47]. The technique is known as RNA interference (RNAi) and may be used in certain genetic disorders, in cancer, HIV, and other harder to treat infections. Recent publish data indicate that mammalian expression vectors expressing short hairpin RNA (shRNA) under the control of specific vascular promoters inhibit gene expression through an RNAi effect [47].

7. Angiogenesis and cancer

The phenomenon of angiogenesis is fundamental in tumor growth, progression, and metastasis [48]. Angiogenesis itself is the result of a highly orchestrated series of molecular and cellular events including a plethora of genes, signal cascades, and transcription factors which are highly organized and work in a systematic way to generate microvessels in normal physiological angiogenesis [49]. However, the tumor angiogenesis is disorganized, irregular, and not systematic at the level of molecular and cellular events and ultimately propagates many tumors into cancers [48]. The cancer cells contain the ability to stimulate angiogenesis by producing a lot of angiogenic factors including cell growth factors, cytokines, and numerous other molecules [48, 49].

Many pro- and anti-angiogenic molecules involved in the induction of angiogenesis and neovascularization, their receptor ligands, and intracellular signaling pathways have been identified within last 30 years [50]. Much work has been done to develop anti-angiogenic treatment strategies for cancer patients [51]. However, numerous preclinical trials show no promise regarding high efficacy and tolerability with classical anti-angiogenic drugs as monotherapy [51]. It spurred the researchers and investigators to design and develop novel anti-angiogenic compounds to be used in combination with classical cytotoxic agents and radiotherapy [52]. FDA-approved angiogenesis inhibitors in combination with chemotherapy have proven their clinical worth regarding improved patient survival time and patient tolerability in certain cancers [52].

In the coming section, we briefly overview molecular mechanisms of major cell signaling pathways involved in the induction of angiogenesis, and at the end, some brief glimpse about the clinical impacts of newly developed angiogenic inhibitors will be described. The cellular events in the regeneration and propagation of tumor angiogenesis are already explained briefly at page 5 and depicted in **Figure 1**.

7.1. VEGF intracellular signaling

Vascular endothelial-derived growth factor (VEGF) is one of the most important and potent angiogenic molecules which play an integral role in tumor angiogenesis [50]. It presents the first in a class of cytokines which induce vascular leakage and therefore also known as vascular permeability factor. Until now, six members (VEGF-A to VEGF-F) of this unique family of cytokines have been discovered [53]. VEGF-A is mainly involved in angiogenesis and vasculogenesis whereas VEGF-B is a survival factor for ECs, SMCs, and pericytes [54]. VEGF-C and VEGF-D are essential for lymphangiogenesis, and PGF also acts as a survival factor for ECs and modulates VEGF cell signaling [55].

Vascular endothelial growth factors activate ECs by binding to a family of class III transmembrane receptor tyrosine kinases (RTKs) expressing at high levels in endothelial cell lineage [53]. VEGF-R1 and VEGF-R2 are located on ECs and activate during angiogenesis while VEGF-R3 induces intracellular signaling in lymphatic cells. VEGF-R1 acts as a decoy receptor as it is RTK defective and acts as a negative regulator of angiogenesis (**Figure 2**) [54]. The angiogenic multiple cell signaling pathways are initiated as VEGF-A binds to VEGF-R2, and the receptor dimerizes and intracellular receptor domains are phosphorylated in ECs and induce overexpression of growth factors, cell proliferation, mitogenesis, chemotaxis, and prosurvival signaling (**Figure 2**) [55]. VEGF-C binds to VEGFR-3 and initiates mitogenesis in lymphatic cells and stimulates hyperplasia in parent lymphatic vessels [53–55]. The production of VEGF is regulated by several growth factors produced by the tumor cells including, endothelial growth factor (EGF), transforming growth factor (TGF-α & β), fibroblast growth factor (FGF), and platelet-derived growth factor (PDGF) [54]. Some hormones (e.g., estrogen, thyroid-stimulating hormone (TSH)) and interleukins (e.g., IL-1 & 6) also stimulate VEGF-induced intracellular events in other types of cells [56].

7.2. Notch signaling pathways

The Notch receptors are located on stromal cells and expressed as a heterodimeric complex of two domains, that is, the Notch extracellular domain (NECD) and Notch intracellular domain (NICD) which are associated with each other via noncovalent interactions (**Figure 3a**) [57]. The Notch cell signaling may mimic direct tumor angiogenesis however actively involved to trigger dormant tumors [1]. Notch ligand Delta-like 4 (DLL4) induces cell signaling pathways to improve vascular functions by endocytosis and nonenzymatic dissociation of Notch heterodimer in host stromal cells (**Figure 3a**) [1]. DLL4 inhibition may promote cell proliferation response in ECs which ultimately increase angiogenic sprouting and vessel branching [58]. Despite increased endothelial cell vascularity, the tumor cells perfuse poorly, which reduces cell oxygen concentrations (i.e., increased hypoxia), and consequently, tumor growth is inhibited [59].

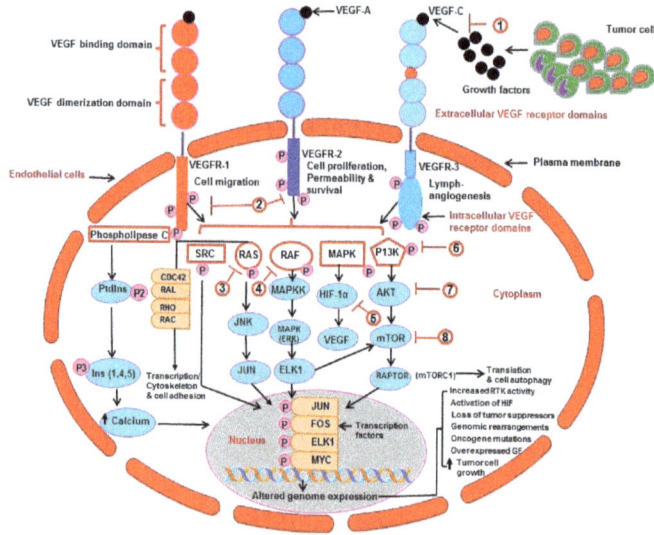

Figure 2. VEGF-induced intracellular signaling in tumor angiogenesis and angiogenic inhibitors with targeted active sites: The binding of vascular endothelial growth factors (VEGF) to respective transmembrane receptors stimulates a plethora of intracellular signaling pathways which regulate nuclear transcription factors for altered gene expressions of normal cell responses including loss of tumor suppression, activation of hypoxia inducible factor (HIF-α), increased receptor tyrosine kinase activity, increased tumor cell growth, and repression of oncogene mutations. Angiogenic inhibitors to their targeted active sites are also shown with numerical circles in the figure. Only anti-angiogenic compounds approved by the US Food and Drug Administration (FDA) for the treatment of numerous solid tumors and carcinomas are depicted where circle 1 represents growth factor inhibitors (bevacizumab, aflibercept); circle 2, growth factor receptor inhibitors (sunitinib, sorafenib); circle 3, RAS inhibitors (tipifarnib, lonafarnib); circle 4, RAF inhibitors (sorafenib); circle 5, HIF-1α inhibitors (geldanamycin, chetomin, echinomycin, 2ME2); circle 6, PI3K inhibitors (wortmannin, LY294002); circle 7, AKT inhibitors (FARA-A); and circle 8, mTOR inhibitors (rapamycin and analogues). JNK = JUN N-terminal kinase; MAPK = mitogen-activated protein serine/threonine kinase, MAPKK = MAPK kinase, PDK1 = phosphoinositide-dependent protein kinase-1; PLC = phospholipase C; PtdInP2 = phosphatidylinositol 4,5-bisphosphate, Ins (1,4,5) = inositol 1,4,5-triphosphates.

In contrast, DLL4 expressed in ECs stimulates Notch 3 receptors located on adjacent cells (e.g., colorectal cancer or T-cell acute lymphoblastic leukemia cells) to activate tumor progression from dormant to active phase [60]. Such findings consider Notch pathways a potential therapeutic target for the design and development of novel anti-angiogenic compounds, although the Notch cell signaling shows a mixed behavior of tumor progression and inhibition in clinical assays [58, 59].

7.3. Transforming growth factor-β (TGF-β)

Transforming growth factor is a ubiquitously expressed paracrine polypeptide of approximately 25 kDa molecular weight [61]. TGF 1 to TGF 3 are three highly homologous isoforms of the polypeptide and discovered in humans and mammals [62]. TGF-β is initially synthesized as a zymogen, and after secretion, an associated peptide is proteolytically sliced to release active form of the growth factor [63].

Active TGF-β binds to constitutively active serine/threonine kinase TGFBR2 receptors to activate TGFBR1 in a heterodimer complex which controls transcription via activation of canonical signal pathways mediated by a family of SMAD proteins (SMAD1-5) (**Figure 3b**) [64]. The

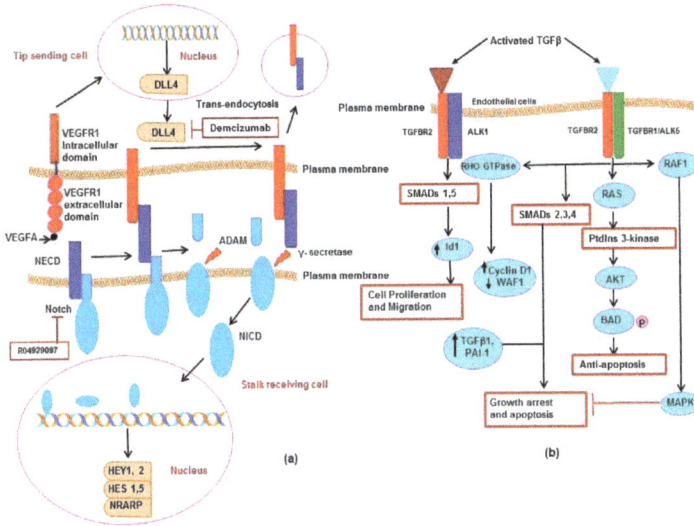

Figure 3. A schematic diagram of Notch and TGF-β induced cell signaling pathways in tumor angiogenesis: (a) Notch cell signaling pathways: The ligand DLL4 dissociates Notch heterodimers by nonenzymatic degradation and cell endocytosis. Notch extracellular domain exposes Notch to ADAM metalloproteases and γ-secretase in sending cells (tip cells) for proteolytic cleavage and the release of Notch intracellular domain which translocates to the nucleus of receiving cells (stalk cells) for the transcriptional activation of Notch target genes (shown in the nucleus of the stalk cells). The DLL4 ligand and Notch inhibitors are also depicted in the red rectangular boxes. (b) Transforming growth factor (TGF-β) induced intracellular signaling pathway: In normal cells, the binding of TGF-β to transmembrane TGFBR2 receptors activates TGFBR1 receptors which upregulate the expression of a series of SMAD proteins (SMAD 2, 3, and 4) and cause cell cycle arrest and apoptosis. However, TGF-β stimulates other molecular pathways in transformed cells to inhibit cell apoptosis and accelerates cell migration and metastasis. In contrast, a second type 1 receptor (ALK1) is expressed in ECs which stimulates cell proliferation and migration via activating SMADs 1 and 5 genes.

activation of SMAD 1 and 5 proteins in transformed cells inhibits apoptosis and mediates cell proliferation and migration via the activation of other cell signaling pathways [65]. However, in normal cells, the stimulation of SMAD 2, 3, and 4 exhibits cell cycle arrests and apoptosis [66]. Similarly, the SMAD 2, 3, and 4 proteins increase the expression of PAI-1which is essential for vessel maturation in angiogenesis (**Figure 3b**) [66].

8. Clinical impact of angiogenic inhibitors

The discovery and development of angiogenic inhibitors have raised the hopes to treat a lot of tumors and carcinomas and ultimately to reduce the morbidity and mortality related to tumors and cancers [67]. Five classes of anti-angiogenic compounds have established and are still under investigation on the basis of potential antitumor drug targeted sites including proteases inhibitors (MMP synthesis inhibitors), ECs proliferation and migration inhibitors, vascular endothelial growth factor inhibitors, cell matrix protein inhibitors, and angiogenic inhibitors with unique mechanisms (**Figure 2**) [68, 69].

Although the anti-angiogenic compounds approved by the FDA show therapeutic efficacy in some categories of cancer as monotherapy, however, sufficient published data recently reveal this fact that angiogenic inhibitors are best therapeutic choices for tumors when used in combination with traditional chemotherapies [70, 71]. However, one would not expect in the first instance that angiogenic inhibitors might reduce the intratumoral delivery of cytotoxic agents (traditional chemotherapy) by decreasing perfused blood vessels with impaired blood flow and decrease drug transport in treated tumor cells [48, 72]. It would also increase tissue hypoxia and inhibit tumor cell proliferation although proliferating cells are an easy target for chemotherapy [48, 72].

To overcome such hurdles and to enhance synergistic therapeutic potential of chemo and anti-angiogenic drugs when used in combination, Kerbel proposed three mechanistic approaches in this scenario to be adopted; first, normalization of tumor microvessels by anti-angiogenic compounds [73, 74]; second, maximum tolerated dose chemotherapy during the break periods of successive courses [72, 75], and third, use of known chemotherapeutic agents having anti-angiogenic effects [72]. The additional advantages of chemotherapy while improving their anti-angiogenic effects may be grabbed by adopting "metronomic chemotherapy" which states that "the administration of chemotherapeutic agents at relatively low, minimally toxic doses on a frequent schedule of administration at regular close intervals, with no prolonged drug-free breaks [76, 77]." By such approaches, endothelial cells are directly killed, and progenitor ECs are suppressed in circulation. Furthermore, minimal use of toxic doses lowers the frequency of adverse events in treated patients [72, 76, 77]. Such treatment strategies may be adopted for a prolonged period of time with angiogenic inhibitors in the treatment of advanced solid tumors with little side effects as validated by phase II clinical trials; however, phase III clinical studies are extensively demanded in this direction [70, 71].

9. Conclusions

In vivo, in vitro, and in ova assays for angiogenesis assessment are the reliable approaches in basic research and to some extent in real-world clinical practices. However, in vivo systems are difficult to perform and time consumable, and the process of quantification is much complicated than in vitro assays. Conversely, these are relatively better due to complex nature of the vascular response to the test compound. In vitro angiogenesis assays may perform in a short period and provide the accurate and reliable outcome of angiogenic processes. Mouse models based angiogenesis assays have also standardized to an improved understanding of tumor angiogenesis and lymphangiogenesis. Similarly, such models are also used to assess vasculogenesis and arteriogenesis in ischemic heart diseases, blindness, psoriasis, and arthritis. Angiogenesis assessment always plays a focal role to determine the pathogenesis and progression of certain challenging diseases in human populations in particular human cancer. An ample understanding of angiogenesis research in tumor progression, by knowing the molecular mechanisms and cellular pathways, also opens the ways to design and develop effective anti-angiogenic inhibitors. The manipulation of the human genome in a precise and predictable manner due to recently developed molecular techniques has opened new gates for the generation of more reliable models for angiogenesis studies and the testing of new therapeutic strategies.

Author details

Imran Shahid[1,2]*, Waleed H. AlMalki[1], Mohammed W. AlRabia[3], Muhammad Ahmed[1], Mohammad T. Imam[4], Muhammed K. Saifullah[5] and Muhammad H. Hafeez[6]

*Address all correspondence to: iyshahid@uqu.edu.sa

1 Department of Pharmacology and Toxicology, College of Pharmacy, Umm Al-Qura University, Makkah, Saudi Arabia

2 Applied and Functional Genomics Laboratory, Center of Excellence in Molecular Biology (CEMB), University of the Punjab, Lahore, Pakistan

3 Department of Medical Microbiology, College of Medicine, King Abdul Aziz University, Jeddah, Saudi Arabia

4 Department of Clinical Pharmacy, College of Pharmacy, Umm Al-Qura University, Makkah, Saudi Arabia

5 Department of Pharmaceutical Chemistry, College of Pharmacy, Umm Al-Qura University, Makkah, Saudi Arabia

6 Department of Gastroenterology and Hepatology, Fatima Memorial College of Medicine and Dentistry, Shadman, Lahore, Pakistan

References

[1] Herbert SP, Huisken J, Kim TN, et al. Arterial-venous segregation by selective cell sprouting: an alternative mode of blood vessel formation. *Science* 2009; 326:294–298.

[2] Fidler IJ, Ellis LM. The implications of angiogenesis for the biology and therapy of cancer metastasis. *Cell* 1994; 79:185–188.

[3] Carmeliet P, Jain RK. Angiogenesis in cancer and other diseases. *Nature* 2000; 407:249–257.

[4] Kerbel RS. Tumor angiogenesis: past, present and the near future. *Carcinogenesis* 2000; 21:505–515.

[5] Carmeliet P. Angiogenesis in health and disease. *Nat Med* 2003; 9:653–660.

[6] Adams RH, Alitalo K. Molecular regulation of angiogenesis and lymphangiogenesis. *Nat Rev Mol Cell Biol* 2007; 8:464–478.

[7] Staton CA, Brown NJ, Reed MW. Current status and future prospects for antiangiogenic therapies in cancer. *Expert Opin Drug Discov* 2009; 4:961–979.

[8] Rouslahti E, Rajotte D. An address system in the vasculature of normal tissues and tumors. *Annu Rev Immunol* 2000; 18:813–27.

[9] Hasan J, Shnyder SD, Bibby et al. Quantitative angiogenesis assays *in vivo*—a review. *Angiogenesis* 2004; 7:1–16.

[10] Auerbach R, Auerbach W, Polakowski I. Assays for angiogenesis: a review. *Pharmacol Ther* 1991; 51:1–11.

[11] Vallee BL, Riordan JF, Lobb RR, et al. Tumor-derived angiogenesis factors from rat Walker 256 carcinoma: an experimental investigation and review. *Experientia* 1985; 41:1–15.

[12] Jain RK, Schlenger K, Höckel M, et al. Quantitative angiogenesis assays: progress and problems. *Nat Med* 1997; 3:1203–8.

[13] Fregene TA, Khanuja PS, Noto AC, et al. Tumor-associated angiogenesis in prostate cancer. *Anticancer Res* 1993; 13:2377–2381.

[14] Weidner N, Carroll PR, Flax J, et al. Tumor angiogenesis correlates with metastasis in invasive prostate carcinoma. *Am J Pathol* 1993; 143:401–409.

[15] Craft PS, Harris AL. Clinical prognostic significance of tumour angiogenesis. *Ann Oncol* 1994; 5:305–311.

[16] Gimbrone MA, Cotran RS, Leapman SB, et al. Tumor growth and neovascularization: an experimental model using the rabbit cornea. *J Natl Cancer Inst* 1974; 52:413–27.

[17] Auerbach R, Kubai L, Knighton D, et al. A simple procedure for the long-term cultivation of chicken embryos. *Dev Biol* 1974; 41:391–4.

[18] Ausprunk DH, Knighton DR, Folkman J. Differentiation of vascular endothelium in the chick choriallantois: a structural and autoradiographic atudy. *Dev Biol* 1974; 38:237–48.

[19] Ausprunk DH, Knighton DR, Folkman J. Vascularization of normal and neoplastic tissues grafted to the chick chorioallantois. Role of host and pre-existing graft blood vessels. *Am J Pathol* 1975; 79:597–628.

[20] Folkman J. Tumor angiogenesis. *Adv Cancer Res* 1974; 19:331–9.

[21] Norrby K, Jakbsson A, Sörbo J. Mast-cell-mediated angiogenesis: a novel experimental model using the rat mesentery. *Virchows Arch. [Cell Pathol.]* 1986; 52:195–206.

[22] Norrby K, Jakobsson A, Sörbo J. Quantitative angiogenesis in spreads of intact rat mesenteric windows. *Microvasc Res* 1990; 39:341–8.

[23] Andrade SP, Fan TP, Lewis GP. Quantitative in-vivo studies on angiogenesis in a rat sponge model. *Br J Exp Pathol* 1987; 68:755–66.

[24] Fajardo L-F, Kowalski J, Kwan HH, et al. The disc angiogenesis system. *Lab Invest* 1988; 58:718–24.

[25] Passaniti A, Taylor RM, Pili R, et al. A simple, quantitative method for assessing angiogenesis and antiangiogenic agents using reconstituted basement membrane, heparin, and fibroblast growth factor. *Lab Invest* 1992;67:519–28.

[26] Anghelina M, Krishnan P, Moldovan L, et al. Monocytes/macrophages cooperate with progenitor cells during neovascularization and tissue repair: conversion of cell columns into fibrovascular bundles. *Am J Pathol* 2006; 168:529–41.

[27] Kragh M, Hjarnaa PJ, Bramm E, et al. *In vivo* chamber angiogenesis assay: an optimized Matrigel plug assay for fast assessment of anti-angiogenic activity. *Int J Oncol* 2003; 22:305–11.

[28] Ley CD, Olsen MW, Lund EL, et al. Angiogenic synergy of bFGF and VEGF is antagonized by angiopoietin-2 in a modified *in vivo* Matrigel assay. *Microvasc Res* 2004; 68:161–8.

[29] Serbedzija GN, Flynn E, Willett CE. Zebrafish angiogenesis: a new model for drug screening. *Angiogenesis* 1999; 3:353–9.

[30] Isogai S, Horiguchi M, Weinstein BM. The vascular anatomy of the developing zebrafish: an atlas of embryonic and early larval development. *Dev Biol* 2001; 230:278–301.

[31] Lawson ND, Weinstein BM. *In vivo* imaging of embryonic vascular development using transgenic zebrafish. *Dev Biol* 2002; 248:307–18.

[32] Jensen LD, Cao R, Cao Y. In vivo angiogenesis and lymphangiogenesis models. *Curr Mol Med* 2009; 8:982–91.

[33] Houdebine L M. The methods to generate transgenic animals and to control transgene expression. *J Biotechnol* 2002; 98:145160.

[34] Emanueli CA, Caporali N, Krankel B, et al. Type-2 diabetic Lepr(db/db) mice show a defective microvascular phenotype under basal conditions and an impaired response to angiogenesis gene therapy in the setting of limb ischemia. *Front Biosci* 2007; 12:3–12.

[35] Ingalls JM, Dickie MM, Snell GD. Obese, a new mutation in the house mouse. *J Hered* 1950; 41:17–18.

[36] Brakenhielm E, Cao R, Gao B, et al. Angiogenesis inhibitor, TNP-470, prevents diet induced and genetic obesity in mice. *Circ Res* 2004; 94:79–88.

[37] Friedman JM, Halaas JL. Leptin and the regulation of body weight in mammals. *Nature* 1998;395:63–70.

[38] Hummel KP, Dickie MM, Coleman DL. Diabetes, a new mutation in the mouse. *Science* 1966; 153:1127–8.

[39] Cao Y. Therapeutic angiogenesis for ischemic disorders: what is missing for clinical benefits? *Discov Med* 2010; 9:179–84.

[40] Lundberg G, Luo F, Blegen H, et al. A rat model for severe limb ischemia at rest. *Eur Surg Res* 2002; 35:430–8.

[41] Xue Y, Religa P, Cao R, et al. Anti-VEGF agent confer survival advantages to tumor-bearing mice by improving cancer-associated systemic syndrome. *Proc Natl Acad Sci U S A*, 2008;105:18513–8.

[42] Melo LG, Gnecchi, AS, Pachori D, et al. Endothelium-targeted gene and cell-based therapies for cardiovascular disease. *Arterioscler Thromb Vasc Biol* 2004;24:1761–1774.

[43] Nagy A. Cre recombinase: the universal reagent for genome tailoring. *Genesis* 2000; 26:99–109.

[44] Mallo M. Controlled gene activation and inactivation in the mouse. *Front Biosci* 2006; 11:313–327.

[45] Houdebine L M. Animal transgenesis: recent data and perspectives. *Biochimie* 2002; 84:1137–1141.

[46] Ryding AD, Sharp MG, Mullins JJ. Conditional transgenic technologies. *J Endocrinol* 2001; 171:1–14.

[47] Brummelkamp TR, Bernards R, Agami R. Stable suppression of tumorigenicity by virus-mediated RNA interference. *Cancer Cell* 2002; 3:243–7.

[48] Folkman J. What is the evidence that tumors are angiogenesis dependent? *J Natl Cancer Inst* 1990; 82:4–6.

[49] Folkman J. Tumor angiogenesis: therapeutic implications. *N Engl J Med.* 1971; 285:1182–1186.

[50] Ohta M, Konno H, Tanaka T, et al. The significance of circulating vascular endothelial growth factor (VEGF) protein in gastric cancer. *Cancer Lett* 2003; 192:215–225.

[51] Mauriz JL, Gonzalez-Gallego J. Antiangiogenic drugs: current knowledge and new approaches to cancer therapy. *J Pharm Sci* 2008; 97:4129–4154.

[52] Benny O, Fainaru O, Adini A, et al. An orally delivered small-molecule formulation with antiangiogenic and anticancer activity. *Nat Biotechnol* 2008; 26:799–807.

[53] Yokoyama Y, Charnock-Jones DS, Licence D, et al. Expression of vascular endothelial growth factor (VEGF)- D and its receptor, VEGF receptor 3, as a prognostic factor in endometrial carcinoma. *Clin Cancer Res* 2003; 9:1361–1369.

[54] Kurahara H, Takao S, Maemura K, et al. Impact of vascular endothelial growth factor-C and -D expression in human pancreatic cancer: its relationship to lymph node metastasis. *Clin Cancer Res* 2004; 10:8413–8420.

[55] Adini A, Kornaga T, Firoozbakht F, et al. Placental growth factor is a survival factor for tumor endothelial cells and macrophages. *Cancer Res* 2002; 62:2749–2752.

[56] Carmeliet P, Ferreira V, Breier G, et al. Abnormal blood vessel development and lethality in embryos lacking a single VEGF allele. *Nature* 1996; 380:435–439.

[57] Li JL, Sainson RC, Shi W, et al. Delta-like 4 Notch ligand regulates tumor angiogenesis, improves tumor vascular function, and promotes tumor growth in vivo. *Cancer Res* 2007; 67:11244–11253.

[58] Noguera-Troise I, Daly C, Papadopoulos NJ, et al. Blockade of Dll4 inhibits tumour growth by promoting non-productive angiogenesis. *Nature* 2006; 444:1032–1037.

[59] Ridgway J, Zhang G, Wu Y, et al. Inhibition of Dll4 signalling inhibits tumour growth by deregulating angiogenesis. *Nature* 2006; 444:1083–1087.

[60] Indraccolo S, Minuzzo S, Masiero M, et al. Cross-talk between tumor and endothelial cells involving the Notch3-Dll4 interaction marks escape from tumor dormancy. *Cancer Res* 2009; 69:1314–1323.

[61] de Larco JE, Todaro GJ. Growth factors from murine sarcoma virus transformed cells. *Proc Natl Acad Sci U S A* 1978; 75:4001–4005.

[62] Laiho M, DeCaprio JA, Ludlow JW, et al. Growth inhibition by TGF-beta linked to suppression of retinoblastoma protein phosphorylation. *Cell* 1990; 62:175–185.

[63] Niles RM, Thompson NL, Fenton F. Expression of TGF-beta during in vitro differentiation of hamster tracheal epithelial cells. *In Vitro Cell Dev Biol Anim* 1994; 30A:256–262.

[64] Filvaroff EH, Ebner R, Derynck R. Inhibition of myogenic differentiation in myoblasts expressing a truncated type II TGF-beta receptor. *Development* 1994; 120:1085–1095.

[65] Le Roy C, Leduque P, Dubois PM, et al. Repression of transforming growth factor beta 1protein by antisense oligonucleotide induced increase of adrenal cell differentiated functions. *J Biol Chem* 1996; 271:11027–11033.

[66] Goumans MJ, Valdimarsdottir G, Itoh S, et al. Balancing the activation state of the endothelium via two distinct TGF beta type I receptors. *EMBO J* 2002; 21:1743–1753.

[67] Cobleigh MA, Langmuir VK, Sledge GW, et al. A phase I/II dose escalation trial of bevacizumab in previously treated metastatic breast cancer. *Semin Oncol* 2003; 30:117–24.

[68] Majima M, Hayashi I, Muramatsu M, et al. Cyclo-oxygenase-2 enhances basic fibrobrast growth factor-induced angiogenesis through induction o vascular endothelial growth factor in rat sponge implants. *Br J Pharmacol* 2000; 268:641–9.

[69] Yang JC, Haworth L, Sherry RM, et al. A randomized trial of bevacizumab, an anti–vascular endothelial growth factor antibody, for metastatic renal cancer. *N Engl J Med* 2003; 349:427–34.

[70] Hurwitz H, Fehrenbacher L, Novotny W, et al. Bevacizumab plus irinotecan, fluorouracil, and leucovorin for metastatic colorectal cancer. *N Engl J Med* 2004; 350:2335–2342.

[71] Giantonio B, Catalano PJ, Meropol NJ, et al. High-dose bevacizumab in combination with FOLFOX-4 improves survival in patients with previously treated advanced colorectal cancer: results from the Eastern Cooperative Group (ECOG) study E2300. *J Clin Oncol* 2005; 23(16S):2.

[72] Kerbel RS. Antiangiogenic therapy: a universal chemosensitization strategy for cancer? *Science* 2006 312:1171–1175.

[73] Jain RK. Normalizing tumor vasculature with antiangiogenic therapy: a new paradigm for combination therapy. *Nat Med* 2001; 7:987–989.

[74] Jain RK. Normalization of tumor vasculature: an emerging concept in antiangiogenic therapy. *Science* 2005; 307:58–62.

[75] Hudis CA. Clinical implications of antiangiogenic therapies. *Oncology* (Willits Park NY) 2005; 19:26–31.

[76] Kerbel RS, Kamen BA. The anti-angiogenic basis of metronomic chemotherapy. *Nat Rev Cancer* 2004; 4:423–436.

[77] Kerbel RS, Klement G, Pritchard KI, et al. Continuous low-dose anti-angiogenic/metro-nomic chemotherapy: from the research laboratory into the oncology clinic. *Ann Oncol* 2002; 13:12–15.

Permissions

The contributors of this book come from diverse backgrounds, making this book a truly international effort. This book will bring forth new frontiers with its revolutionizing research information and detailed analysis of the nascent developments around the world.

We would like to thank all the contributing authors for lending their expertise to make the book truly unique. They have played a crucial role in the development of this book. Without their invaluable contributions this book wouldn't have been possible. They have made vital efforts to compile up to date information on the varied aspects of this subject to make this book a valuable addition to the collection of many professionals and students.

This book was conceptualized with the vision of imparting up-to-date information and advanced data in this field. To ensure the same, a matchless editorial board was set up. Every individual on the board went through rigorous rounds of assessment to prove their worth. After which they invested a large part of their time researching and compiling the most relevant data for our readers.

The editorial board has been involved in producing this book since its inception. They have spent rigorous hours researching and exploring the diverse topics which have resulted in the successful publishing of this book. They have passed on their knowledge of decades through this book. To expedite this challenging task, the publisher supported the team at every step. A small team of assistant editors was also appointed to further simplify the editing procedure and attain best results for the readers.

Apart from the editorial board, the designing team has also invested a significant amount of their time in understanding the subject and creating the most relevant covers. They scrutinized every image to scout for the most suitable representation of the subject and create an appropriate cover for the book.

The publishing team has been an ardent support to the editorial, designing and production team. Their endless efforts to recruit the best for this project, has resulted in the accomplishment of this book. They are a veteran in the field of academics and their pool of knowledge is as vast as their experience in printing. Their expertise and guidance has proved useful at every step. Their uncompromising quality standards have made this book an exceptional effort. Their encouragement from time to time has been an inspiration for everyone.

The publisher and the editorial board hope that this book will prove to be a valuable piece of knowledge for researchers, students, practitioners and scholars across the globe.

List of Contributors

Norika Mengchia Liu
University of California, Los Angeles, CA, USA

Susumu Minamisawa
The Jikei Medical University, Tokyo, Japan

Cheryl G. Pfeifer
The Michael Smith Laboratories, University of British Columbia, Vancouver, Canada

Wilfred A. Jefferies
The Michael Smith Laboratories, University of British Columbia, Vancouver, Canada
Department of Microbiology & Immunology, University of British Columbia, Vancouver, Canada
Department of Medical Genetics, University of British Columbia, Vancouver, Canada
Department of Zoology, University of British Columbia, Vancouver, Canada
Centre for Blood Research, University of British Columbia, Vancouver, Canada
Djavad Mowafaghian Centre for Brain Health, University of British Columbia, Vancouver, Canada

Chaahat Singh
The Michael Smith Laboratories, University of British Columbia, Vancouver, Canada
Department of Medical Genetics, University of British Columbia, Vancouver, Canada

Nicolás F. Renna and Roberto M. Miatello
Department of Pathology, School of Medicine, National University of Cuyo, Mendoza, Argentina
Institute of Experimental Medicine and Biology of Cuyo (IMBECU), CONICET, Mendoza, Argentina

Rodrigo Garcia
Institute of Experimental Medicine and Biology of Cuyo (IMBECU), CONICET, Mendoza, Argentina

Jesica Ramirez
Genetics Institute, School of Medicine, National University of Cuyo, Mendoza, Argentina

Lamia Heikal and Gordon Ferns
Brighton and Sussex Medical School, University of Sussex, Brighton, United Kingdom

Scott T. Robinson
Department of Surgery, University of Michigan School of Medicine, Ann Arbor, MI, USA

Luke P. Brewster
Department of Surgery, Emory University of Medicine, Atlanta, GA, USA
Atlanta VA Medical Center, Surgical and Research Services, Decatur, GA, USA

Sepehr Feizi
Ophthalmic Research Center and Department of Ophthalmology, Labbafinejad Medical Center, Shahid Beheshti University of Medical Sciences, Tehran, Iran

Bhamini Patel, Peter Hopmann, Mansee Desai, Kanithra Sekaran, Kathleen Graham, Liya Yin and William Chilian
Department of Integrative Medical Science, Northeast Ohio Medical University, Rootstown, Ohio, USA

Paola A. Guerrero and Joseph H. McCarty
Department of Neurosurgery, University of Texas MD Anderson Cancer Center, Houston, TX, USA

Lucia Napione, Maria Alvaro and Federico Bussolino
Laboratory of Vascular Oncology, Candiolo Cancer Institute – IRCCS, Candiolo, Italy
Department of Oncology, University of Torino, Candiolo, Italy

Marina M. Ziganshina, Lyubov V. Krechetova, Lyudmila V. Vanko, Zulfiya S.Khodzhaeva, Ekaterina L. Yarotskaya and Gennady T. Sukhikh
Federal State Budget Institution "The Research Center for Obstetrics, Gynecology and Perinatology" of the Ministry of Healthcare of the Russian Federation, Moscow, Russia

Waleed H. AlMalki and Muhammad Ahmed
Department of Pharmacology and Toxicology, College of Pharmacy, Umm Al-Qura University, Makkah, Saudi Arabia

Imran Shahid
Department of Pharmacology and Toxicology, College of Pharmacy, Umm Al-Qura University, Makkah, Saudi Arabia
Applied and Functional Genomics Laboratory, Center of Excellence in Molecular Biology (CEMB), University of the Punjab, Lahore, Pakistan

Mohammed W. AlRabia
Department of Medical Microbiology, College of Medicine, King Abdul Aziz University, Jeddah, Saudi Arabia

Mohammad T. Imam
Department of Clinical Pharmacy, College of Pharmacy, Umm Al-Qura University, Makkah, Saudi Arabia

Muhammed K. Saifullah
Department of Pharmaceutical Chemistry, College of Pharmacy, Umm Al-Qura University, Makkah, Saudi Arabia

Muhammad H. Hafeez
Department of Gastroenterology and Hepatology, Fatima Memorial College of Medicine and Dentistry, Shadman, Lahore, Pakistan

Index

www.ingramcontent.com/pod-product-compliance
Lightning Source LLC
Chambersburg PA
CBHW061954190326
41458CB00009B/2866